THERE IS A

CURE FOR

DIABETES

THERE IS A
CURE FOR
DIABETES

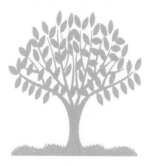

The Tree of Life
21-Day+ Program

GABRIEL COUSENS, MD
with David Rainoshek

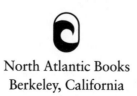

North Atlantic Books
Berkeley, California

Published by
North Atlantic Books
P.O. Box 12327
Berkeley, California 94712

Cover and book design by Suzanne Albertson
Printed in the United States of America

There Is a Cure for Diabetes: The Tree of Life 21-Day+ Program is sponsored by the Society for the Study of Native Arts and Sciences, a nonprofit educational corporation whose goals are to develop an educational and crosscultural perspective linking various scientific, social, and artistic fields; to nurture a holistic view of arts, sciences, humanities, and healing; and to publish and distribute literature on the relationship of mind, body, and nature.

MEDICAL DISCLAIMER: The following information is intended for general information purposes only. Individuals should always see their health care provider before administering any suggestions made in this book. Any application of the material set forth in the following pages is at the reader's discretion and is his or her sole responsibility.

North Atlantic Books' publications are available through most bookstores. For further information, call 800-733-3000 or visit our website at www.-northatlanticbooks.com.

Library of Congress Cataloging-in-Publication Data

Cousens, Gabriel, 1943–
    There is a cure for diabetes : the tree of life 21-day+ program / by Gabriel Cousens ; with David Rainoshek.
        p. cm.
    Summary: "Presents a breakthrough approach that reverses diabetes to a physiology of health and well-being by resetting the genetic expression of a person's DNA through green juice fasting and a 100% organic, nutrient-dense, vegan, low-glycemic, low-insulin-scoring, and high-mineral diet of living foods in the first 21 days"—Provided by publisher.
    Includes bibliographical references and index.
    ISBN 978-1-55643-691-8
    1. Diabetes—Diet therapy. 2. Vegetable juices. 3. Low-calorie diet. 4. Glycemic index. I. Rainoshek, David. II. Title.
    RC662.C68 2008
    616.4'620654—dc22   2007039056

3   4   5   6   7   8   9   United   12   11   10   09   08

CONTENTS

CHAPTER 3
A Comprehensive Theory of Diabetes 95

CHAPTER 4
The Tree of Life 21-Day+ Program 159

Contents

CHAPTER 5

Happy Continuation: Living in the Culture of Life and Juice Feasting 241

CHAPTER 6
Culture of Life Cuisine 281

APPENDIX 1
About the Tree of Life 361

Contents

ACKNOWLEDGMENTS

There Is a Cure for Diabetes has been an interesting collective effort over thirty-five years, of input mostly from clients who have been my main teachers, and of inspiration from the pioneers of the live-foods movement, each illuminating another aspect of the live-food approach to healing diabetes naturally. These people include: **David Wolfe,** who was personally and directly supportive in the creation of this book; **Viktoras Kulvinskas,** who specifically offered his insights in the importance of enzyme therapy for diabetes; **Brian Clement** of Hippocrates Health Institute; and **Reverend George Malkmus** of Hallelujah Acres. All expressed their experience in confirming the viability of a live-foods approach to diabetes reversal.

Dr. Edmond Bordeaux Szekeley, over a period of thirty years (1940–1970), healed all manner of diseases including diabetes with a live-food diet. **Max Gerson, MD,** made some of the earliest and best publicized public healings with live foods, including healing Dr. Albert Schweitzer of diabetes. I also want to acknowledge **Paavo Airola, ND, PhD,** who shared his insights on healing diabetes. We appreciate the pioneering work of **Neal Barnard, MD,** the research of **T. Colin Campbell, PhD,** and the practice of **John McDougall, MD,** in clinically supporting the efficacy of a plant-sourced diet for diabetes reversal.

To my two inspiring and guiding spiritual teachers, **Swami Prakashananda** and **Swami Muktananda Paramahansa** from India, who both had diabetes and showed how it could be managed with a simple vegan diet. With gratitude to my research assistant, **David Rainoshek, MA.** His research, collaboration, and detailed reference work allowed this book to be accomplished more quickly and thoroughly than I could have done on my own. I also thank him for his addition of the Four Means to Get Your Greens approach to a live-foods diet; and thank David and his colleague **John Rose** for the Juice Feasting concept, which a back-up part of the support phase of this program. **Katrina Rainoshek,** who assisted David and me in research and compilation of materials, and provided nutritional support. The **Tree of Life staff,** specifically café manager and co-manager **Tim** and **Michela Casey,** who put together the diabetic food training program over the last two years, and provided the Rainbow Green Live-Food World Cuisine recipes in Chapter 6.

To my wonderful partner, **Shanti Golds-Cousens,** whose love and support for this book is greatly appreciated, and who leads the yoga aspect of our 21-Day+ Program both in the U.S. and in Israel. The program in Israel now serves Europe, Greece, Turkey, and the rest of the Middle East. We also want to thank the Tree of Life Israel staff for their tremendous effort in putting together this program in Israel.

With gratitude to the Tree of Life program in the U.S. and the support of Tree of Life physician **Helen Ross, MD,** who conducted client evaluations for our 21-Day+ Program. Thank you to **Nurse Carol Saghir,** who helped compile much of the client data.

Finally, the collaborators in the film *Raw for 30: Reversing Diabetes Naturally:* **Mark Perlmutter,** who brought the idea of *Raw for 30* to me to be done at the Tree of Life and was open to my idea of doing *Raw for 30* with diabetics, an inspirational film that has led to this book; **Keith Lyons,** who provided essential support through the birth of the film; and **Michael Bedar,** my personal assistant, who helped this process.

To the service of God, who inspired me to write this book and to carry on the teachings of Genesis 1:29 as the spiritual and nutritional blueprint for the healing of diabetes:

> "See, I give you every seed-bearing plant that is upon all the earth, and every tree that has seed-bearing fruit; they shall be yours for food."

And the inspiration of God through Moses Rabineau in Devarim (Deuteronomy) 30:19–20:

> "I call heaven and earth to witness this day against you, that I have set before thee life and death, blessing and cursing: therefore choose

life, that both thou and thy seed may live: that thou mayest love the Lord thy God, and that you mayest obey God's voice and cleave to the Divine: for the Divine Presence is thy life and length of days."

Please note: Nothing in this book is intended to constitute medical advice or treatment. For development of an individualized diet or the use of fasting cycles, it is advised that any person first consult his or her wholistic physician. It is important that he or she remain under the doctor's supervision throughout any major shift in diet or while fasting.

We have referred to a variety of studies, a few of which have involved animals. In no way does this mean that we endorse the use of animal studies for scientific purposes, and when data were available to illustrate points without using these studies, we have done so. Animal studies, particularly studies in which the animals have been sacrificed, interfere with the peace between the animal world and the human world.

FOREWORD

by Brian R. Clement, PhD, NMD, LNC
Director, Hippocrates Health Institute

There is a Cure for Diabetes is a well-written, concise compilation of
sound research, common sense suggestions, and clinical experience that
demonstrates a proven way to prevent and eradicate diabetes. This
book is undoubtedly one of the most-if not the most—significant books
ever written to address this disease. Gabriel Cousens, MD, is a caring
professional who delivers a heartfelt, inspiring message and a practical
plan that, based on my own experience over the past forty years, results
in the swift and permanent elimination of Type-2 diabetes for those
who choose to take responsibility for their lifestyle. The plan may also
produce potentially significant reductions in insulin dosages for people
with Type-1 diabetes. Type-2 diabetes is directly linked to lifestyle
choices; it does not deserve the status of billions of dollars spent on it
for research and drug development, marketing, and institutions that
protect corporate and government interests and their industry profits.
Diabetes and the promotion of a drug-dependent "cure" by multi-
national pharmaceutical companies and the medical community are
the real global epidemics that are destroying the possibility of a healthy,
drug-free life for millions worldwide. Maintaining health is much simpler than is purported in the journals of medicine and mainstream media,
and Dr. Cousens is a leader in showing us how. *There is a Cure for
Diabetes* is essential reading for anyone who desires life-long health
and a saving grace for current and future generations who wish to be
free from diabetes.

FOREWORD

by Brian M. Connolly
Founder and CEO, Healthful Communications, Inc.

For those of us most directly affected by diabetes (all 250 million of us on the planet), we are fortunate that a book whose time has indeed come has finally arrived, a book that affirms in clear and precise language that *there is in fact a cure for diabetes.* For those millions more of you flirting with developing this fast-spreading illness, you have been given a gift of prevention in the form of this book, a prescription that, if followed, will ensure the maintenance of your health and well-being far into the future.

It is written by an extraordinary physician, Gabriel Cousens, MD, who has been walking his talk for decades as a leader in the health care field. Thanks to his life's work, and the steps he has outlined within this book, I was able to go from a dangerously high Type-2 diabetic condition, with a blood glucose reading of 292, down to a diabetes-free reading of 113 in just nine days. I know this sounds astonishing, if not unbelievable. But let me assure you that it not only happened, it is in fact documented. More importantly, it is possible for you to accomplish what I did and make a similar transformation in the quality of your life, whether it is in nine days or in twenty-one days, as recommended in the steps within these pages.

For each one of us there are pivotal days, signposts along the road of our lives that stick with us forever. For me that day was September 14, 2006, when I received what for most is a life sentence. It was 4:30 in the afternoon and I was on the phone with a diabetes expert, the esteemed Dr. William Kaye, a Harvard medical school graduate and the founder and director of one of the largest private practices in the United States for diabetes treatment. Dr. Kaye informed me that I had officially joined the ranks of his approximately 18,000 patients as a newly diagnosed Type-2 diabetic.

A funny thing happens when you hear this for the first time. It creates a pause in one's life—and hopefully a wake-up call. When you let family members, friends, and loved ones know that you have diabetes, there is usually an even longer pause. You can practically smell their fear, as if they just found out someone they care about is going to die. In my case I even felt embarrassed about contracting diabetes, as I considered myself a minor expert in the field of the disease.

I had been vice president of the Diabetes Research and Wellness Foundation, a national not-for-profit that had raised thirty million dollars, 90 percent of which went directly into research and education programs. I had also served a tenure on the board of directors of the University of Miami School of Medicine's Diabetes Research Institute, which had an annual budget of twenty million dollars. During this time I worked daily with all the major pharmaceutical and diabetic supply companies and associations, including the American Diabetes Association, the Juvenile Diabetes Research Foundation, Bayer, Elli Lilly, and Pfizer as well as with certified diabetes educators. These groups provided diabetics with insulin, pharmaceuticals, syringes, glucose meters, magazines, newsletters, books, and nurses certified to treat the disorder. What seems so interesting to me now is how back then everyone appeared more intent on selling their wares, their services, or raising money than on promoting the cause and urgency of diabetes prevention and reversal as Dr. Cousens outlines in this book.

The University of Miami School of Medicine's Diabetes Research Institute was focused on creating a new Frankenstein's monster, performing cell transplants from a pig into a human at an extremely high cost to society and patients, both financially and health-wise. One can only wonder what the more than fifty million diabetic Jews and Muslims who cannot consume pork think of this protocol.

What was particularly insidious about this decades-old failing protocol was that they were patting themselves on the back for taking patients off of insulin, yet they were doing something far more harmful: performing an invasive surgery that brings pig parts into human organs and then inundating the patients with immune-suppressing drugs that prevented the body from its natural response of killing off the implanted pig cells. These cells would then kill off the body's healthy cells, weakening the patient's immune system and putting them at risk for multiple maladies. They actually had the audacity to refer to this procedure as a cure. That was my first day—and my last—serving on their board, as I could not in good conscience support them in any way whatsoever.

From firsthand experience I can tell you that a whole lot of people have been making a tremendous amount of money at the expense of those innocent guinea pigs called diabetics. Is it any wonder that when it comes to producing positive results—actually turning this deadly disease around and having fewer people diagnosed with it each year—all these companies, research institutes, foundations, and associations have failed miserably? When I opened the Palm Beach office for the Diabetes Research and Wellness Foundation in 2000, an estimated 200 million people had been diagnosed with the disease internationally. In just seven years that number increased by approximately fifty million people. This is what the Centers for Disease Control and Prevention refers to as an epidemic. The real tragedy is that it is an entirely preventable epidemic, as you will learn for yourself in the following pages. And when you follow the steps recommended by Dr. Cousens, you will not only become a healthier person, you will most likely become diabetes-free for life.

You would think that these diabetes organizations, representing billions of dollars, would have figured out by now that their approach to this disease has not worked. During my tenure on the board of one such organization, I came to realize that these institutions are more interested in self-perpetuation and in raising money than in finding a prescription for prevention or a non-invasive, cost-efficient cure. Diabetics are over-medicated, strained financially, and subjected to more amputations than patients with any other illness. They often become blind and die early, all because the money-making incentives are too seductive for the diabetes establishment to do the right thing.

In sharp contrast, Dr. Gabriel Cousens wastes no money, exerts zero strain on taxpayers, and has a nearly 100 percent success rate without drugs or side effects. It is safe to say that if the diabetes establishment stopped wasting all their money and resources on useless research and antiquated, failing protocols and simply adopted the techniques and protocols in this book, Type-2 diabetes, which represents nearly 99 percent of all diabetics, could be eradicated forever!

So once again, congratulations to you on time and money well spent purchasing *There Is a Cure for Diabetes*. Make this book your friend, write notes on it, clip pages of interest, share your favorite quotes and statistics with your family and friends. And after you cure yourself, or integrate its preventive measures into your lifestyle, please take the next and most important step: tell your diabetic friends and professionals that there is now a cure—and that you are living proof.

INTRODUCTION

Healing Diabetes Is a Shift
in Consciousness

Society is always taken by surprise by any new example of common
sense.

RALPH WALDO EMERSON

No physician can ever say that any disease is incurable. To say so blasphemes God, blasphemes Nature, and depreciates the great architect
of Creation. The disease does not exist, regardless of how terrible it
may be, for which God has not provided the corresponding cure.

PARACELSUS

It's supposed to be a professional secret, but I'll tell you anyway. We
doctors do nothing. We only help and encourage the doctor within.

ALBERT SCHWEITZER

Yes ... Type-2 diabetes is a curable disease. From my thirty-five years
of clinical experience as a wholistic medical doctor, and that of live-
food therapeutic centers since the 1920s when Max Gerson, MD, healed
Albert Schweitzer of diabetes with live foods, the fact that diabetes is
a curable disease is common knowledge in the live-food community.
Diabetes is not a fixed sentence; it is not our natural condition, and has
only become a problem of pandemic proportions since the 1940s. The
word *pandemic* comes from the Greek *pan-*, meaning "all," plus *demos*,
meaning "people or population." Thus, "pandemos" or "all the people."
A pandemic is an epidemic that becomes very widespread and affects
a whole region, a continent, or the world. This book is about looking
deeply at the underlying causes of diabetes on both the pandemic-global
and the personal level, and supplying readers with a way to achieve

rapid reversal from the misery of a diabetic physiology to a joyous and healthy physiology.

Although many people have a genetic susceptibility to Type-2 diabetes, the true causes (which activate the genetic potential physiology of diabetes) lie in a personal and world lifestyle and diet that pulls the trigger on the diabetes gun. This *diabetogenic* personal and world lifestyle and diet includes on the level of individual responsibility: a diet high in refined carbohydrates such as white sugar and white flour; high amounts of cooked animal saturated fats; trans-fatty acids produced from cooking (and especially frying oils at high temperatures); low-fiber food; coffee and caffeinated beverages; smoking; a lifestyle devoid of love and exercise; high stress; watching TV programming. Diabetogenic contributing factors on a planetary level include living in a degraded environment in which the air, earth, and water are, according to the Environmental Protection Agency, filled with 70,000 different toxic chemicals, heavy metals, agrochemicals, and other toxic substances—65,000 of which are potentially hazardous to our health. The Environmental Defense Council reports that more than four billion pounds of toxic chemicals are released into the environment each year, including seventy-two million pounds of known carcinogens. In addition, we live in a mental and emotional environment filled with messages of stress and death from the media, including news of constant wars and terrorism infecting the planet. The degenerate conditions, lifestyle, and diet that create diabetes emanate from these modern human-created realities, which, taken together, we are calling the Culture of Death.

The cure, on the most profound level, is to move away from a global and personal Culture of Death, to embrace the Culture of Life. On a personal level this means choosing to live in a way that promotes life and well-being for oneself as well as the planet. It means creating a diet and lifestyle in which there is minimal or no incidence of diabetes. Individually, this means a diet that is organic, vegan, at least 80 percent live-food, high in mineral content, 15–20 percent plant-only fat (no animal fat), high-fiber, low-glycemic, low-insulin index, well hydrated, individualized, and prudent food intake—a cuisine that is sustainable for the duration of one's life, and prepared and eaten with love. Collectively, it means creating a world culture where all people have access to healthy, organic food and water, decent shelter, and a living environment free of chemicals and pollutants. Healing diabetes in this personal and global context is an act of love for oneself and the living planet. This love is an expression of the Culture of Life.

The teaching of this book is that humanity is created to be vibrant, alive, and healthy. As it says in Deuteronomy 30:19 from 3,400 years ago: "Today, I have set before you life and death and a blessing and a curse. You must choose life in order that you and your children shall live." Things have not changed. We still have that choice. This book is about empowering you, health professionals, and national and global policymakers to have that choice. Even in the most adverse circumstances, it still is possible for motivated individuals and nations to heal on the Tree of Life 21-Day+ Program as an act of love and consciousness.

The inspiration for this book began with a movie on diabetes and live foods that was made at the Tree of Life Rejuvenation Center in Patagonia, Arizona. The original idea was to do a film on the effect of being raw for thirty days. I strongly suggested that it would be more interesting to the general public to witness on film the effect of live foods on diabetic, McDonald's-Culture-of-Death individuals. Based on my clinical experience in healing diabetes naturally with motivated people, I was confident that these principles and approach would work with this new group of diabetic people. It seemed like an interesting exploration of how it would work for a group of people totally unfamiliar with live-food cuisine and way of life. The results were amazing. Of the six who started the program, only one dropped out. By the fourth day, four were off their insulin or oral hypoglycemic medications, and one Type-1 diabetic was down from 70 units of insulin per day to moving toward the 5 units he reached by the end of the month. One of the two Type-1 diabetics, whose fasting blood sugar (FBS) chart appears later in the book, and who was diagnosed with Type-1 diabetes by doctors in a hospital setting, dropped to a normal blood sugar after two weeks, and has remained there ever since. As of this writing, two years later, he remains cured of Type-1 diabetes. Another participant, who had severe neuropathy in his lower limbs, numbness in his scrotum and feet, was suffering from mental deterioration and confusion, and was preparing to have a foot amputated, recovered completely from the neuropathy and became mentally clearer. The tissue of his foot also healed and his blood sugar dropped to normal range in the first two weeks. Two of the women who had been living with a blood sugar of 300-plus while on medications dropped to blood sugars of 111 and 130 by the end of the month *without medications*. Most of the other blood chemistries of all of them became normal after one month. Mental state became clear and joyous in all participants.

On realizing the powerful effect of thirty days of live food with specific diabetic supplements and herbs on participants' physical and mental states, and on their diabetes in particular, it became clear that we had a program that could be applicable and successful for everyone, as this group was representative of the Western populace. The Tree of Life 21-Day+ Program is more powerful than the thirty-day raw approach seen in the film. It includes a minimum seven-day green juice fast in the first week, which greatly accelerates the reversing of the diabetic degenerative physiological process. Based on research by Dr. Stephen Spindler, it is our theory that calorie restriction turns on the anti-aging and theoretically the anti-diabetic genes. In our dietary approach, there is actually no restriction, but the participant is invited to enjoy a delicious, healthy cuisine. This is the powerful secret of the success of this program. In the second week, a four-day course shows people how to let go of their belief that diabetes is incurable. It also shows people how to let go of all the psychological programming and habits that create the diabetes lifestyle. In the third week, people learn how to prepare low-glycemic foods and a healthy healing cuisine. We then have a one-year follow-up that supports people in staying on the program, which includes, if needed, supervised Juice Feasting, a powerful at-home practice for those who need to continue to lose weight and heal the complications associated with a diabetic physiology that develops over many years and takes some time to reverse.

This book is divided into two parts. The first part (Chapters 1 through 5) presents the global diabetes pandemic, the causes of diabetes, the program for curing it, and the follow-up support program. The second part (Chapter 6) includes Rainbow Green World Cuisine recipes, an infinitely variable menu, and a live "fast food" preparation section called the Four Means to Get Your Greens.

There Is a Cure for Diabetes contains 530-plus references. Most are primary sources of information, which include hundreds of other researchers' scientific publications, spanning many decades, that support a nutritional approach to diabetes reversal. Some of the statistics on diabetes and research findings vary. For example the Centers for Disease Control estimates 21 million pre-diabetics in the U.S. and the American Diabetic Association estimates 54 million. I have chosen to include the variances, rather than to average. The variations show the state of the knowledge and should not be interpreted as contradictions.

Make no mistake: To liberate ourselves from the cultural, nutritional, and personal habits that contribute to the manifestation of diabetes is to not only heal ourselves and realize better health, but it is an act of love and consciousness that contributes to a multi-level positive transformation of society.

Only one question is left to the reader: Do you love yourself and the planet enough to want to heal yourself of diabetes and help the world switch from the Culture of Death, which is the ultimate cause of diabetes, to the Culture of Life, which brings love, peace, abundance, and health to the planet?

With blessings to your health and joy,

GABRIEL COUSENS, MD

CHAPTER 1

Diabetes Pandemic: World, Nations and Cultures, Cities

The World

Worldwide, diabetes has reached pandemic proportions. Data published in December 2006 in the International Diabetes Federation's *Diabetes Atlas* show that the disease now affects a staggering 246 million people worldwide, with 46 percent of all those affected in the 40-to-59 age group. Previous figures underestimated the scope of the problem, while even the most pessimistic predictions fell short of the current figure. The new data predict that the total number of people living with diabetes will skyrocket to 380 million within twenty years if nothing is done.[1] Diabetes, mostly Type-2, now affects 5.9 percent of the world's adult population, with almost 80 percent of the total in developing countries. The regions with the highest rates are the Eastern Mediterranean and Middle East, where 9.2 percent of the adult population is affected, and North America (8.4 percent). The highest numbers, however, are found in the Western Pacific, where some 67 million people have diabetes, followed by Europe with 53 million.

The World Health Organization (WHO) warns that deaths due to diabetes will increase globally by as much as 80 percent in some regions over the next ten years.[2] Professor Pierre Lefèbvre, president of the International Diabetes Federation (IDF), explains: "It is estimated that over 3.8 million deaths can be attributed to diabetes each year. That is 8,700 deaths every day; or six deaths every minute." He adds that "the dramatic rise in diabetes prevalence that can be found mainly in low and middle income countries is of particular concern." According to the WHO in 2007, by 2025, the largest increases in diabetes prevalence will take place in developing countries, where the number of people with diabetes will increase by 150 percent.[3] With no action to defuse this increase, it is estimated that total direct health care expenditures on diabetes worldwide will be up to 396 billion international dollars (ID) in 2025. This means that the proportion of the world's health care budget spent on diabetes care in 2025 will be between 7 percent and 13 percent.[4]

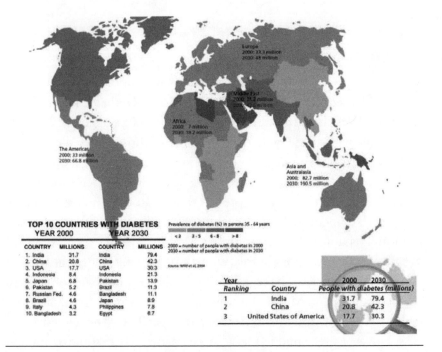

Figure 1: Diabetes prevalence by region, current and projected. (The graph shows 2000 data for the top ten countries, and projected data for 2030.)

According to a WHO report,[5] deaths from diabetes will increase by 80 percent in the Americas, by 50 percent in the Western Pacific and the Eastern Mediterranean regions, and by more than 40 percent in Africa over the next ten years. It may seem strange that the developing world, which is often associated with hunger and inadequate nutrition for children, is now experiencing an epidemic of Type-2 diabetes, a disease related to wealth and unhealthy lifestyle. This can be explained by the high degree of urbanization in some countries such as India that has brought adaptation to the lifestyles from industrialized countries, resulting in diseases such as diabetes related to this new lifestyle.[6] Epidemiologically, diabetes mellitus has been linked to the Western lifestyle and is uncommon in cultures consuming a more historical and indigenous diet.[7,8] As populations switch from their native diets to the "foods of commerce," their rate of diabetes increases, eventually reaching the same proportions seen in Western societies.[9]

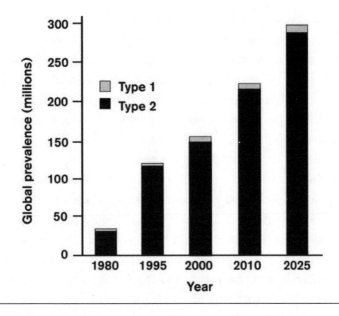

Figure 2: Estimated global prevalence of Type-1 and Type-2 diabetes

As we look at this pandemic, we need to be clear that it is worldwide. In short, we can call it a metabolic time bomb: Of the estimated 41 million people diagnosed with pre-diabetes in the U.S. alone,[10] about 10 percent will develop full-blown diabetes each year, shortening life spans by ten to nineteen years and accounting for about 210,000 deaths per year from diabetes. An infant born in 2000 in the U.S. has a one-in-three chance of developing diabetes. For those in certain ethnic groups such as Native American, Puerto Rican, Mexican, and Chinese, that projection may even be increased to one in two. African Americans and Latinos have about twice the risk of developing Type-2 diabetes. Type-2 diabetics are about three-four times more likely to develop clinical depression than non-diabetics.

There is explicit hope for Type-2 diabetes being completely reversed in a relatively short time. The good news is that Type-2 diabetes is not necessarily a death sentence; rather, it is a *benign* disease if it is appropriately addressed.

The message is apparent. Uncontrolled diabetes is a forced death march for those who are not willing to make the effort to heal themselves and a disaster in progress for the cultures and economies of nations worldwide. This book outlines a clear and safe approach to addressing the individual and global issue of diabetes, and in that context is a way forward for policymakers and all people who want to reverse this preventable trend. Type-2 diabetes is a pandemic wake-up call to the world to change its diet and lifestyle relying on junk food and high-sugar and high-saturated-animal-fat, trans-fatty-acid, pesticide- and herbicide-laden food. First, we must understand the full extent of the problem among nations and cultures. An obvious result of this discordant diet and lifestyle is obesity. We need to be clear: Obesity does not cause diabetes, but is a symptom of the diet and lifestyle that create diabetes. It is an indicator that is easy to associate with diabetes, and helps us track the diabetic trend, as up to 90 percent of Type-2 diabetics are overweight.

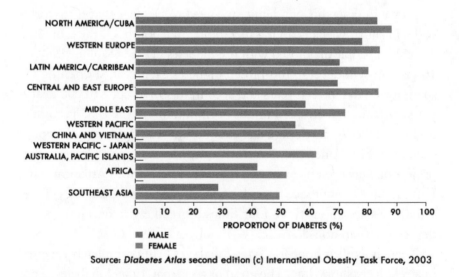

Source: *Diabetes Atlas* second edition (c) International Obesity Task Force, 2003

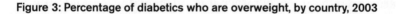

Figure 3: Percentage of diabetics who are overweight, by country, 2003

Nations and Cultures

In 2007, the three countries with the most diabetics are India (40.9 million), China (39.8 million), and the United States (19.2 million), followed by Russia (9.6 million) and Germany (7.4 million). Below is a chart of sugar consumption in the "top three." Notice a pattern?

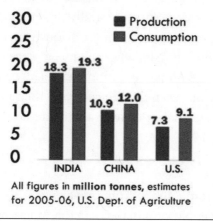

All figures in **million tonnes,** estimates for 2005-06, U.S. Dept. of Agriculture

Figure 4: Sugar production and consumption in India, China, and the U.S., 2005–2006

ASIA

India has the largest diabetic population in the world, with an estimated 40.9 million Type-2 diabetics, or 8 percent of the adult population. The WHO predicts that deaths from diabetes in India will increase by 35 percent over the next ten years. In China, the number of people with Type-2 diabetes is likely to reach 50 million in the next twenty-five years. What we are looking at is a trend toward diabetes in Asian countries.

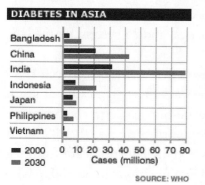

We do not have to look far to understand why. About 14 percent of Asian children are obese. That's

about twice the normal obesity rate of their parents. In Japan, the prevalence of Type-2 diabetes among junior high school children has almost doubled, from 7.3 per 100,000 in 1976–80 to 13.9 per 100,000 in 1991–95. Type-2 diabetes now outnumbers Type-1 diabetes in Japanese children.[11] In China, the number of obese people has tripled since 1992 to 90 million as Western fast-food cuisine has become more popular and people are becoming more materially prosperous.

This is pointing to a problem that is obviously very serious throughout the world, including Asia, where people in nations such as Korea, China, and Japan are 60 percent more genetically susceptible to diabetes than Caucasians, even though currently their national rates may be lower because they have not fully assimilated the Western cultural diet.

THE AMERICAS

Based on 1994 extrapolations from prevalence studies, there are now about 33 million people with diabetes in the Americas (approximately 20 million in the United States and 13 million in Latin America and the Caribbean). This accounts for one-quarter of the world's total population suffering from diabetes. This estimate for the Americas is projected to increase 45 percent by the year 2010, with Latin America and the Caribbean surpassing the U.S. and Canada. According to projections, however (estimates vary—we are providing what we consider reasonable estimates from the literature), the most dramatic increase will be seen in Central America, with an increase close to 100 percent. In the Caribbean islands, prevalence is expected to increase by 74 percent, compared to 40 percent for South America, and 25 percent for the U.S. and Canada.[12]

Recent changes in mortality profiles in the Americas (between 1980 and 1990) indicate that diabetes is the seventh leading cause of death and the third most common chronic condition leading to high mortality. Hispanics are the fastest-growing minority group in the U.S., with one out of two Hispanic women developing diabetes. Data from the Third National Health and Nutrition Examination Survey (NHANES

III) showed that minority persons with diabetes in the U.S., particularly Mexican Americans, were more likely to have poorer glycemic control than African Americans and non-Hispanic whites.[13]

> Organic and nutritious foods make a meaningful impact on children's health that lasts throughout life.
>
> **JORGE VALENZUELA, SAVE THE CHILDREN**

There is a growing awareness in Spanish-speaking communities of the importance of prudent nutrition and of the disastrous Type-2 diabetes. I am working with John David Arnold, PhD, president of the League of United Latin American Countries (LULAC) and with Jorge Valenzuela, head of Save the Children and Mexico Executive Director, FIA, on these issues.

> Diabetes is the unnecessary scourge of humanity that, unless prevented, will continue to evolve in future generations until it wipes us off the face of the planet.
>
> **JOHN DAVID ARNOLD, PHD, PRESIDENT OF LULAC**

D. Z. Jackson, in the pages of the January 11, 2006 edition of the *Boston Globe,* aptly commented on the tidal wave of diabetes cases in the United States: "Type 2 diabetes is sweeping so rapidly through America we need not waste time giving children bicycles. Just roll them a wheelchair."[14]

In the United States, estimates by the Centers for Disease Control and Prevention (CDC) are 20.8 million diabetics diagnosed and about 20 million who are considered pre-diabetic. In 2004, about 1.4 million adults in the U.S. between ages 18 and 79 were diagnosed with diabetes. From 1997 through 2004, the number of new cases of diagnosed diabetes increased by 54 percent.[15] This means there was an increase from 4.8 to 7.3 percent of the population. Diabetes *was* a very rare illness in 1880, with only 2.8 persons out of every 100,000 having diabetes. The prevalence of diabetes in the Native American population in 2002 was 15.3 percent, which is an increase of 33.2 percent from 1994. This is more than 50 percent greater than the general U.S.

population. From 1990 to 1998 the number of newly diagnosed diabetics among people younger than 34 increased by 71 percent in the U.S. Native American populations. Diabetes-related deaths have jumped 45 percent since 1987, while death rates from heart disease, stroke, and cancer have actually decreased. Diabetes deaths are independent of those general trends.

In response to a study published in the January 1, 2003, issue of the *Journal of the American Medical Association* (*JAMA*), which used Behavioral Risk Factor Surveillance System (BRFSS) data to show a recent increase in diagnosed diabetes as well as a significant association between overweight and obesity and diabetes, CDC director Dr. Julie L. Gerberding stated: "These increases are disturbing and are likely even underestimated. What's more important, we're seeing a number of serious health effects resulting from overweight and obesity." Dr. Gerberding added: "If we continue on this same path, the results will be devastating to both the health of the nation and to our healthcare system."[16]

Why we are overweight is a no-brainer. Americans at the beginning of the twenty-first century are consuming more food and several hundred more calories per person per day than did their counterparts in the late 1950s (when per capita calorie consumption was at the lowest level in the last century), or even in the 1970s. The U.S. food supply in 2000 provided 3,800 calories per person per day, 500 calories above the 1970 level and 800 calories above the record low in 1957 and 1958. Of that 3,800 calories, the USDA's Economic Research Service (ERS) estimates, roughly 1,100 calories are lost to spoilage, plate waste, and cooking and other losses, putting dietary intake of calories in 2000 at just under 2,700 calories per person per day. ERS data suggest that average daily calorie intake increased by 24.5 percent, or about 530 calories, between 1970 and 2000. Of that increase, grains (mainly refined grain products) contributed 9.5 percentage points; added fats and oils, 9.0 percentage points; added sugars, 4.7 percentage points; fruits and vegetables together (which are our Culture of Life anti-diabetogenic foods) only 1.5 percentage points.[17]

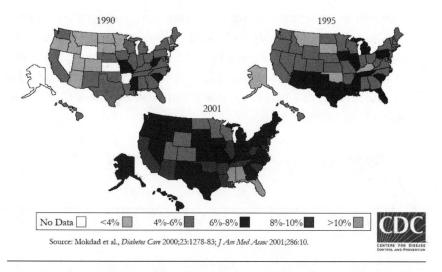

| No Data ☐ | <4% ■ | 4%-6% ■ | 6%-8% ■ | 8%-10% ■ | >10% ■ |

Source: Mokdad et al., *Diabetes Care* 2000;23:1278-83; *J Am Med Assoc* 2001;286:10.

Figure 5: Diabetes trends among adults in the U.S., 1990, 1995, 2001

DIABETES AS A CAUSE OF DEATH

According to the CDC, diabetes was the sixth leading cause of death listed on U.S. death certificates in 2002 (other reports suggest it is fifth—regardless, we need to pay attention). This ranking is based on the 73,249 death certificates in which diabetes was listed as the underlying cause of death. According to death certificate reports, diabetes contributed to a total of 224,092 deaths.

Still, diabetes is likely to be underreported as a cause of death. Studies have found that only 35–40 percent of decedents with diabetes had it listed anywhere on the death certificate and only 10–15 percent had it listed as the underlying cause of death. Overall, the risk for death among people with diabetes is about twice that of people without diabetes of similar age.

Diabetes mortality and family income show a strong relationship, according to data from the National Longitudinal Mortality Study for 1979 to 1989. For people 45 and older, the age-adjusted death rate in the U.S. from diabetes decreased as family income increased. The relationship between family income and death from diabetes was similar for men and women; for both sexes, mortality from diabetes decreased at each higher level of family income. The diabetes death rate among women in families with incomes below $10,000 was three times the death rate of those with incomes of $25,000 or more; among men, the death rate among the lowest income group was 2.6 times that of the highest income group.[18]

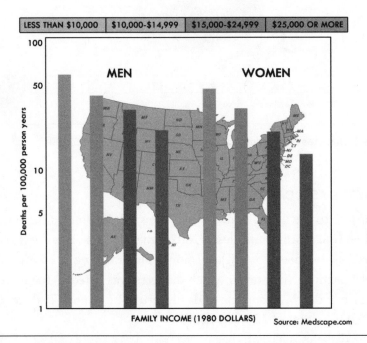

Figure 6: Diabetes death rates among adults 45 and over, by family income and gender

Diabetes is strongly associated with economic factors that differ from industrialized nations to developing nations. In developed countries, "low-income" means poor access to healthy foods, the most affordable diet being one that actually creates a diabetic physiology—nutrient-poor foods high in calories from processed sugar and hydrogenated oils. These cheap calories come at a high price for the lower class, as seen in Figure 7.

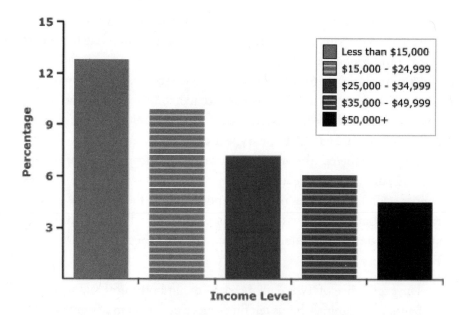

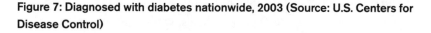

Figure 7: Diagnosed with diabetes nationwide, 2003 (Source: U.S. Centers for Disease Control)

In England, as in the U.S., the poor are 2.5 times more likely to develop Type-2 diabetes than the general population, and 3.5 times more likely to develop serious complications. In these societies obesity is nearly 50 percent higher among poor women and they are 50 percent more likely to be smoking. In Northeastern England diabetes is 45 percent higher in women and 28 percent higher in men than the national average. People from black and minority ethnic groups are up to six times higher.

AFRICA

In Africa, the current figure of 13.6 million people with diabetes is expected to almost double in the next 25 years, reaching just under 27 million, according to Professor Jean-Claude Mbanya, vice-president of the International Diabetes Federation (IDF). "Of concern is also the early onset of diabetes, particularly in sub-Saharan Africa, where more and more people in their thirties and early forties are developing Type-2 diabetes. They run a high risk of diabetes complications such as heart disease and foot ulcers at an early age."[19]

Until recently, there was a lack of data on the epidemiology of diabetes mellitus in Africa. Over the past decade, information on the prevalence of Type-2 diabetes has increased, albeit still limited, but there is still a lack of adequate data on Type-1 diabetes in sub-Saharan Africa. For Type-2 diabetes, although the prevalence is low in some rural populations, moderate and even high rates have been reported from other countries. In low diabetes prevalence populations, the moderate to high rates of impaired glucose tolerance is a possible indicator of the early stage of a diabetes epidemic.[20] According to the African Diabetes Federation:

> The prevalence of Type-2 diabetes is low in both rural and urban Bantu communities, but is ten times more prevalent in Muslim and Hindu communities in Tanzania and South Africa, and in the Chinese community in Mauritius. Type-1 diabetes, while still rare, is becoming increasingly prevalent. [Diabetes prevalence is higher in urban, migrant and African-origin populations living abroad.] Diabetes is already a major public health problem in Africa and its impact is bound to increase significantly if nothing is done to curb the rising rate of impaired glucose tolerance (IGT), which now exceeds 16 percent in some countries.[21]

THE MIDDLE EAST

In Israel, mostly among the large non-European immigrant population, the diabetes rate is already 7 percent of the population, with some 400,000 people diagnosed with diabetes. Another 600,000 suffer from some form of pre-diabetes or the metabolic syndrome (Syndrome X), which is strongly associated with insulin resistance among Jewish immigrant populations such as Yemenites, Kurds, and Ethiopians who, in their indigenous environment, had extremely low rates of diabetes. Upon arrival in Israel, they took on the more European junk-food culture, stopped exercising, and began experiencing skyrocketing incidence of diabetes. Yemenites are the ethnic group with the highest incidence of the disease.

In one study of Arab men and women from the Galilee in Israel, Dr. Mohammed Abdul-Ghani, a family physician and diabetes expert in the town of Nahf, discovered that 26 percent of his patients were diabetic and didn't know it, while 42 percent had impaired glucose tolerance and were at risk. Only 31 percent had no diabetic symptoms. This isn't just about Israeli Arabs; in Saudi Arabia 25 percent of the population have diabetes, and in Bahrain, about 32 percent have diabetes. Something in the Arab genetics makes them more susceptible to diabetes.

In the Arab countries, high levels of overweight and obesity exist particularly among women, in countries as diverse as Egypt and the Gulf states including Saudi Arabia. Obesity rates are 25–30 percent in Saudi Arabia and Kuwait, with the United Arab Emirates and Bahrain not far behind. In Iran, obesity rates vary from rural to urban populations, rising to 30 percent among women in Tehran. In northern Africa the prevalence of obesity among women is high. Half of all women are overweight (body mass index, or BMI, greater than 25), with rates of 50.9 percent in Tunisia and 51.3 percent in Morocco, and obesity rates (BMI > 30) in women of 23 percent in Tunisia and 18 percent in Morocco, representing a threefold increase over twenty years.[22]

EUROPE

The World Health Organization estimates 53 million diabetes cases in Europe as of 2007, and projects 64 million by 2025. In England, there are 1.4 million diabetics, and the number of people in the UK with diabetes is predicted to reach 3 million by 2010.

Diabetes has been known to the world for thousands of years; it was also noted by Hippocrates. The Sanskrit term for diabetes mellitus, *madhumeda,* appeared in Ayurvedic texts from thousands of years ago. Madhumeda translates as "honey urine" because the ancient practitioners first diagnosed the disease by testing the patient's urine to see if it, like honey, attracted ants.[23] It was portrayed in ancient Egyptian wall paintings showing somebody having what we call a muscle wasting disease and urinating copiously. One of the earliest known records of diabetes spoke of frequent urination, or "polyuria," as a symptom on papyrus written by Hesy-Ra, a Third Dynasty Egyptian physician.[24] During the first century AD, Arateus described diabetes as "the melting down of flesh and limbs into urine," and Galen of Pergamum, a Greek physician, felt diabetes was a form of kidney failure.[25] Then, it was rare; today, it is pandemic. What we are seeing today is a commentary on the state of mind and consequent lifestyle of our world culture. The behavior and lifestyle habits that create Type-2 diabetes are a Crime Against Wisdom. It is this lifestyle and diet of refined white sugar, saturated animal fat, and junk food that causes a metabolic disorder of carbohydrate, lipid, and protein metabolism.

Yes, diabetes has a very clear genetic component, especially for Type-2 diabetes. Type-1 diabetes also has a genetic component, but the genetic component is a less important factor. Both of these may be associated with gestational diabetes (diabetes during pregnancy). Type-2 is also associated with vitamin and mineral deficiencies. The key deficient minerals are: magnesium, chromium, vanadium, manganese, and potassium. It is associated with lack of exercise and obesity. It has become a pandemic, because people are not living in a way that brings them into balance with themselves. They are living the lifestyle of the Culture of Death and not the Culture of Life. This is why we call it a *Crime Against Wisdom,* an ancient Ayurvedic term that describes the situation.

CULTURES

Type-2 diabetes seems to have the highest rates in indigenous cultures where they have minimal genetic defense. When indigenous cultures come in contact with processed, adulterated, high-white-sugar and white-flour foods, and move from an active to a more passive lifestyle with its concomitant obesity, they are at serious risk for diabetes.

The association between poor diet and obesity is strong. Obesity is secondary to a diet high in saturated cooked animal fats and high in sugar. Americans have become conspicuous consumers of sugar and sweet-tasting foods and beverages. Per capita consumption of caloric sweeteners, mainly sucrose (table sugar made from cane and beets) and corn sweeteners (notably high-fructose corn syrup, or HFCS) increased 43 pounds, or 39 percent, between 1950–1959 and 2000. In 2000, each American consumed an average 152 pounds of caloric sweeteners. That amounted to more than two-fifths of a pound, or *52 teaspoons per person per day.*[26] This is something unheard of in human history. Dr. Thomas Cleave did a historical survey after World War II of indigenous cultures to which white sugar and white flour had been introduced. He found that in every culture in which there was an outbreak of Type-2 diabetes, the disease occurred approximately twenty years after white sugar and white flour were introduced. That's a very clear statement. Although it is commonly thought that diabetes is a blood sugar imbalance, it is actually a metabolic disorder that affects protein metabolism, fat metabolism, and carbohydrate metabolism. This metabolic imbalance is interwoven with diet and lifestyle characterized by obesity and lack of exercise, combined with high-processed-sugar, high-animal-fat, and low-fiber foods.

A much greater percentage of the uneducated and lower classes develop diabetes, and more specifically, a great many Native Americans, African Americans, Asians, and Hispanics suffer from it.

We only have to go back a little bit in history to see that this pandemic is relatively new. We have been on the planet for perhaps 3.2 million years. The Pima Indians had only one single documented case of diabetes by 1920. Their cousins the Tarahumaras, who have stuck with a natural diet, have only 6 percent incidence of diabetes, while their genetic relatives the Pimas have up to 51 percent incidence. In 1970 the Pimas' ability to fish was compromised by some river dams and they turned more to Western culture junk foods. The rate skyrocketed when genetics and a diabetogenic Western diet collided. The rate of diabetes is dramatically affected by the genetics for diabetes in a particular culture, and many scientists believe genetics may explain the obesity problem among Native Americans. The first U.S. researcher to learn about the Mexican Pimas was Leslie O. Schulz, professor of health sciences

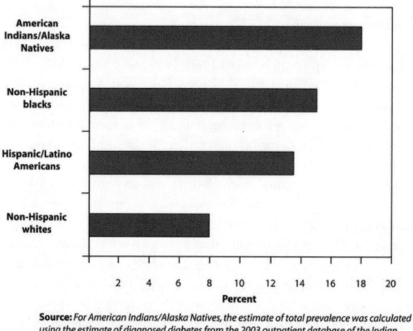

Source: *For American Indians/Alaska Natives, the estimate of total prevalence was calculated using the estimate of diagnosed diabetes from the 2003 outpatient database of the Indian Health Service and the estimate of undiagnosed diabetes from the 1999-2002 National Health and Nutrition Examination Survey. For the other groups, 1999-2002 NHANES estimates of total prevalence (both diagnosed and undiagnosed) were projected to year 2006.*

* Graph and information obtained from CDC (Center for Disease Control and Prevention) website at http://www.cdc.gov/diabetes/pubs/estimates05.htm#prev4 on December 1, 2006.

Figure 8: Estimated age-adjusted total prevalence of diabetes in people age 20 years or older by race/ethnicity, United States, 2005

at the University of Wisconsin-Milwaukee. With the cooperation of the tribe, she has established a clinic and research site to test several hypotheses about this contrast in diabetes rates. Since 1991, she has made some fifteen trips to Maycoba, as well as many visits to the Gila River reservation. Her "thrifty gene" theory is related below.[27]

Before food preservation and transportation methods were developed in the United States, indigenous populations in North America relied exclusively on locally produced food, in the same way indigenous Mexican populations such as the Pimas do today. When the harvest was poor, people ate less. Long periods of drought and famine were especially common in desert regions, such as the area the Pimas inhabit.

"The theory is that Native Americans have what is called the 'thrifty gene,'" Schulz explains. "They're genetically geared to conserving and being thrifty in terms of their calories, so that they don't waste it in case a famine comes along. They're going to be the ones to survive."

The continual availability of food in the United States today appears to have contributed to the Pimas' problems with obesity, Schulz says. The thrifty gene, which allows Indians to survive long periods of famine in Mexico, works against them on the Gila River reservation. "All of a sudden, there's this constant food supply, like we have now, 24 hours a day. We never have the famine, so that's why they become so much more overweight. Then, being overweight, they develop the Type-2 diabetes that goes with that."

TOTAL PREVALENCE OF DIABETES BY RACE/ETHNICITY[28]

Non-Hispanic Whites: 13.1 million, or 8.7 percent of all non-Hispanic whites age 20 years or older have diabetes.

Non-Hispanic Blacks: 3.2 million, or 13.3 percent of all non-Hispanic blacks age 20 years or older have diabetes. After adjusting for population age differences, non-Hispanic blacks are 1.8 times as likely to have diabetes as non-Hispanic whites.

Hispanic/Latino Americans: After adjusting for population age differences, Mexican Americans, the largest Hispanic/Latino subgroup, are 1.7 times as likely to have diabetes as non-Hispanic whites. If the prevalence of diabetes among Mexican Americans is applied to the total Hispanic/Latino population, according to the Centers for Disease control in 2006, about 13.5 percent of Hispanic/Latino Americans age 20 years or older would have diabetes. Sufficient data are not available to derive estimates of the total prevalence of diabetes (both diagnosed and undiagnosed diabetes) for other Hispanic/Latino groups. However, residents of Puerto Rico are 1.8 times as likely to have diagnosed diabetes as U.S. non-Hispanic whites.

American Indians and Alaska Natives: 99,500, or 12.8 percent of American Indians and Alaska natives age 20 years or older who received care from Indian Health Service (IHS) in 2003 had diagnosed diabetes. Some 118,000 (15.1 percent) American Indians and Alaska natives age 20 years or older have diabetes (both diagnosed and undiagnosed). Taking into account population age differences, American Indians and Alaska natives are 2.2 times as likely to have diabetes as non-Hispanic whites.

Asian Americans and Pacific Islanders: The total prevalence of diabetes (both diagnosed and undiagnosed) is not available for Asian Americans or Pacific Islanders. However, in Hawaii, Asians, native Hawaiians, and other Pacific Islanders age 20 years or older are more than twice as likely to have diagnosed diabetes as Caucasians after adjusting for population age differences, and are more susceptible than Caucasians to being overweight. Similarly, in California, Asians are 1.5 times as likely to have diagnosed diabetes as non-Hispanic whites. Other groups in these populations also have increased risk for diabetes.

Cities

New York City is an amplified microcosm of this information. There are 800,000 people with diagnosed diabetes in New York City—one in eight people. It is the only major disease in the city that is growing. The percentage of diabetics in New York City is about a third higher than the rest of the nation and cases have been increasing about twice as fast as nationally. In the past ten years, New York City has seen a 140 percent increase in diabetes. The proportion of diabetics is higher than that of Los Angeles, Chicago, or Boston. In New York, the diabetic rate is highest where there are ethnic groups with high genetic tendencies.

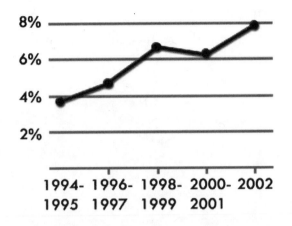

8%

6%

4%

2%

1994- 1996- 1998- 2000- 2002
1995 1997 1999 2001

Sources: NYC Dept. of Health & Mental Hygiene;
US Centers for Disease Control and Prevention;
World Health Organization

Figure 9: Diabetes rates in New York City (Source: NYC Dept. of Health & Mental Hygiene)

It is worst in East Harlem, where the health department survey shows that 16–20 percent, or up to one in five, adults have diabetes. The only place that is higher is among the Pima Indians in Arizona, where approximately 50 percent suffer from diabetes. In East Harlem diabetes-related amputations are also higher than in any other part of the city. And of course that is also the location of the highest percentage of people who are overweight—people who have bad food habits, exercise very little, and have significant poverty.

According to the U.S. Centers for Disease Control, one in three children born in the U.S. are expected to become diabetic in their lifetimes. New York is not the only place where diabetes is epidemic. As quoted in *The Daily Texan* in 2005: "In President George W. Bush's home state of Texas, state health services commissioner Dr. Eduardo Sanchez said, 'Half of Texas children born after the year 2000 will develop diabetes.'"

AGE AS A FACTOR

Diabetes also increases with age. It could be considered a marker of accelerated aging.

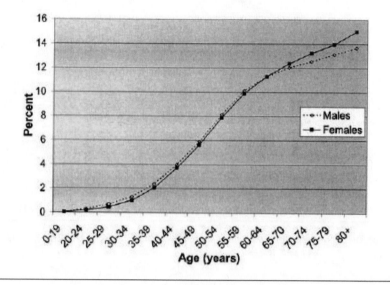

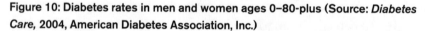

Figure 10: Diabetes rates in men and women ages 0–80-plus (Source: *Diabetes Care,* 2004, American Diabetes Association, Inc.)

Today one in five New Yorkers 65 years and older have diabetes. New York is not even the most overweight. In New York, 20 percent are overweight, while 20–30 percent are overweight in the rest of the country. But it is in New York, as in England, that Type-2 diabetes is very much connected with race, genetics, and money. It seems to have an inverse relationship to income. Poverty seems to be associated with less access to fresh fruits and vegetables, exercise, and health care. New York's poverty rate is approximately 20 percent, which is higher than the nation's 12.7 percent.

African Americans, Latinos, Mexican Americans, and Puerto Ricans have a diabetes rate close to twice that of white people. In England, we see the same kinds of racial ratios. Asian Americans and Pacific Islanders also appear more susceptible, and they seem to develop diabetes at lower comparative weights. There is no question that genetics plays a role, but our lifestyle is the determining factor. Our collective world lifestyle is one big Crime Against Wisdom.

In New York City—home to a pretty educated group—a 2002 health department survey found that 89 percent of diabetics didn't know their HgbA1c levels.[29] The HgbA1c is called the glycosylated hemoglobin test; this important test measures the level of sugar that binds non-enzymatically to hemoglobin and thus helps monitor the degree of diabetes. Any HgbA1c result above 6.0 is considered diabetic. In New York City, half the grade schoolers are overweight, and roughly one in four are obese (more than 20 pounds overweight). While the state was trying to promote more exercise, the city actually passed a school budget with less exercise. According to the Centers for Disease Control, nationwide daily participation in gym class has dropped to 28 percent in 2003, from 42 percent in 1991. The federal government of the U.S. had actually made proposals to cut the exercise time even less. Diabetes reflects the imbalance of the culture.

American kids are watching 20,000 hours of commercials for junk food. They can buy junk food readily from machines in their schools. We act as if this is not really happening, but data of the diabetes pandemic show the hard-core reality. The dramatic increase in Type-2 diabetes among children is an ominous symptom of the Culture of Death lifestyle. How much more suffering and disability do we need to wake up from this deadly lifestyle and diet of the Culture of Death?

COSTS TO SOCIETY

By 2025, the largest increases in diabetes prevalence will take place in developing countries. Each year an additional 7 million people worldwide develop diabetes. An even greater number die from cardiovascular disease made worse by diabetes-related lipid disorders and hypertension.[30] People with diabetes face the near certainty, and in many poor countries the stark reality, of premature death. Type-1 diabetes is particularly costly in terms of mortality in poor countries, where many children die because access to life-saving insulin is not subsidized by governments (in some countries, there even is a high tax on purchased insulin), and is often not available at any price. Recent studies in Zambia, Mali, and Mozambique highlight a stark reality: A person requiring insulin for survival in Zambia will live an average of eleven years; a person in Mali can expect to live for thirty months; in Mozambique a person requiring insulin will be dead within twelve months.[31] In Tanzania, mortality of patients with insulin-dependent diabetes was found to be 40 percent after a mean of five years.[32] The main causes of death in those dying in hospital were ketoacidosis (50 percent) and infection (32 percent)—mirroring the patterns observed in Europe and the United States in the pre-insulin era.[33] Using World Health Organization figures on years of life lost per person dying of diabetes, this translates into more than 25 million years of total life lost each year to the disability and to reduced quality of life caused by the preventable complications of diabetes.[34]

ECONOMIC IMPACT

The estimated economic impact of diabetes is considerable, and is becoming most noticeably felt in the poorest countries, where people with diabetes and their families bear almost the entire cost of whatever medical care they can afford. In Latin America, families pay 40–60 percent of diabetes care costs out of their own pockets, and in India, the poorest people with diabetes spend an average of 25 percent of their income on private care. Most of this money is used to stay alive by avoiding fatally high blood sugar levels.

Because diabetes is increasing faster in the world's developing economies than in its developed ones, it is the developing world that will bear the brunt of the future cost burden. More than 80 percent of expenditures for medical care for diabetes are made in the world's economically richest countries. Less than 20 percent of expenditures are made in the middle- and low-income countries, where 80 percent of people with diabetes will soon live. The United States is home to about 8 percent of the world's population living with diabetes, and spends more than 50 percent of all global expenditure for diabetes care.

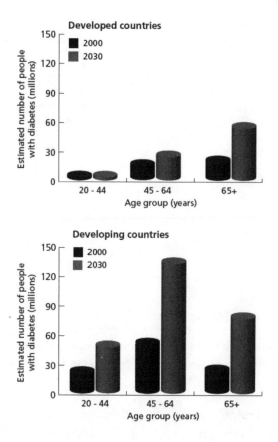

In the U.S. in 1997, the total medical expenditures incurred by people with diabetes was $77.7 billion, or $10,071 per capita annually for medical products and services, compared with $2,669 for people without diabetes.[35] Related ailments are costly, as well: $30,400 for a heart attack or amputation, $40,200 for a stroke, and $37,000 for end-stage kidney disease. The CDC estimated that the annual cost of diabetes in the United States by 2002 was in the range of $264 billion.[36] Listed below are key cost elements:

- $132 billion total (direct and indirect)
- $92 billion direct medical costs
- $40 billion indirect costs (disability, work loss, premature mortality)

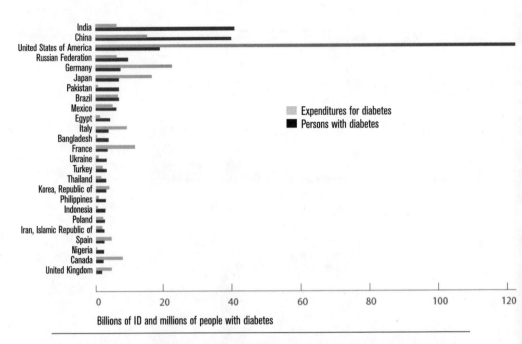

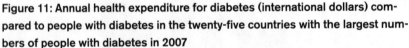

Billions of ID and millions of people with diabetes

Figure 11: Annual health expenditure for diabetes (international dollars) compared to people with diabetes in the twenty-five countries with the largest numbers of people with diabetes in 2007

Government budgets worldwide will face the immense strain of diabetes care on disability payments, pensions, social and medical service, and revenue loss.

Diabetes affects all people in society, not just those who live with the disease. WHO estimates that mortality from diabetes, heart disease, and stroke costs about 250 billion international dollars (ID) in China, ID225 billion in the Russian Federation, and ID210 billion in India in 2005. Much of the heart disease and stroke in these estimates was linked to diabetes. WHO estimates that diabetes, heart disease, and stroke together will cost approximately:

- $555.7 billion in lost national income in China over the next ten years
- $303.2 billion in the Russian Federation
- $333.6 billion in India

- $49.2 billion in Brazil
- $2.5 billion even in a very poor country like Tanzania

These estimates are based on lost productivity, resulting primarily from premature death. Accounting for disability might double or triple these figures.

Diabetes also has a negative impact upon a person's general health condition and work performance. In 2003, the CDC found: 33.6 percent of U.S. adults with diabetes reported at least one day of poor mental health for each thirty days; 53.9 percent reported at least one day of poor physical health; and 62.8 percent reported at least one day of either poor mental or physical health. Also, 32.6 percent of adults with diabetes were unable to perform their usual activities at least one day per month due to either poor mental or physical health.

If we actually followed the diet of prevention we could probably save hundreds of billions in direct and indirect costs, *but are we going to do that*—that is the question. Why not do the obvious? Roughly $40 billion in federal subsidies are going to pay corn growers, so that corn syrup is able to replace cane sugar. Corn syrup has been singled out by many health experts as one of the chief culprits of rising obesity, because corn syrup does not turn off appetite. Since the advent of corn syrup, consumption of all sweeteners has soared, as have people's weights.

According to a 2004 study reported in the *American Journal of Clinical Nutrition,* the rise of Type-2 diabetes since 1980 has closely paralleled the increased use of sweeteners, particularly corn syrup. Data collected from the study of 51,603 nurses in the United States found that women who drank one serving of non-diet soda or fruit punch daily, which was sweetened with either sugar or high-fructose corn syrup, gained more weight, an average of 10.3 pounds, than women who drank less than one per month. The study was conducted over four years. In addition, the sugar consumers had an 82 percent increased risk of developing Type-2 diabetes. "The message is: Anyone who cares about their health or the health of their family would not consume these beverages," said Walter C. Willett of the Harvard School of Public

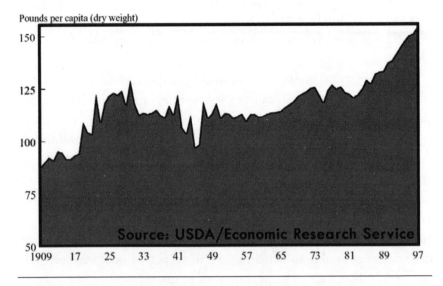

Pounds per capita (dry weight)

Source: USDA/Economic Research Service

Figure 12: Sugar consumption among Americans, 1909–1997

Health, who helped conduct the study. "Parents who care about their children's health should not keep [processed-sugar beverages] at home."[37] Dr. Willett's statement makes the point clearly: The profits made from the Culture of Death lifestyle are in direct conflict with our ability to care for our children and ourselves. The ability to love and care for our children and ourselves is a healthy characteristic of the Culture of Life. Do we choose life or do we choose death?

Research also indicates that high-fructose corn syrup interferes with the heart's use of key minerals like magnesium, copper, and chromium, in addition to being implicated in elevated blood cholesterol levels and the creation of blood clots. All of these factors contribute to cardio-vascular disease—the leading cause of death among diabetics. High-fructose corn syrup has also been found to inhibit the action of white blood cells so that they are unable to defend the body against harmful foreign invaders.[38]

There are not any real accidents here. This is very straightforward, and is a clear and ongoing tragedy. The American Diabetes Association estimates that diabetes is costing about $132 billion a year. To put this cost in perspective: all the cancers together in United States cost about $171 billion a year. We have a major epidemic, and we are only making the problem worse.

There are many secondary causes to this pandemic. Some doctors are a little concerned, as increasing numbers of children are given anti-psychotic drugs for anxiety and conditions like autism. This is because these drugs can promote weight gain and therefore elevate the risk of diabetes. The anti-psychotic Zyprexa, for example, has been implicated in causing weight gain and diabetes. With increased weight, there is increased diabetes. Little research has been done on the long-term impact of Type-2 diabetes on children, over their life span. The chronic complications that follow tend to happen ten to fifteen years after the onset. This means that life-limiting complications such as kidney disease, heart disease, stroke, and blindness are now hitting people in the prime of their lives, in the middle of their most productive years. The projections by the Centers for Disease Control for children with Type-2 diabetes is that their life span will be shortened by nineteen years.

The treatment of diabetes is further complicated by a belief system stated by the *New York Times* and backed by most doctors treating diabetes: "Diabetes has no cure. It is progressive and fatal." Even the preliminary results of our research are showing this to be a myth. It is a myth because we did not previously have widespread knowledge of how to reverse it naturally, although as early as 1920, Max Gerson, MD, healed Albert Schweitzer, MD, of diabetes with a live-food diet.

Diabetes is clearly a pandemic created by the world lifestyle of the Culture of Death. The statistics are overwhelming. Nothing less than the health of whole societies is at stake. What is needed is to help the world transition into the Culture of Life, which must be done on a personal basis. Before we talk about how we can easily reverse our current pandemic to a world without diabetes, we need to scientifically investigate personal lifestyle habits that create diabetes and, from this science-based approach, develop a program that can help us choose prudent lifestyle habits that will create a nondiabetic, healthy physiology.

CHAPTER 2

Diabetic Lifestyle Habits
and Risk Factors

When we break the natural laws, they break us. In this chapter, you are going to read about some things that you may hold very dear as part of what you see as your identity. It is very important that you acknowledge the healthy part of yourself that does not want diabetes, or the diet and lifestyle that create it, to be your life experience anymore. Any attachment we had to the diabetic that we were, and the diet and lifestyle we lived that created it, need to be transformed. "My precious burdens," Walt Whitman said, "My precious burdens I carry them wherever I go."

What we will investigate now are our precious burdens, and in Chapter 4, we will develop a mental space and life practices that will help us let go of these for a life that draws in the best things possible. Chapter 5 will show you how to eat a Culture of Life anti-diabetogenic diet that is accessible and tasty, no matter what your busy life schedule may bring. If you are having any doubt as you read this book cover to cover, *see the client results in Chapter 4.* What you will see is the reality that you want for yourself, for your family, and for society. Hold in your mind the potential that you can be one of the healthiest, most vibrant people you know. We are going to guide you to achieving just that. With this in mind, let's look at these precious burdens, these lifestyle attachments that need to be transformed to help reverse Type-2 diabetes.

Risk factors associated with the Culture of Death are listed below. We'll look at them one by one in this chapter, along with other issues of diabetes as an accelerated aging reality, genetics, diabetes in children, insulin resistance, gestational diabetes, Alzheimer's associated diabetes, and cancer associations. The personal lifestyle habits, choices, and predisposing diseases that are diabetogenic include:

- Inactivity, especially television watching
- Overweight and obesity—including the causal behaviors of eating a processed-cooked-pasteurized-irradiated food diet, a

high-glycemic and high-insulin index diet, a low-fiber diet, meat
eating, high-fat diet, and food-borne environmental toxicity—
including that found in fish
- Dairy consumption
- Blood cholesterol
- High-stress lifestyle and hypertension
- Candida
- Depression
- Metabolic syndrome (Syndrome X)
- Toxicity of heavy metals and drinking water
- Vaccinations
- Coffee and caffeinated beverages
- Smoking

Inactivity

According to the U.S. Centers for Disease Control (CDC), 37.7 percent
of diabetics report being physically inactive. Inactivity promotes Type-
2 diabetes, and even increases insulin needs in Type-1 by not accessing
the benefit of special proteins that transport glucose into the cells.
Essentially, exercise works like taking an insulin shot, because it reduces
blood glucose levels. Working your muscles more often and making
them work harder improves their ability to use insulin and absorb glucose. This puts less stress on your insulin-making pancreatic beta cells.

   A new theory on how exercise serves to work like insulin stems from
the special proteins called GLUT-4 transporters that usher glucose into
the muscle cells. Exercise causes GLUT-4 transporters to rise to the surface of the cellular membrane, where they can shuttle circulating glucose into the cell, increasing insulin sensitivity and decreasing insulin
needs. Findings from the Nurses' Health Study and Health Professionals
Follow-Up Study suggest that walking briskly for a half hour every day
reduces the risk of developing Type-2 diabetes by 30 percent. The benefits of exercise, with suggestions and data, will be presented at greater
length in Chapter 3.

Television Programming

Let's look at television watching specifically. A study by the American Diabetes Association followed 41,811 men ages 40 to 75 over a ten-year period. A direct association was observed between television watching and risk of developing diabetes. The men who reported sitting in front of a TV more than nineteen hours per week were more than 150 percent more likely to become diabetic than those who watched less than three hours a week. "Bubble gum for the eyes," Steve Allen called it. Television watching is another form of inactivity, and increasing evidence suggests that exercise is protective against the development of Type-2 diabetes mellitus.

Every two hours per week you spend watching TV instead of pursuing something more active increases the chances of developing diabetes by 14 percent.[1]

Overweight and Obesity

It is important to understand overweight and obesity, taken together or separately, as a reflection of the Culture of Death diet and lifestyle, as an underlying cause of insulin resistance and diabetes. Data from the CDC shows that among diabetics, 82.1 percent are overweight or obese, and 48.1 percent are obese based on self-reported height and weight. Overweight or obesity is a precondition for many of the preventable causes of death now experienced in the developed world. A special report in the *New England Journal of Medicine* found that obesity is now such a significant factor that "it is larger than the negative effect of all accidental deaths combined (e.g., accidents, homicide, and suicide), and there is reason to believe that it will rapidly approach and could exceed the negative effect that ischemic heart disease or cancer has on life expectancy."[2] They continue: "From our analysis of the effect of obesity on longevity, we conclude that the steady rise in life expectancy during the past two centuries may soon come to an end."

Let's look at some of the theoretical underlying causes of overweight and obesity.

PROCESSED, COOKED, PASTEURIZED, AND IRRADIATED FOOD

There is no necessity to sell out our health and shorten our lives so that someone else can profit from marketing longer-shelf-life, so-called "convenient" foods. To continue to eat these foods is to reaffirm membership in the Culture of Death.

When you cook food, according to the Max Planck Institute, you coagulate 50 percent of the food's protein. Other research shows that 70–90 percent of vitamins and minerals and up to 100 percent of phytonutrients are destroyed when food is cooked. Processing, cooking, pasteurization, and irradiation are all food handling methods that destroy the anti-diabetogenic qualities of our foods given to us in their natural state. Because of these processes that destroy the nutritional value of the food by at least 50 percent, we end up needing to eat more food to get the nutritional value that we would have gotten with the uncooked food in its whole state. This additional eating leads to overweight. This has significant implications for why we use a nutrient-dense live-foods diet, as discussed in Chapter 4. In addition, the junk food diet fills us with empty calories, leaving us more hungry and further craving food.

For example, to make this point crystal clear, shopping the center of the supermarket (where the processed foods are) *can* create diabetes. Adam Drewnowski, an obesity researcher at the University of Washington, wanted to figure out why it is that the most reliable predictor of obesity in America is a person's low economic status. Drewnowski gave himself a hypothetical dollar to spend, using it to purchase as many calories as he could. He discovered that he could buy the most calories per dollar in the *middle aisles of the supermarket,* among the towering canyons of processed food and soft drinks. Drewnowski found that a dollar could buy 1,200 calories of cookies or potato chips, but only 250 calories of carrots; that his dollar bought 875 calories of soda but only 170 calories of orange juice.[3] This is a potential insight into why people of low economic means have the highest rates of diabetes in Western cultures.

Going deeper into the psychospiritual level, as we contrast the Culture of Death with the Culture of Life, it is my teaching that "there is never enough food for the hungry soul." The Culture of Death creates a hungry, empty soul experience, which we try to fill with food as a substitute for love and connection. The Culture of Life fills our souls with love.

GLYCEMIC INDEX AND INSULIN INDEX

A high-glycemic diet is one that includes any white sugar, any white flour, white rice, honey, maple syrup, alcohol, coffee, wheat, any junk food, and most fruit (some fruit, such as berries and cherries, is moderate to low on the glycemic index). A high-glycemic diet also includes cooked beets and carrots, rutabaga, summer squash, cooked yams, pumpkin, parsnips, white potatoes, apricots, figs, grapes, raisins, melons, mangos, bananas, papaya, pears, peaches, plums, pineapple, kiwi, sapote, cherimoya, rambutian, durian, dates, and dried fruits. All fruit juices, carrot juice, and beet juice are also high-glycemic foods. High insulin index foods, which are low on the glycemic index but still diabetogenic, include meat, fish, chicken, and dairy.

We recommend against fruit for three to six months until the fasting blood sugar (FBS) stabilizes at 85 or below, and then only low-glycemic fruit such as berries, cherries, citrus, goji berries, cranberries, and an occasional apple.

LOW FIBER

Fiber is the part of the plant that cannot be digested or absorbed by the body. It is a carbohydrate that is obtained from vegetables, fruits, nuts, and seeds. Fiber is either water soluble or water insoluble. Water-soluble fiber is especially good for people with diabetes, because it delays the pace at which food passes through the stomach. This allows a slower rate of absorption of glucose into the bloodstream, which reduces the glycemic roller-coaster. It also improves insulin sensitivity, combating insulin resistance and helping insulin do its job of ushering glucose into the cells.

According to Dr. Julian Whitaker, MD:

One of the earlier studies demonstrating the power of dietary fiber in the treatment of diabetes was conducted by Perla M. Miranda, RD, MS, and David L. Horwitz, MD, PhD, FACp, and published in the *Annals of Internal Medicine* in 1978. Each of eight subjects who had insulin-dependent diabetes consumed either 20 grams of dietary fiber per day in the form of high-fiber bread or a mere 3 grams of fiber. All other factors of the diet were kept constant, as was the patients' insulin dosage. On the low-fiber intake, the average blood glucose level of the patients was 169.4 mg/dl. During the period of higher fiber intake, the mean blood sugar level was 120.8 mg/dl.[4]

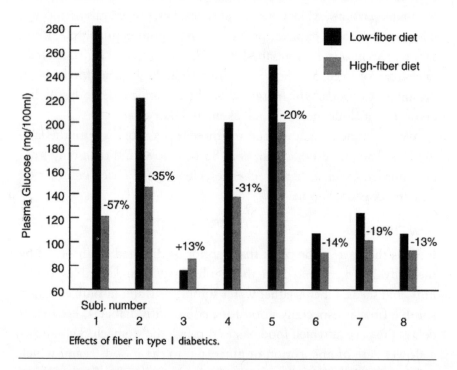

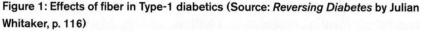

Effects of fiber in type I diabetics.

Figure 1: Effects of fiber in Type-1 diabetics (Source: *Reversing Diabetes* by Julian Whitaker, p. 116)

HIGH ANIMAL FAT: MEAT EATING

A potential diabetic can be transformed into a completely diabetic individual by administration of the time-honored carbohydrate-free meal of meat and fat.

DR. I. M. RABINOWICH, 1930

A quarter pound of beef raises insulin levels in diabetics as much as a quarter pound of straight sugar.

DIABETES CARE 7, 1984, P. 465

Cheese and beef elevate insulin levels higher than "dreaded" high-carbohydrate foods like pasta.

AMERICAN JOURNAL OF CLINICAL NUTRITION 50, 1997, P. 1264

A single burger's worth of beef, or three slices of cheddar cheese, boost insulin levels more than almost two cups of cooked pasta.

AMERICAN JOURNAL OF CLINICAL NUTRITION 50, 1997, P. 1264

We have been hinting that a successful reversal of diabetes takes us back to high-enzyme live food and unprocessed food, which is part of the Culture of Life. This is a diet similar to what the human organism has been eating for perhaps 3.2 million years. A shift happened about 10,000 years ago, when farming and herding came into the forefront of the tribal cultures and we began to switch to a grain-based and herding civilization. Herding meant the introduction for the first time in history of high amounts of flesh food on a regular basis. Before that the human species really did not eat a lot of meat. According to Robert Leakey, one of the leading medical anthropologists in the world, the human diet was primarily a vegan chimpanzee diet with an occasional bite of meat. Through simple logic, we can see that a brown bear is clearly more carnivorous than a human by looking at its claws and teeth, and yet a brown bear eats a diet of 95–97 percent raw plant food. The longest-living Hunza people of northern Pakistan live on a diet that contains less than 1 percent meat. Consider that between 1840 and 1974, the quantity of meat eaten per person in the United States increased *five times over*. During roughly the same time, the United States went from being the healthiest nation in world in 1900, out of 100 surveyed, to dead last in 1990.[5]

The diet that historically has been best for health and prevention of Type-2 diabetes really is one that is high-complex-carbohydrate, non-animal-fat, and moderately low-plant-fat (15–20 percent); low-glycemic and low-insulin; and high in fiber. In World War II, Professor H. P. Himsworth noted that when food shortages removed the white flour, white sugar, and excessive meat protein and fats from the typical British diet, *the death rate from diabetes fell 50 percent.*

Studies have shown that Seventh-Day Adventist men who ate meat six or more days a week had 3.8 times greater risk of having diabetes mentioned on the death certificate as compared with those Seventh-Day Adventists who were lacto-ovo-vegetarians.[6] This would not be unexpected since meat contains considerable cholesterol and saturated fat, which would result in higher risk of atherosclerosis, the major cause of death among diabetics. However, the unexpected finding was that twenty years prior, at the outset of the study, those who were nondiabetic were more apt to get diabetes if they were customarily in the habit of consuming meat.

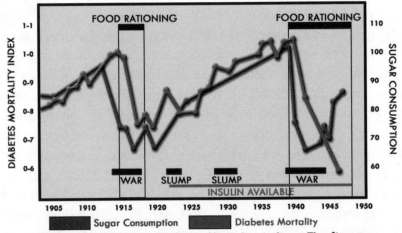

England and Wales. Diabetic Mortality indices. The figures for 1946 and 1947 supplied by Dr. Percy Stocks. Drawn by Thomas L. Cleave in *The Saccharine Disease.*

In *The China Study,* T. Colin Campbell, PhD, relates a study that measured diets and diabetes in a population of Japanese American men in Washington state. These men, sons of Japanese immigrants to the U.S., remarkably had more than four times the prevalence of diabetes than the average rate found in similar-age men who stayed in Japan. For Japanese Americans, the ones who developed diabetes also ate the most animal protein, animal fat, and dietary cholesterol, each of which is only found in animal-based foods.[7] Total fat intake also was higher among the diabetics. These same dietary characteristics also resulted in excess weight. These second-generation Japanese Americans ate a meatier diet with less plant-based food than men born in Japan. The researchers wrote: "Apparently, the eating habits of Japanese men living in the United States resemble more the American eating style than the Japanese." The consequence: four times as much incidence of diabetes.[8]

The benefits of a diet of plant foods is professionally recognized. The American Dietetic Association (ADA), the world's largest organization of professional dieticians, published the following statements in June 2003 on a vegetarian diet and lifestyle:[9]

> Vegetarians have been reported to have lower body mass indices than nonvegetarians, as well as lower rates of death from ischemic heart disease; vegetarians also show lower blood cholesterol levels; lower blood pressure; and lower rates of hypertension, type 2 diabetes, and prostate and colon cancer. Well-planned vegan and other types of vegetarian diets are appropriate for all stages of the life cycle, including during pregnancy, lactation, infancy, childhood and adolescence.
>
> Vegetarian diets offer a number of nutritional benefits, including lower levels of saturated fat, cholesterol, and animal protein as well as higher levels of carbohydrates, fiber, magnesium, potassium, folate, and antioxidants such as vitamins C and E and phytochemicals. ...
>
> It is the position of the American Dietetic Association and Dietitians of Canada that appropriately planned vegetarian diets

are healthful, nutritionally adequate, and provide health benefits in the prevention and treatment of certain diseases.

Meat eating is diabetogenic on all accounts, and meat is by no means an ideal food or protein source for humans. Meat eating creates the preconditions for diabetes, and accelerates the complications of the condition once it has manifested. Research cited in *Spiritual Nutrition* shows that meat protein can increase insulin resistance, a precondition for diabetes and the diabetic degenerative process. Let's investigate the negative aspects of meat eating, and consider whether these realities should be included or excluded from a Culture of Life antidiabetogenic diet and lifestyle designed to completely reverse diabetes.

According to T. Colin Campbell, PhD, numerous studies have shown that vegetarians and vegans are slimmer than their meat-eating counterparts. People in these studies who are vegetarian or vegan are anywhere from 5 to 30 pounds slimmer than their fellow citizens.[10,11,12,13,14,15,16] Our results in the Tree of Life 21-Day+ Program bear this out. During the thirty-day program for the film, participants, who were meat eaters, lost between 20 and 32 pounds.

Cardiovascular disease is significantly higher in meat eaters. In 1961 the AMA stated that 97 percent of heart disease would be eliminated if people gave up eating meat and ate a vegetarian diet.

Udo Erasmus reports in his book *Fats That Heal, Fats That Kill* that several species of fish actually contain toxic fats and oils. An example is the toxic cetoleic fatty acid, found in herring, capelin, menhaden, anchovetta, and even in cod liver oil!

Younger women who regularly eat red meat appear to face an increased risk for a common form of **breast cancer,** according to a large, well-known Harvard study of women's health published in the *Archives of Internal Medicine* November 2006. The study of more than 90,000 women found that the more red meat the women consumed in their twenties, thirties, and forties, the greater their risk for developing breast cancer fueled by hormones in the next twelve years. Those who consumed the most red meat had nearly twice the risk of those who ate red meat infrequently.[4217]

Men whose mothers have low beef intake, compared to men of mothers with high beef intake, are more virile. Sons of mothers with low beef consumption have sperm concentrations 24.3 percent higher than those of high-beef-consumption mothers. Eighteen percent of sons of mothers with high beef consumption had sperm levels lower than what the World Health Organization considers the lower limit of subfertility—this rate of infertility is three times higher than sons of mothers with low beef consumption. Extrapolating, we have two theoretical potentials: sons of vegan mothers are more virile, and vegan men are more virile.

Research has also shown that removing meat from your diet and eating a plant-sourced diet can reduce or eliminate **asthma.** Thirty-five patients who had suffered from bronchial asthma for an average of twelve years, all receiving long-term medication, twenty including cortisone, were subject to a plant-source-only diet for one year. In almost all cases, medication was able to be withdrawn or drastically reduced. There was a significant decrease in asthma symptoms. Twenty-four patients (69 percent) fulfilled the treatment. Of these, 71 percent reported improvement at four months and 92 percent at one year.[18]

Osteoporosis is significantly higher in meat eaters or even women who drink three or more glasses of milk per day. Research suggests that the higher amounts of protein create an acidity that forces the bones to give up calcium to neutralize the acidity.

The high phosphorus content in meat actually pulls calcium from the bones. In essence, from the perspective of health and diabetes in particular, animal flesh sourced protein—fish included—is inferior to vegetable protein as a quality protein source. This undisputed scientific fact is confirmed by the China Study by T. Colin Campbell and the epidemiological evidence of 6,500 Chinese across 65 provinces. A meat-based protein is a poorer quality protein source than a plant-based protein, as evidenced by cancer data from that study showing that the more animal protein was consumed, the higher the rates of cancer. According to the Max Planck Institute, cooking coagulates approximately 50 percent of the protein, making the food less digestible, more coarse, and more inflammatory. In essence, cooking meat protein creates a situation in which one actually gets one-half the protein that is eaten and the other half acts as an inflammatory toxin.

The best and most assimilable sources of protein are the algaes (about 70 percent protein), nuts and seeds, bee pollen, and greens, grains, and beans. Spirulina, blue-green algae, chlorella, hemp seeds, olives, durian, all sprouts (including sprouted grains and beans), bee pollen, green vegetables (especially spinach, watercress, arugula, kale, broccoli, brussel sprouts, collard greens, and parsley), powdered grasses, and green superfood powders are examples of relatively high-protein live foods.

ENVIRONMENTAL TOXICITY IN FOODS

Animals concentrate plant foods to form their tissues. And if there is toxicity in their air, water, and/or food environment—such as chemicals, pesticides, herbicides, larvicides, fungicides, detergents, bleaches, toxic solvents—then these toxins accumulate in the animal. Dairy products contain five times as many pesticides as commercial fruits and vegetables. And flesh foods, such as fish or chicken, which are higher up on the food chain, contain fifteen times as many pesticide residues as commercial fruits and vegetables.

From a practical point of view, eating fish is potentially dangerous because of the widespread, ever-increasing pollution of the waters of the world. The biggest water contaminants are PCBs and mercury. PCBs, along with dioxin, DDT, and dieldrin, are among the most toxic chemicals on the planet. According to John Culhane, in his 1980 article "PCBs: The Poisons That Won't Go Away," only a few parts per billion of these substances can cause cancer and birth defects in lab animals.[19] The tenth annual Council on Environmental Quality, sponsored by the U.S. government, reported PCBs in 100 percent of all human sperm samples. According to a *Washington Post* article in 1979, PCBs are considered one of the main reasons that the average sperm count of the American male is approximately 70 percent of what it was thirty years ago. This same article also points out that 25 percent of college students were sterile at the time as compared to 0.5 percent thirty-five years earlier. Most toxicity experts agree that the main source of human contamination comes from eating fish from waters in which the PCB levels are high, which today can be almost anywhere. The Environmental Protection Agency estimates that fish can accumulate up to *nine million times* the level of PCBs in the water in which they live. PCBs have been found in fish from the deepest and most remote parts of the world's oceans.

Fish and shellfish are natural accumulators of toxins, because they live and are flushed by the water in which they dwell. Shellfish such as oysters, clams, mussels, and scallops filter ten gallons of water every hour. In a month, an oyster will accumulate toxins at concentrations that are 70,000 times greater than the water they are living in. The problem isn't solved by not eating fish—after all, half the world's fish catch is fed to livestock. According to *Diet for a New America* by John Robbins, more fish are consumed by U.S. livestock than by the entire human population of all the countries in Western Europe. Periodic testing in the U.S. has found eggs and chickens highly contaminated with PCBs after being fed fish contaminated with PCBs.

Mercury toxicity from ingesting fish is another well-known source of illness. Two forms of mercury are the most dangerous: quicksilver mercury and methylmercury, which is about fifty times more toxic. Although there is general agreement that mercury in plants is a less toxic form, experts do not agree on whether the mercury in fish is stored primarily in the form of the more toxic methylmercury. In any case, children and adults who ate fish from mercury-contaminated waters in Minamata Bay, Japan, in 1953, along the Agano River in Niigata, Japan, in 1962, and other locations in Iraq, Pakistan, and Guatemala, all have suffered death, coma, or a variety of brain and neurological damage.

Researchers in Taiwan say they have established for the first time that the mercury compound present as a contaminant in some seafood can damage the insulin-producing cells in the pancreas. In their experiments, Shing-Hwa Liu and colleagues exposed cell cultures of insulin-producing beta cells to methylmercury. They used concentrations of methylmercury at about the same levels as people would consume in fish under the U.S. Food and Drug Administration's recommended limits.[20]

Contamination of fish is widespread. According to Rudolph Ballentine, MD, mercury toxicity is being reported with increasing frequency by physicians as well as dentists. The two main contributing factors seem to be a diet high in fish and the common use of silver-mercury amalgams for dental work. Fish consumption alone may be enough to cause mercury toxicity. An article by the Canadian Medical Association in 1976 reported that Indians in Northern Canada, who ate more than a pound of fish per day, had symptoms of mercury poisoning. A 1985 study in West Germany of 136 people who regularly consumed fish from the Elbe River found a correlation between the blood levels of both mercury and pesticides and the amount of fish eaten.

In a study published in the *Diet and Nutrition Letter* of Tufts University, it was reported that the more fish pregnant mothers ate from Lake Michigan, the more their babies showed abnormal reflexes, general weakness, slower responses to external stimuli, and various signs of depression. They found that mothers eating fish only two or three times a month produced babies weighing seven to nine ounces less at birth and with smaller heads.[21] Jacobsen, in a 1986 follow-up study reported in *Child Development,* found that there was a definite correlation between the amount of fish the mothers ate and the child's brain development, even if fish was eaten only once a month. He found that the more fish the pregnant mothers ate, the lower was the verbal IQ of the children.[22] These children also had lower SAT scores seventeen to eighteen years later. Children are usually the most sensitive to toxins, and they are prime indicators of what may be happening to adults on a more subtle level. A Swedish study in 1983 found that the milk of nursing mothers who regularly ate fatty fish from the Baltic Sea had higher levels of PCBs and pesticide residues than even meat-eaters. *Lactovegetarians were found to have the lowest pesticide residues in this study.*

Dairy Consumption

For everyone who lives on milk, being still an infant, is unskilled in the word of righteousness. But solid food is for the mature, for those whose faculties have been trained by practice to distinguish good from evil.

HEBREWS 5:13–14

Children with diabetic genetic tendencies who drink cow's milk have an 11–13 times higher rate of juvenile diabetes than children who are breastfed by their own mothers for at least three months. Although many are not aware of it, milk consumption is directly associated with juvenile diabetes. The American Academy of Pediatrics made a decision, based on this data, in 1994 to strongly encourage families with a diabetic history not to give their children cow's milk or cow's milk products for at least two years. The key to understanding this is that there are more than 100 antigens found in milk. The reason for the increase in juvenile diabetes is that the children have much higher formation of antibodies to the cow's milk antigens. According to a 1999 study reported in the journal *Diabetes* by Outi Vaarala, researchers found up to eight times the number of antibodies against milk protein in dairy-product-consuming children who also developed juvenile diabetes.[23] Finland, which has the world's highest milk consumption, also has the world's highest per capita rate of insulin-dependent diabetes.[24] The problem is that the antibodies to the milk antigens cross-react with the beta cells of the pancreas, creating inflammation and scarring. This consequently blocks or destroys beta cell production of insulin.

This is not new information. In 1992 the *New England Journal of Medicine* reported a study done in Finland on children ages 4–12. They measured the antibodies in these children against BSA (bovine serum albumin). Of the 142 children with juvenile diabetes every one one had an antibody titer greater that 3.55 and not one of the 79 nondiabetic children had an antibody titer greater than 3.55. The complete lack of overlap of serum antibodies of these two populations lead to some very productive studies in understanding the relationship of cow's milk intake and incidence of juvenile diabetes. One study in Chile[25] found that genet-

ically susceptible children who were weaned too early onto cow's milk—
before three months of age—had a risk factor for juvenile diabetes of
13.1 times greater than children who did not have a genetic proclivity,
or who were breastfed for at least three months. Another significant
study in the U.S.[26] found that children with a genetic tendency who
were weaned onto cow's milk before three months had a Type-1 diabetes incidence of 11.3 times greater than those who did not have a
genetic tendency and who were breastfed for at least three months. The
general statistical view is that anything more than 3–4 times higher is
considered a significant finding.

Charting the degree of milk consumption from ages 0 to 14 against
the onset of Type-1 diabetes reveals the correlation between milk consumption and Type-1 diabetes.[27] It is no accident that Japanese children, who have the lowest milk consumption, have 1/36th the incidence
of Type-1 diabetes than do the children from Finland, who had the
highest consumption of milk.

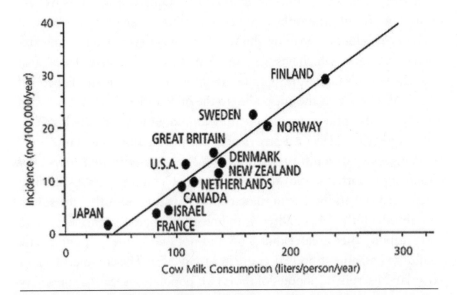

Figure 2: Association of cow's milk consumption and incidence of Type-1
diabetes in different countries (Source: T. Colin Campbell, *The China Study*)

When the data for both the genetically susceptible and non-susceptible are merged, there is an increased risk for children who are weaned and put on cow's milk before three months of approximately 1.5 times, which is approximately a 50 percent increase in incidence of Type-1 diabetes. One additional study in Finland showed that the consumption of cow's milk increased the rate of Type-1 diabetes by 500–600 percent.[28]

The overall results strongly suggest that cow's milk, especially in children who are genetically susceptible and who are weaned before three months, significantly increases the risk of developing Type-1 diabetes. Milk consumption has many other health and spiritual problems, which are beyond the scope of this book.

ALLERGIES AND LACTOSE INTOLERANCE

Cow's milk is the number one cause of food allergies among infants and children, according to the American Gastroenterological Association.[29] Most people begin to produce less lactase, the enzyme that helps with the digestion of milk, when they are as young as 2 years old. This reduction can lead to lactose intolerance.[30] Millions of Americans are lactose intolerant, and an estimated 90 percent of Asian Americans and 75 percent of Native- and African Americans suffer from the condition, which can cause bloating, gas, cramps, vomiting, headaches, rashes, and asthma.[31] Studies have also found that autism and schizophrenia in children may be linked to the body's inability to digest the milk protein casein; symptoms of these diseases diminished or disappeared in 80 percent of the children who were switched to milk-free diets.[32] A UK study showed that people who were suffering from irregular heartbeats, asthma, headaches, fatigue, and digestive problems "showed marked and often complete improvements in their health after cutting milk from their diets."[33]

OSTEOPOROSIS

Walter Willett is chairman of the Nutrition Department at the Harvard School of Public Health, and co-authored a major study of more than

75,000 American nurses, which found that women with the highest calcium consumption from dairy products actually had substantially more fractures than women who drank less milk. Citing a 1980 study in the journal *Clinical Orthopedics and Related Research,* Mark Hegsted of Harvard University makes the point that people in the U.S. and Scandinavian countries consume more dairy products than anywhere else in the world, yet they have the highest rates of osteoporosis.[34] As pointed in out in *Conscious Eating* and the *American Journal of Clinical Nutrition,* there is a problem of excessive protein in the diet. This excessive animal protein creates acidity and a high phosphorus content that pulls calcium out of the bones, and therefore is a plausible explanation for why those with the highest dairy intake have the highest rates of osteoporosis. A 1985 study in *The American Journal of Clinical Nutrition* suggests that dairy products offer no protection against osteoporosis, probably due to the high protein content of milk.[35]

The bottom line is that calcium deficiency is not a threat to someone eating a plant-source-only cuisine. In fact, inadequate calcium intake appears not to be a problem at all. A scholarly review of the subject in the *Postgraduate Medical Journal* in 1976 revealed that calcium deficiency caused by an insufficient amount of calcium in the diet is not known to occur in humans at all.[36]

CANCERS

T. Colin Campbell did a twenty-seven-year study, published as *The China Study,* jointly arranged by Cornell, Oxford, and the Chinese Academy of Preventive Medicine. Funded by the National Institutes of Health, the American Cancer Society, and the American Institute for Cancer Research, the study was called by the *New York Times* the "Grand Prix of Epidemiology." His research team investigated the role of protein in promoting cancer. They found one protein that consistently and strongly promoted cancer—casein in cow's milk. Casein is 87 percent of the proteins in dairy, and it promotes all stages of the cancer process.

What were the safe proteins? Those from plant sources. In fact, their research found that the people who ate the most plant-based foods were the healthiest and tended to avoid chronic disease. More important, they discovered through the findings of other researchers and clinicians worldwide, as we have, that "the diet that has time and again been shown to reverse and/or prevent [diseases caused by animal protein consumption] is the same whole-foods, plant based diet found to promote optimal health in laboratory research and in the China Study. *The findings are consistent.*"[37]

LYMPHOMA

In Norway, 15,914 individuals were followed for eleven and a half years. Those drinking two or more glasses of milk per day had 3.5 times the incidence of cancer of the lymphatic organs.[38] One of the more thoughtful articles on this subject is from Allan S. Cunningham of Cooperstown, New York, writing in *The Lancet,* November 27, 1976 (page 1184), in an article entitled "Lymphomas and Animal-Protein Consumption." Cunningham tracked the beef and dairy consumption in terms of grams per day for a one-year period, 1955–1956, in fifteen countries. New Zealand, United States, and Canada had the highest consumption, respectively. The lowest meat and dairy consumption was in Japan. The difference between the highest and lowest was nearly thirty-fold: 43.8 grams/day for New Zealanders versus 1.5 for Japan. Cunningham found a highly significant positive correlation between deaths from lymphomas and beef and dairy ingestion in the fifteen countries analyzed. The reason for the role of dairy is that the dairy intake creates a chronic immunological stress that tends to cause lymphomas in laboratory animals and also possibly in humans. We know that ingestion of cow's milk can produce generalized lymphopathy, swollen liver, swollen spleen, and significant adenoid hypertrophy. It can be hypothesized that meat protein adds its general carcinogenic effect to the specific carcinogenic effect on the lymph from dairy.

OVARIAN CANCER

Drinking more than one glass of milk a day, or its equivalent, has been shown to give women a 3.1 times greater risk of ovarian cancer than non-milk drinkers. Harvard Medical School did a study and analyzed data from twenty-seven different countries, to find the same increased amount of ovarian cancer associated with dairy.

A positive relationship between ovarian cancer and dairy products was first reported in *The Lancet* by Cramer et al. in 1989, when it was suggested that lactose consumption may be a dietary risk factor for ovarian cancer.52[39] More recently, data collected from the Harvard Nurses Health Study was used to assess the lactose, milk, and milk product consumption in relation to ovarian cancer risk in more than 80,000 women. Over sixteen years of follow-up, 301 cases of one particular type of ovarian cancer were confirmed in this study group. Results showed that women who consumed the most lactose had twice the risk of this type of ovarian cancer than women who drank the least lactose. It was suggested that galactose (a component of lactose) may damage ovarian cells, making them more susceptible to cancer.[40]

In 2004, Susanna Larsson and colleagues of the Karolinska Institute in Stockholm, Sweden, published a study[41] in the *American Journal of Clinical Nutrition* that examined the association between intake of dairy products and lactose and the risk of ovarian cancer. In this study of 61,084 women age 38 to 76 years, the diet was assessed over three years. After 13.5 years 266 participants had been diagnosed with ovarian cancer. Results showed that women consuming four or more servings of dairy a day had double the risk of ovarian cancer, compared to those consuming low or no dairy. Milk was the dairy product with the strongest positive association with ovarian cancer.

LUNG CANCER

A study by Curtis Mettlin, funded by the American Cancer Society and cited in the *International Journal of Cancer,* April 15, 1989, showed that people drinking three or more glasses of whole milk a day had a twofold increase in lung cancer.[42]

BREAST AND PROSTATE CANCERS

The journal *Cancer* in 1989 reported that men drinking three or more glasses a day of whole milk were shown to have a 2.49 times increase in prostate cancer.[43] A 2001 Harvard review of the research put a finer point on it:

> Twelve of … fourteen case-control studies and seven of … nine cohort studies [have] observed a positive association for some measure of dairy products and prostate cancer; *this is one of the most consistent dietary predictors for prostate cancer in the published literature* [italics added]. In these studies, men with the highest dairy intakes had approximately double the risk of total prostate cancer, and up to a fourfold increase in risk of metastatic or fatal prostate cancer relative to low consumers.[44]

We see this data corroborated in world data for breast and prostate cancer rates in China, Japan, England, Scotland, and Canada (by the International Agency for Research), and in the U.S. (by the Surveillance Epidemiology and End Results Program of the National Cancer Institute). Figure 15 illustrates that the lowest rates of breast and prostate cancer are consistently in China and Japan, where dairy and animal meat are rarely consumed. As Jane Plant, PhD, remarks in *The No Dairy Breast Cancer Prevention Program*:

> The Japanese cities of Hiroshima and Nagasaki have similar rates of breast cancer: and remember, both cities were attacked with nuclear weapons, so in addition to the usual pollution-related cancers, one would also expect to find some radiation-related cases. If, as a North American woman, one was living a Japanese lifestyle in industrialized, irradiated Hiroshima, you would slash your risk of contracting breast cancer by a half to a third. The conclusion is inescapable. Clearly, some lifestyle factor not related to pollution, urbanization, or the environment is seriously increasing the Western woman's chance of contracting breast cancer.[45]

Looking at the chart below, you can see that a black man in the United States is 280 times more likely to develop prostate cancer than a man in rural Quidong, China, and 70 times more prone than a man in urban Tianjin, China.

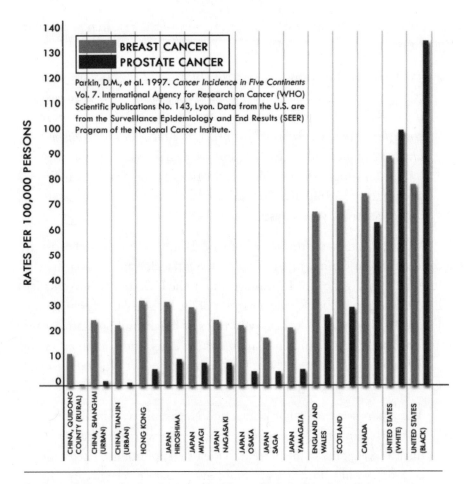

Figure 3: Age-standardized rates of incidence for breast and prostate cancer

Plant continues:

We know ... that whatever causes the huge difference in breast and prostate cancer rates between Eastern and Western countries, it isn't genetic. Migration studies show that when Chinese or Japanese people move to the West, within one or two generations their rates of incidence and mortality from breast and prostate cancer approach those of their host community.[46]

Over the next couple of years, Plant and her husband Peter examined the results of the China-Cornell-Oxford Project of T. Colin Campbell, and credited the fact that Easterners do not eat dairy products for their low rates of breast and prostate cancer. Pick up an Asian recipe book at the store—you'll find no mention of dairy products.

PUS CELLS

One cubic centimeter (cc) of commercial cow's milk is allowed to have up to 750,000 somatic cells (common name, "pus") and 20,000 live bacteria before it is kept off the market. That amounts to a whopping 20 million live, squiggly bacteria and up to 750 *million* pus cells per liter. According to Robert Cohen, author of *Don't Drink Your Milk,* the average liter of milk in Florida has 633 million pus cells, the highest in the nation. Montana is the lowest, with 236 million pus cells per liter. This is not a healthy thing, whether it is 236 or 633 million. Besides pus cells and blood, which are now normal in milk produced during machine suckling, the milk is also high in pesticides, herbicides, antibiotics, hormones, radioactive iodine, and disease factors such as mad cow prion and bovine leukemia virus. In addition, research cited by Robert Cohen has made the point that there is up to a gallon of extra mucus in the body created as a result of drinking dairy. The mucus problem is associated with the fact that 87 percent of milk protein is casein, the main ingredient of Elmer's Glue.

High Blood Cholesterol

All animal foods raise the blood cholesterol; that includes beef, fish, chicken, dairy, and eggs. Plant-source foods do not contain cholesterol. Caldwell B. Esselstyn, MD, author of *Prevent and Reverse Heart Disease,* in a private communication in July 2007 said that an LDL of greater than 80 increases your risk for heart disease, and levels lower than 80 are safe. Dr. Esselstyn said that LDL levels are the most important cholesterol indicator for propensity to heart disease. According to the Centers for Disease Control, 55.9 percent of diabetics reported that their cholesterol was high, placing them at an increased risk for heart disease and poor glucose control.

In our Tree of Life program, which includes the moderate use of healthy, raw nuts and seeds and a 100 percent live-food diet, we had dramatic drops in 21–30 days in LDL cholesterol. For example, one person went from 148 to 86, another from 86 to 46, a third from 216 to 88, a fourth from 153 to 105, and a fifth from 142 to 85, for an average 67-point drop in LDL cholesterol on a plant-sourced live cuisine including nuts and seeds in just 21–30 days. This is an average drop of 44 percent of LDL in one month. There is no other diet that comes anywhere close to these dramatic drops in LDL, which is why we recommend a 100 percent live-food plant-based diet. To place these numbers in perspective, at the University of Toronto Dr. David Jenkins applied a vegan diet with standard cooked vegan elements such as nuts, seeds, oat bran, soy products, and plant sterols. In a four-week period, he achieved a 29.6 percent drop in LDL cholesterol. On a natural live-food vegan diet, our results in four weeks were 50 percent better, *without the use of oats or soy.*

High-Stress Lifestyle and Hypertension

When the body is under stress, many hormones are released that indirectly increase insulin excretion and indirectly create insulin resistance, a precursor to a diabetic physiology. These hormones release energy in the form of glucose and fat, which is made available to the cells of the body. This provides fuel for what has been traditionally referred to as the "fight or flight" response. With stress, one sees increases in the secretion of catecolamines, especially from the adrenals, resulting in an increased glucose release from the liver into the blood stream, and glucocorticoid or steroid hormones secreted by the adrenal glands and growth hormone produced by the pituitary gland. Extreme stress for months at a time has been known to trigger the onset of a diabetic physiology.

In the U.S., 62.5 percent of adults with diabetes reported having **hypertension** (source: CDC). Hypertension is part of the basket of symptoms seen in Syndrome X, discussed below.

Candida

Candida is also commonly associated with diabetes and is a larger symptom of a Culture of Death diabetogenic diet and lifestyle. Candida is a fungal parasite that excretes toxic waste that can get into the bloodstream and cause symptoms of bloating, clouded thinking, depression, diarrhea, exhaustion, halitosis (bad breath), menstrual pains, thrush, unclear memory recall, recurring vaginal or bladder infections, anxiety, constipation, diarrhea (or both), depression, environmental sensitivities, fatigue, feeling worse on damp or muggy days or in moldy places, food sensitivities, insomnia, low blood sugar, mood swings, premenstrual syndrome, ringing in the ears, and sensitivities to perfume, cigarettes, or fabric odors. Diets high in cooked starches (bread, baked potato, cakes, cookies, pasta) and diets loaded with refined or hybridized (seedless) fruit sugars both feed candida. Diabetes with its higher blood sugar levels makes people good candidates for candida.

Rainbow Green Live-Food Cuisine examines the pathogenic microorganism candida and how its presence in the body pushes the recycling button or "composting button" as the candida functions to recycle the organism it inhabits back to the soil. In essence, candida accelerates the rate of fermentation of the system. At the turn of the nineteenth century, candida yeast was primarily seen in people who were dying of cancer and other very serious diseases, as *fungation* is the seventh stage of disease (we will discuss the Seven Stages of Disease in Chapter 3). Depending on the degree of toxicity, this composting process leads to chronic disease, misery, and ultimately death. The key to restoring health is minimizing or eliminating the toxic conditions so that the composting button is turned off. A low-sweet, live-food, non-acidic diet and healthy lifestyle are the key factors to reversing the aging-degenerative process of chronic candidiasis. The diet and lifestyle to do this is exactly the anti-diabetogenic diet and lifestyle of the Culture of Life that we are outlining in this book.

Depression

According to an evaluation of twenty studies over the past ten years, the prevalence rate of diabetics with major depression is three to four times greater than in the general population. While depression affects 3–5 percent of the population at any given time, the rate is 15–20 percent in patients with diabetes, according to the American Diabetic Association. Women in particular are at greater risk, according to other studies.[47]

For many years it has been hypothesized that depression is a diabetic complication, which is almost certain given that the diabetogenic diet and lifestyle is the same diet and lifestyle that creates a biologically altered brain, fatty-acid and amino-acid deficiencies, and toxemia, and thus gives rise to depression. More recent research, however, points to depression as a possible cause or trigger for diabetes. Researchers at Kaiser Permanente's Center for Health Research in Portland, Oregon, looked at 1,680 diabetic members of its health maintenance organization. They found that when compared with nondiabetics, those with diabetes were more likely to have been treated for depression within six months before their diabetes diagnosis. About 84 percent of those diabetics also reported a higher rate of earlier depressive episodes than those in the control group. Gregory Nichols, a Kaiser researcher who conducted the study, said the study suggests depression frequently precedes the onset of diabetes, rather than vice versa.[48]

A major study in 2004 by Johns Hopkins and other centers tracked 11,615 initially nondiabetic adults age 48–67 over six years, and found that "depressive symptoms predicted incident Type-2 diabetes." In prospective analyses, after adjusting for age, race, sex, and education, individuals in the highest quartile of depressive symptoms had a 63 percent increased risk of developing diabetes compared with those in the lowest quartile.[49]

The good news is that I have developed a five-step program for treating depression naturally that seems to work in about 90 percent of patients. It is detailed in my book, *Depression-Free for Life.*

Metabolic Syndrome (Syndrome X)

Syndrome X was first coined as a term by Gerald Reaven, MD, at Stanford University to describe a group of symptoms that arise from an overall metabolic disorder. These symptoms may include Type-2 diabetes, obesity with an inability to lose weight, high cholesterol, high blood pressure, high triglycerides, low HDL cholesterol, and coronary heart disease. Some 655,000 people are newly diagnosed each year, and it is estimated that an equal 655,000 cases are not diagnosed. Some estimates cite some 47 million people with the basket of symptoms known as Syndrome X. A classic symptom and hint of the metabolic syndrome is the accumulation of fat in the abdomen and the inability to lose fat and weight. Dr. Simeon Margolis, co-author of a Johns Hopkins report on Syndrome X, says that abdominal obesity is often the first outward sign of Syndrome X. It seems to be associated with insulin resistance. Some long-term studies have suggested that the higher the fasting blood insulin levels and the greater the amount of abdominal fat, the greater likelihood of death from Syndrome X.

The metabolic disorder that we've created through unnatural ways of living from the lifestyle and diet of the Culture of Death has a significant effect on people's health. Some researchers estimate that we age one-third faster when blood sugar levels are high. Some of the negative impact is related to the glycation process, in which glucose fuses with protein. It disorganizes the protein function, creating cross linkages and disrupting the protein function in the cell membrane and enzymes. The glycation process also results in greatly increased free radical production. Untreated or even poorly managed Syndrome X and diabetes produce an accelerated aging and death process.

Syndrome X and diabetes also create a chemical change in the nerves. These changes impair the nerves' ability to transmit signals. Symptoms of nerve damage include numbness, tingling, increased sensitivity to touch, insensitivity to pain and temperature, and loss of coordination. The excess sugar also damages blood vessels that carry the oxygen and nutrients to the nerves. People with Syndrome X are more likely to develop obstruction to the arteries and therefore increased or decreased blood flow to the extremities, which creates increased rates of amputations. Up to 70 percent of people with Syndrome X have some form of nerve damage. It is even worse in smokers. Some people feel the metabolic syndrome is not reversible, but with the Tree of Life program, we have seen a high frequency of the reversal of this syndrome over a three-week cycle.

Toxicity of Heavy Metals and Drinking Water

> The development of insulin-dependent diabetes mellitus is thought to be dependent on the interaction of environmental agents with the pancreatic beta cells.[50]
>
> **UNIVERSITY OF CALGARY**

Just as consuming organic foods is a way to avoid ingesting toxins, becoming aware of the quality of water one drinks and uses is increasingly essential in today's polluted world, since water can be a major source of toxins. According to *Diet for a Poisoned Planet,* less than 1 percent of the Earth's surface water is safe to drink. In some places in the United States and other countries, the term "drinking water" for tap water should be considered nothing more than a euphemism.

The water that the general public uses comes from two sources: underground sources, such as springs and wells, and surface water, such as rivers and lakes. Presently, both these sources are becoming more and more polluted as toxic chemicals, acid rain, raw sewage, agricultural herbicides, pesticide runoff, chlorination, fluoridation, sewage landfills, and radioactive wastes are either dumped into or seep into them. One of the best-known examples of toxic water pollution to date is the infamous Love Canal, where according to the *New York Times* in 1984, thousands of tons of toxic chemicals were dumped, including 60 pounds of the deadly poison dioxin.

The pollution situation is so out of control that in monitoring cancer rates in Philadelphia, one researcher was able to correlate the different rates and types of cancer in the population with the specific river the people lived near. According to Steve Meyerowitz, in his book *Water,* the Environmental Cancer Prevention Center found that residents drinking from the west side of the Schuylkill River had 67 percent more deaths from esophagus cancer than those on the east side. Those drinking from the Delaware River on the east side suffered 59 percent more deaths from cancer of the brain, 83 percent more malignant melanoma, and 32 percent more colorectal cancers than those on the west side. This is just one of many studies linking specific water pollution to an increase in cancer rates.

Medical science has discovered how sensitive the insulin receptor sites are to chemical poisoning. Metals such as cadmium, mercury, arsenic, lead, fluoride,[51] and possibly aluminum may play a role in the actual destruction of beta cells through stimulating an auto-immune reaction to them after they have bonded to these cells in the pancreas. It is because mercury[52] and lead attach themselves at highly vulnerable junctures of proteins that they find their great capacity to provoke morphological changes in the body. Changes in pancreatic function are among the pathogenetic mechanisms observable during lead intoxication.[53]

CADMIUM

Cadmium, a widespread heavy metal contaminant found in air, soil, and water, can accumulate in the pancreas and exert diabetogenic effects in animals. In a large cross-sectional study, urinary cadmium levels are significantly and dose-dependently associated with both impaired fasting glucose and diabetes.[54] Such accumulations increase the likelihood of kidney damage and failure, spur free radical activity, and exacerbate neuromuscular complications of Type-2 diabetes.[55,56,57,58] Cadmium sources include tap water, fungicides, marijuana, processed meat, rubber, seafood (cod, haddock, oyster, tuna), sewage, tobacco, colas (especially from vending machines), tools, welding material, evaporated milk, airborne industrial contaminants, batteries, instant coffee, incineration of tires/rubber/plastic, refined grains, soft water, galvanized pipes, dental alloys, candy, ceramics, electroplating, fertilizers, paints, motor oil, and motor exhaust.

MERCURY

Because mercury is increasingly becoming elevated in all forms of life, we can assume that more people will have some defects in pancreatic function. Pancreatic support is increasingly necessary for optimal health.

FROM A PERSONAL COMMUNICATION WITH DR. GARRY GORDON

In August 2006, the American Chemical Society published research that showed conclusively that methylmercury induces pancreatic cell apoptosis and dysfunction.[59] Mercury is a well-known toxic agent that produces various types of cell and tissue damage, yet billions of people are exposed to levels of mercury harmful to pancreatic health. In the case of diabetes mercury is especially telling, for it affects the beta cells, the insulin itself, and the insulin receptor sites, setting off a myriad of complex disturbances in glucose metabolism.[60]

Mercury leads the pack in the potency of its toxicity and in the pervasiveness of it presence in the environment through fish, air, and water, medicine through vaccines, and dentistry with dental amalgams. Some say we are all receiving, just through our air, water, and food about a microgram of mercury a day. Sounds like a little until you calculate that a microgram contains 3,000 trillion atoms with each of them holding the potential to deactivate insulin and the receptor sites crucial to their function.[61]

ARSENIC

Studies out of Taiwan and Bangladesh show that individuals who are exposed to higher amounts of arsenic—in their soil and/or drinking water—have a higher independent risk of developing Type-2 diabetes.[62,63] Arsenic in tap water is common; this hormone disruptor is suspected of playing a role in diabetes. Arsenic interferes with the action of glucocorticoid hormones, which belong to the same family of steroid hormones as estrogen and progesterone. Glucocorticoids turn on many genes that help regulate blood sugar and even ward off cancer. Repeatedly drinking water containing certain amounts of arsenic has been linked to increased rates of cancer and diabetes. The underlying mechanism is now thought to be hormone disruption.[64]

LEAD

Lead exposure has been associated with an increased risk of hypertension, and is a well-established risk factor for kidney disease. Lead either affects blood pressure indirectly through alterations in kidney function or via more direct effects on the vasculature or neurologic blood pressure control. Researchers at Harvard Medical School state:

> Our findings support the hypothesis that long-term low-level lead accumulation (estimated by tibia bone lead) is associated with an increased risk of declining renal function particularly among diabetics or hypertensives, populations already at risk for impaired renal function.[65]

FLUORIDE

According to "Fluoride in Drinking Water: A Scientific Review of EPA's Standards," made public by the National Research Council in 2006:

> The conclusion from the available studies is that sufficient fluoride exposure appears to bring about increases in blood glucose or impaired glucose tolerance in some individuals and to increase the severity of some types of diabetes. In general, impaired glucose metabolism appears to be associated with serum or plasma fluoride concentrations of about 0.1 mg/L or greater in both animals and humans. In addition, diabetic individuals will often have higher than normal water intake, and consequently, will have higher than normal fluoride intake for a given concentration of fluoride in drinking water. An estimated 21 million people in the U.S. have diabetes mellitus; therefore, any role of fluoride exposure in the development of impaired glucose metabolism or diabetes is potentially significant.[66]

FILTERING YOUR WATER

Compressed, activated, charcoal block filters are an inexpensive way to get protection from the carbon-based organic pollution, pesticides, herbicides, insecticides, PCBs, cysts, heavy metals, asbestos, VOCs (volatile organic chemicals), and THMs in our water. They also eliminate chlorine and foul odors. They do not, however, absorb inorganic mineral salts such as chloride, fluoride, sodium, nitrates, and soluble minerals. For this reason, they are best for city water systems but not for well water systems, which have a potential to be polluted with high amounts of nitrates from agricultural wastes. A concern regarding granular charcoal filters is their tendency to be a gathering ground for bacteria, yeasts, and molds, and their inability to remove pollutants found in some drinking water. Some of the more sophisticated charcoal filters do have a reverse wash system in an attempt to compensate for this. Another problem with charcoal filters is that the charcoal can break down with age or from hot water and release the contaminants back into our drinking water. The best way to avoid this is to pay attention to any change in taste, smell, or color of the water, or a reduction in water flow rate. Duane Taylor, a water expert from North Coast Waterworks in Sonoma County, California, suggested in a personal communication that the main problem with charcoal filters is that the user does not replace the filter often enough. He recommends purchasing a filter unit that will stop the flow and make the user change the filter when its filtering capacities are used up. If one does not have such a filter, then he recommends changing the filter at 75 percent of the manufacturer's suggested lifetime. If one waits until there is a taste change, decrease in rate of flow, or smell to the water, the filter may already be dumping contaminants back into the water. Activated carbon is rated on its ability to remove iodine and phenols. The iodine number should be greater than 1,000 on the measuring scale, and the phenol number should be 15 or less. Another important consideration for carbon filter effectiveness is the contact time of water with the filter. The slower the flow rate and the more carbon there is in the filter, the better job the filter does.

Reverse osmosis (RO) is one of the best methods to get pure water without using up a lot of energy. RO units remove bacteria, viruses, nitrates, fluorides, sodium, chlorine, particulate matter, heavy metals, asbestos, organic chemicals, and dissolved minerals. They do not remove toxic gases, chloroform, phenols, THMs, some pesticides, and low-molecular-weight organic compounds. When combined with an activated carbon filtration system, however, they can remove the entire spectrum of impurities from the drinking water, including organic and inorganic chemicals. Many RO units now have pre- and post-filters to take care of any residual impurities that the RO unit does not remove.

In RO, the water to be filtered is forced through a semi-permeable membrane by the moving elements from more-concentrated to less-concentrated solutions. The membrane is permeable to pure water but not to most of its impurities. If conditions are right for sufficient water pressure and the water is not excessively hard, almost no energy is needed for the operation of RO systems. A pressure pump is needed if the total dissolved solids are greater than one thousand parts per million. The water is as pure as distilled, yet it is not heated as in distilled water and therefore not destructured, which is a great advantage. Sometimes a pressure pump is needed for extremely hard water, and this does require electrical energy. The main problem with an RO unit is the fragility of the semi-permeable membrane. Some membranes can be destroyed by chlorinated water, highly alkaline water, or temperatures above 100° Fahrenheit. If the water is chlorinated, a cellulose membrane is needed. A polymer membrane can be used if the water is not chlorinated.

Some people have had the membrane break in less than the expected three years. For this reason, it is good to check the water purity regularly. Newer and stronger membranes are now available on the market, but we are still in the habit of checking the water purity every four months and/or whenever there is a change in the taste. While RO units are similar in appearance and claimed performance, there are many complex, interdependent choices regarding pre-treatment, membrane selection, and post-treatment. To select a system that fits your water filtration needs and to develop the best maintenance plan, it is best to talk with someone who has in-depth knowledge of the many factors involved. If properly selected and maintained, an RO unit may be the most energy-efficient and best way to protect your water. In the past, RO units required a lot of water to work properly, which is a disadvantage, particularly during times of drought. Some of the newer models have been designed to operate with minimal water usage.

Water distillers, although generally more expensive, remove most everything from the water, including bacteria, fluoride, nitrates, radionuclides, and/organic and inorganic toxins, as well as heavy metals such as lead, mercury, and cadmium, and soluble minerals such as calcium and magnesium. Some toxic organic compounds, such as THMs and dioxin, have the same as or a lower boiling point than water and therefore are not filtered out by the distillation process. The heating of the water also disrupts potential homeopathic patterns of toxins that are left in the water in reverse osmosis filtration. Some of the more expensive distillers have built-in pre-boiler or post-boiler filters as options to eliminate this problem.

There are two major drawbacks to water distillers. One is that they are energy-intensive and expensive unless one has a solar water distiller. The other problem is that distilled water is dead, unstructured water so foreign to the body that one actually gets a temporarily high white blood cell count in response to drinking it. It is, however, possible to revive this dead, destructured water by the use of a product called Crystal Energy. I feel that the water distiller is the safest way to approach the water toxicity problem and have outlined in detail how to reactivate distilled water in my book *Spiritual Nutrition.*

Vaccinations and Increased Juvenile Diabetes Rates[67]

In the May 24, 1996 *New Zealand Medical Journal,* J. Bart Classen, MD, a former researcher at the National Institutes of Health, reported a 60 percent increase in Type-1 diabetes following a massive campaign in New Zealand from 1988 to 1991 to vaccinate babies six weeks of age or older with hepatitis B vaccine. His analysis of a group of 100,000 New Zealand children followed since 1982 showed that the incidence of diabetes before the hepatitis B vaccination program began in 1988 was 11.2 cases per 100,000 children per year, while the incidence of diabetes following the hepatitis B vaccination campaign was 18.2 cases per 100,000 children per year.[68]

In the October 22, 1997 *Infectious Diseases in Clinical Practice,* Dr. Classen presented more data further substantiating his findings of a vaccine-diabetes connection. He reported that the incidence of diabetes in Finland was stable in children under 4 years of age until the government made several changes in its childhood vaccination schedule. In 1974, 130,000 children age 3 months to 4 years were enrolled in a vaccine experimental trial and injected with hepatitis B vaccine or meningococcal vaccine. Then, in 1976, the pertussis vaccine used in Finland was made stronger by adding a second strain of bacteria. According to the National Vaccine Information Center's (NVIC) report, "Juvenile Diabetes and Vaccination: New Evidence for a Connection," during the years 1977–1979, there was a 64 percent increase in the incidence of Type-1 diabetes in Finland compared to the years 1970–1976.[69]

Doctors started reporting in the medical literature as early as 1949 that some children injected with pertussis (whooping cough) vaccine (now part of the DPT or DTaP shot) were having trouble maintaining normal glucose levels in their blood. Lab research has confirmed that pertussis vaccine can cause diabetes in mice.

As diabetes research progressed in the 1960s, 70s, and 80s, there were observations that viral infections may be a co-factor in causing diabetes. The introduction of live virus vaccines, such as live MMR vaccine made from weakened forms of the live measles, mumps, and rubella viruses, has raised questions about whether live vaccine virus could be a co-factor in causing chronic diseases such as diabetes.

In 1982, another vaccine was added to the childhood vaccination schedule in Finland. Children age 14 months to 6 years were given the live MMR (measles-mumps-rubella) vaccine. This was followed by the injection of 114,000 Finnish children 3 months and older with another experimental Hib vaccine. In 1988, Finland recommended that all babies be injected with the hepatitis B vaccine.

The introduction of these new vaccines in Finland was followed by a 62 percent rise in the incidence of diabetes in the 0–4 years age group and a 19 percent rise of diabetes in the 5–9 years age group between the years 1980 and 1982 and 1987 and 1989. As shown in the NVIC report, Classen concluded:

> The net effect was the addition of three new vaccines to the 0–4 year old age group, and a 147 percent increase in the incidence of IDDM. The addition of one new vaccine to the 5–9 year olds resulted in a 40 percent rise in diabetes incidence. With no new vaccines added to the 10 to 14 year olds, a rise in the incidence of IDDM was seen by only 8 percent between the intervals 1970–1976 and 1990–1992. The rise in IDDM in the different age groups correlated with the number of vaccines given.[70]

The Centers for Disease Control published data supporting a link between timing of immunization and the development of diabetes.[71] The data from the CDC's preliminary study supports published data that immunization starting after 2 months is associated with an increased risk of diabetes. The U.S. government study showed that hepatitis B immunization starting after two months was associated with an almost doubling of the risk of IDDM.

Coffee and Caffeinated Beverages

According to Hal Huggins in *It's All in Your Head,* one cup of coffee can elevate the glucose level enough to need three units of insulin to counteract it. Researchers at Queen's University in Ontario investigated the effect of caffeine ingestion on insulin sensitivity in sedentary lean men and obese men with and without Type-2 diabetes. They also examined whether chronic exercise (a three-month aerobic exercise program) influences the relationship between caffeine and insulin sensitivity in these individuals. Their results showed that caffeine ingestion was associated with a significant reduction in insulin sensitivity by a similar magnitude in the lean (33 percent), obese (33 percent), and diabetic (37 percent) groups in comparison with those given placebo. After exercise training, caffeine ingestion was still associated with a reduction in insulin sensitivity by a similar magnitude in the lean (23 percent), obese (26 percent), and Type-2 diabetic (36 percent) groups in comparison with those given placebo.

Figure 16 shows that with exercise, insulin sensitivity did go up, but in all groups, whether lean, obese, or Type-2 diabetic, caffeine intake significantly reduced insulin sensitivity. The researchers concluded that caffeine consumption is associated with a substantial reduction in insulin-mediated glucose uptake independent of obesity, Type-2 diabetes, and chronic exercise.[72]

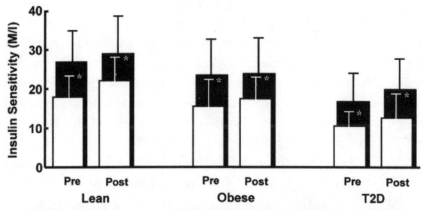

Insulin sensitivity in the lean, obese, and type 2 diabetic (T2D) groups before and after 3 months of exercise. Insulin sensitivity is expressed as the ratio of the amount of glucose metabolized to the prevailing plasma insulin levels [M (mg · kgSM−1 · min−1)/I (µU/ml) x 100] during the last 30 min of the euglycemic clamp. *Glucose uptake is significantly lower (P < 0.05) in the caffeine trial (black bar) compared with the placebo trial (white bar), independent of group and exercise training.

Source: SoJung Lee, PHD1, Robert Hudson, MD, PHD2, Katherine Kilpatrick, MD3, Terry E. Graham, PHD4 and Robert Ross, PHD. "Caffeine Ingestion Is Associated With Reductions in Glucose Uptake Independent of Obesity and Type 2 Diabetes Before and After Exercise Training." Diabetes Care 28:566-572, 2005

Figure 4: Insulin sensitivity in lean, obese, and Type-2 diabetic groups with and without caffeine intake, before and after three months of exercise

Thank You for Not Smoking

According to the CDC, 17.7 percent of U.S. adults with diabetes smoke, and the dangers are very real for diabetics. Smoking affects both carbohydrate and lipid metabolism. In one study of diabetics, 114 smokers were compared to 49 nonsmokers. The smokers had a 15–20 percent higher insulin requirement and serum triglyceride concentration. In heavy smokers the insulin requirement was 30 percent higher. Researchers have found that chronic smokers were likely to be more insulin resistant, hyperinsulinemic, and dyslipidemic compared to matched groups of nonsmokers. It is believed that catecholamines, a type of hormone, are produced in greater quantity in smokers and act as an antagonist to insulin action.[73] A study of forty patients with Type-2 diabetes found insulin resistance was markedly aggravated among those who smoked.[74]

A contributing factor to insulin resistance is nicotine-containing products. Please understand that insulin resistance is a precursor to diabetes, so anything that contributes to insulin resistance encourages a move from pre-diabetes to diabetes, or makes an existing diabetic condition worse. Chronic cigarette smoking has been found to markedly aggravate insulin resistance for Type-2 diabetics.[75] Lack of exercise certainly helps to activate the expression of Type-2 diabetes.[76] The good news is that even mild exercise can help stave off cigarette cravings and withdrawal symptoms as well as decrease a smoker's chance of reaching for a cigarette, according to a study published in the journal *Addiction*. Researchers from the University of Exeter and the University of Toronto reviewed fourteen previously published studies and compared the results. They found that twelve of the studies demonstrated that a session of exercise caused a rapid decrease in cigarette cravings, withdrawal symptoms, and other negative effects of cigarette addiction. As little as five minutes of simple exercises such as walking, isometrics, or muscle flexing proved as effective as a nicotine patch in decreasing an immediate craving.[77] Not only does exercise reduce cravings for cigarettes, but it seems to dramatically improve endurance and fitness, decreases body fat stores, and decrease insulin resistance.

A prospective study of Japanese men concluded that age of smoking initiation and number of cigarettes smoked were major risk factors for developing diabetes.[78] Similarly, data from the U.S. Cancer Prevention Study found that as smoking increased so the rate of diabetes increased for both men and women.[79]

Nicotine has also been associated with decreasing peripheral circulation and thus increasing the tendency for amputation. Smoking increases adrenaline secretions by 23 percent and thus increases blood sugar. Obviously, smoking decreases lung function, and therefore oxygen in the system, and this lack of oxygenation to the tissues decreases peripheral circulation and leads to a greater tendency for gangrene and amputation. Smoking is a documented risk factor for both the development and progression of various types of neuropathy (damage to the peripheral nervous system). A retrospective study of Type-1 and Type-2 diabetic patients found that current or ex-smokers were significantly more likely to have neuropathy than individuals who never smoked (64.8 percent compared to 42.8 percent).[80] A later study found that cigarette smoking was associated with a twofold increase in risk.[81] Studies also show that smoking increases the chances of developing gum disease, a contributing factor in poor glycemic control. In fact, smokers are five times more likely than nonsmokers to have gum disease. For smokers with diabetes, the risk is even greater. If you are a smoker with diabetes, age 45 or older, you are twenty times more likely than a person without these risk factors to get severe gum disease.[82]

Diabetes as an Accelerated Aging Reality

Often diabetes doesn't get diagnosed until its complications begin to arise. Major chronic complications include: retinopathy, which leads to blindness; neuropathy, degeneration of the nervous system; nephropathy, or kidney disease; atherosclerotic coronary disease; and atherosclerotic vascular disease. About 85 percent of all diabetics develop retinopathy, 20–50 percent develop kidney disease, and 60–70 percent have mild to severe forms of nerve damage. Diabetics are two to four times more likely to develop cardiovascular disease (which is a factor in 75 percent of diabetes-related deaths) and two to four times more likely to suffer stroke. Multiple studies show that insulin resistance doubles the risk of heart attack as early as fifteen years before diabetes is diagnosed, along with risk of stroke. Middle-age people with diabetes have death rates and a heart disease rate two times higher than those without diabetes. Diabetics are also three-four times more likely to develop clinical depression than nondiabetics.

The National Institute of Diabetes and Digestive and Kidney Diseases (NIDDK) reported in 1993 that diabetes is the leading cause of new cases of blindness among adults 20 to 74. Somewhere between 12,000 and 24,000 new cases of blindness per year are caused by diabetic retinopathy. About 60–70 percent of the people with diabetes have mild symptoms to severe forms of diabetic nerve damage. Neuropathy is the major cause of nontrauma lower limb amputation, and studies suggest that as many as 70 percent of amputees die within five years.[83] Many people with diabetes have a "slow stomach" or gastric paresis. These conditions all seem to be associated with hyperinsulinemia (high blood insulin) and hyperglycemia (high blood sugar).

Diabetes, in essence, is an accelerated aging. So hyperinsulinemia becomes a part of the continuum of developing diabetes. It is a tip-off point before we get to diagnosable diabetes and the accelerated aging pattern known as chronic disease. Hyperinsulinemia is telling us that we have a higher risk of developing chronic degenerative diseases. Our carbohydrate metabolism requires attention and is one of the most important life extension factors. The diet and lifestyle we are suggesting helps us maintain healthy blood sugar levels.

Proper management of carbohydrate metabolism is key to a healthy life and longevity. A normal fasting blood sugar, according to ADA data, is 100. However, as we have already pointed out, the latest research shows that if you have a blood sugar of 86 or higher you are already entering into the first stages of an abnormal metabolism, an accelerated aging process, and are beginning to lose control of a healthy carbohydrate metabolism.

A major twelve-year study at Harvard University of 42,500 male health professionals ages 40 to 75 who did not initially have diabetes, cardiovascular disease, or cancer found two dietary patterns. One diet was characterized as prudent, with medium to higher concentrations of vegetables, fruit, fish, poultry, and whole grains. The other, characterized as Western, had a high consumption of red meat, processed foods, fat, dairy products, refined grains, sweets, and desserts. The researchers found that the Western dietary pattern was associated with substantially increased risk of Type-2 diabetes. They found that high blood sugar levels led to complications such as blindness, kidney failure, and heart disease. The key factors were being overweight and physically inactive, as well as having a diet that was not prudent. They concluded that all three were important and it was difficult to separate the risk of diet from the risk of being overweight and physically inactive. The study made crystal clear the importance of all three in creating Type-2 diabetes.[84]

Hyperinsulinemia, a metabolic time bomb, is associated with a whole series of chronic degenerative diseases. Not only is it a major risk factor for coronary heart disease, but is linked with the rise in plasma free radicals associated with oxidative stress, which contributes to heart disease and actually decreased brain function. Cell damage resulting from elevated insulin and blood sugar levels can lead to degenerative diseases such as hypertension and cancer.

Chronically elevated blood sugar contributes also to the formation of advanced glycation end products, also known as AGEs. These result from the non-enzymatic glycosylation of proteins. Once the proteins become glycosylated, they lose their function and contribute further to chronic disease including atherosclerotic cardiovascular disease (ASCVD) and renal failure. They cause part of what we call cross linkages, which are, in essence, an accelerated aging process. This glycosylation also produces sugar alcohols. The AGEs in sugar alcohols are associated with nerve damage to blood vessels, kidneys, lenses of the eyes, and the pancreas, and generally accelerate the aging process. The sugar alcohol formation is associated with cataract development and diminished nerve function. Therefore at a minimum, what we want to do is to try to control the high blood sugar.

Genetics

Type-2 has a much stronger genetic component than Type-1. A lot of research on diabetes was done in England, where they have 1.9 million diabetics. Findings explain up to 70 percent of the genetics involved. In Type-2 diabetes, family histories and obesity are major risk factors for the condition. One genetic mutation has been identified as a possible cause of Type-2 diabetes. The mutation was a particular zinc transporter, known as SLC 30 A8, which is involved in regulating insulin secretion.

In another genetic study, a UK team found that people with two copies of the mutant TCF7L2 gene were twice as likely to develop Type-2 diabetes.[85] According to Professor Stephen Humphries, the gene "seems to be causing as many cases of diabetes in the UK as obesity." The researchers discovered that those who carry one variant of the TCF7L2 gene were 50 percent more likely to develop Type-2 diabetes. But those men who carried two copies of the gene were 100 percent more likely to develop diabetes. Professor Humphries, lead researcher on the study for the University College of London Center for Cardiovascular Genetics, said, "Although being overweight is a major risk factor for the development of diabetes, it is clear that an individual's genetic makeup has a big impact on whether or not they will develop diabetes." Professor Humphries said 40 percent of the population carries one mutation of the gene while 10 percent carry both. Again, the message is clear: The genes load the gun, and our lifestyle pulls the trigger. We are not determined by our genes. We are affected by our genes. Our genes have a certain tendency to make us more susceptible to our lifestyles. It is our lifestyle that makes the difference.

Another gene, ENPP-1, disrupts the way the body stores energy and handles sugar by blocking the hormone insulin. Research by a French and UK team showed that children with a faulty version of ENPP-1 often were obese as young as 5 years old.

The gene called SUMO-4 helps regulate the body's immune system, which defends against infection. It was found in the U.S. at the Medical College of Georgia. The gene enables more cytokines to be made and directs the revved-up immune response in the cells of the pancreas that make insulin. In other words, it amplifies inflammation.

Although there is a genetic component, we do not need to use that as an excuse and move into fatalism. We have control of our destiny and need the courage to live a lifestyle that makes us immune to diabetes. This is what this book is about.

Type-2 diabetes, which we have been describing, is self-inflicted, manifesting in an ever-increasing proportion of young people. Because of poor diet and lifestyle, we are seeing Type-2 diabetes in more and more 5-year-olds and 10-year-olds. The Culture of Death diet and lifestyle is obviously accelerating the expression of a poor genotypic tendency for diabetes. In Type-1 diabetes, 85 percent of the people do not have a genetic predisposition, but a genetic predisposition still does play some role. The Type-1 diabetes is called insulin-dependent diabetes mellitus (IDDM) because the beta cells of the pancreas are destroyed by some sort of inflammatory process. Research has suggested that 75–90 percent of the people with Type-1 diabetes have a much raised antibody titer against their own beta cells. These B-cell antibodies seem to be associated with cow's milk. Two specific proteins in the milk cause the cross-reaction with the beta cells of the pancreas. The drinking of milk in the first few months has been associated with eleven to thirteen times higher rates of Type-1 diabetes than those people who don't drink milk in genetically predisposed children who are weaned before three months.

The symptoms of diabetes may come on very quickly. High levels of sugar in the blood and urine, frequent urination, and/or bedwetting may be seen readily in children. Other symptoms include extreme hunger, extreme thirst, weight loss, weakness, tiredness, irritability, mood swings, and nausea. Type-1 has also been associated with a variety of viral infections. This is in contrast to Type-2 diabetes, which is slow to develop with many of the same symptoms, but with hard-to-heal infections, blurred vision, itchy skin, candida, and the mind not working so clearly. Cases of Type-1 can arise from exposure to viruses that have been documented, including measles, mumps, infectious mononucleosis, infectious hepatitis, Coxsackie virus, and cytomegalovirus. These viruses cause an immune inflammation response that destroys the beta cells of the pancreas in an infant. Infant research suggests that exposure to German measles in the womb may have a 40 percent greater chance of developing Type-1 diabetes.

Type-1 diabetes can run in families, but there is a weak association. About 85 percent of people who develop Type-1 diabetes do not have an immediate family member who is diabetic. If you're a twin with diabetes, you have a one-in-three risk factor for Type-1. Figure 17 shows the risk factors associated with other family member diabetics.

FAMILY RISK FACTORS FOR DIABETES

If:	Your risk factor is:
Your twin has diabetes	1 in 3
Your sibling has diabetes	1 in 14
One parent has diabetes	1 in 25
Your mother has diabetes	1 in 40–50
Your father has diabetes	1 in 20
No relative has diabetes	1 in 500

Figure 5: Family risk factors for diabetes (Source: Rotter, J I, Anderson, C E, Rubin, R, Congleton, J E, Terasaki, P I, and Rimoin, D L. "HLA genotypic study of insulin-dependent diabetes the excess of DR3/DR4 heterozygotes allows rejection of the recessive hypothesis." *Diabetes,* Feb. 1983, 32(2):169–174.)

Type-2 Diabetes Cometh

In the early stages, Type-2 diabetics or NIDDM diabetics, do produce insulin, but the cells are unable to use it properly as they are resistant to the signaling of the insulin. Normal insulin production is about 31 units per day on average in the blood. In insulin-resistant diabetes, the pancreas may overwork to produce about 114 units of insulin.[86] The underlying cause of insulin resistance is a breakdown in the communication between the insulin, a chemical messenger, and the receivers of that signal called GLUT-4 transporters. GLUT-4 transporters are proteins within the cell that rise to the cell's membrane, take hold of the glucose, and bring it inside the cell. Insulin resistance means that the cells do not receive the message. Because the cells are not hearing the message from the insulin and thus receiving the sugar, blood glucose levels remain high, causing the pancreatic beta cells to pump out more insulin to "knock" louder on the cell walls. Early in this disease process, the glucose is let in. This is called *compensated insulin resistance,* as the pancreas has put out more insulin and glucose levels stabilize for a while. As this continues, over time the beta cells of the pancreas wear out from producing up to four times the normal insulin levels. Glucose levels remain elevated in this state of *uncompensated insulin resistance,* and over time the person experiences an advanced case of Type-2 with beta cell inflammation and eventually "beta cell burnout." About 30 percent of the people with Type-2 diabetes do inject insulin on a daily basis because their insulin-producing cells become burned out from excessive use. Then these Type-2 (NIDDM) diabetics become insulin-dependent diabetics (IDDM).

There are multiple reasons for insulin resistance. Insulin receptors on the outside of the cells may not accept insulin, or there are too few receptors as the glucose enters the cells, or the cells don't use it properly, or excess dietary fat accumulates in the cell and disrupts glucose absorption. Part of the issue is that the ability to move from glycogen to glucose is blocked within the cells and there is a backup.

This whole system is somewhat affected by free radical production associated with hyperinsulinemia. This elevated free radical production activates Nuclear Factor kB, which is a DNA regulator that acts within the cell nucleus. NFkB activation intensifies inflammatory responses, resulting in more production of free radicals and eventually beta-cell death. So we begin to see that diabetes is also associated with inflammation. In essence inflammation occurs, not only through the autoimmune inflammation that we get in Type-1 but also as the more chronic low-level inflammation we may see in Type-2.

N-acetyl cysteine is a precursor to glutathione (GSH) and is a powerful antioxidant to moderate cell metabolism and gene expression.

GSH is thought to prevent the oxidation that causes beta cell damage, and it does this by inhibiting NFkB activation. So it's possible that the inflammation from the NFkB activation plays an important role in the development of diabetes. And if that's the case n-acetyl cysteine, which inhibits NFkB activation, has the potential to prevent or delay the onset of the disease. In the presence of other oxidants, NFkB can activate the vascular cell adhesion molecules (VCAM-1). This molecule helps these plasma cells attached to the endothelium and therefore creates more clogged arteries. The VCAM-1 increase has been shown to be one of the most important events initiating atherosclerosis. Type-2 diabetes and glucose intolerant hypertensive patients have been found to have elevated levels of plasma VCAM-1.[87] In diabetics n-acetyl cysteine may synergize with the antioxidant vitamins C and E; these three together seem to reduce blood glucose levels in mice. They also increase beta cell mass and preserve insulin content.

Diabetes in Children

Type-1 diabetes is rising alarmingly worldwide, at a rate of 3 percent per year. Some 70,000 children age 14 and under develop Type-1 diabetes annually.

Increasingly, children are also developing Type-2 diabetes, in both developed and developing nations, with reports of Type-2 diabetes in some children as young as 8 years old. Approximately 2 million children ages 12–19 have a Type-2 diabetic condition directly related to obesity and inactivity. About one in fourteen boys seem to have this condition.

In a study reported in the November 2005 issue of *Pediatrics,* based on data involving 950 children in a 1999–2000 national health survey, researchers found that among roughly 177,000 Americans under age 20, both Type-1 and Type-2 have increased. About 25 percent of the diabetic children now have Type-2, compared with just 4 percent ten years ago. Approximately 7 percent of the children in the study were pre-diabetic—that translates to 2 million children. About 16 percent

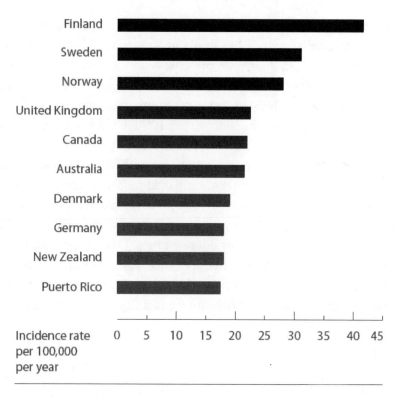

Diabetic Lifestyle Habits and Risk Factors

Incidence rate per 100,000 per year

Only countries where studies have been carried out in that country have been included

Figure 6: Top ten countries for incidence rate of Type-1 diabetes in children, 0–14 years (Source: *Diabetes Atlas,* third edition, International Diabetes Federation, 2006)

of the kids in the study were obese. The study supports the idea that our children are heading more seriously in the direction of a diabetes disaster.

About 5 million children are overweight in the U.S. Overweight is being described as a new epidemic in the American pediatric population, with an overall 33 percent increase in diabetes incidence and prevalence seen in the last ten years. Type-2 diabetes has changed from a disease of our grandparents and parents to a disease of our children. In 1994 Type-2 diabetes accounted for 16 percent of new cases of pediatric diabetes, and by 1999, it accounted for 8 percent to 45 percent, from state to state.[88] In Ohio and Arkansas, African American children with Type-2 diabetes represented 70–75 percent of new pediatric diabetes cases.[89] In Ventura, California, 31 percent of new adult-onset diabetes were Mexican American youths. Among the Pima tribe, pediatric diabetes is seen in 20 to 40 per 1000. Unlike Type-1 diabetes, most children with Type-2 diabetes have a family member with Type-2 diabetes; 45 to 80 percent have a parent with Type-2 diabetes[90] and 70 to 90 percent report at least one affected first- or second-degree relative. Up to 60 to 90 percent of youth who develop diabetes have ancanthosas, a thickening and hyperpigmentation of skin at the neck. This seems to be associated with insulin resistance. Once Type-2 diabetes is established, the persistence of obesity exacerbates the complications of hypertension, dyslipidemia, atherosclerosis, and polycystic ovarian syndrome, which start to appear despite the fact that these patients are still young.[91]

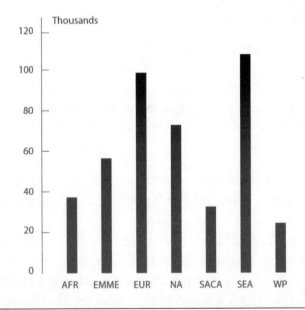

Figure 7: Estimated number of prevalent cases of Type-1 diabetes in children (0-14 years) by region (Source: *Diabetes Atlas*, third edition, International Diabetes Federation, 2006)

Investigators reviewed national health surveys of more than 6,000 U.S. children ages 6 to 18 between 1988 and 1994. They also looked at the data from 3,000 children in China and 7,000 in Russia. In the U.S. about 11 percent of the children were obese and slightly more than 14 percent were overweight, compared to 6 percent in Russia obese and 10 percent overweight. In China 3.6 percent were obese and 2.4 percent were overweight.[92] In contrast to the U.S. and England, the Chinese and Russian children from the wealthiest families tended to be more heavy.

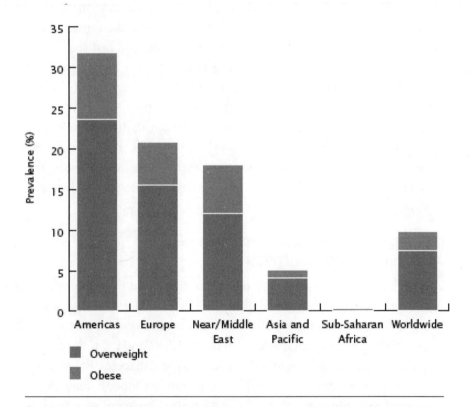

Figure 8: Overweight and obesity among school-age children (5–17 years) worldwide (Source: *Diabetes Atlas,* second edition, International Obesity Task Force, 2003)

Our children are fed daily propaganda to eat foods that are causing them harm. A Kaiser Family Foundation study analyzed more than 8,000 advertisements using detailed data about the viewing habits of children in three age groups. Researchers found that children of all ages are bombarded with promotions for fast food, junk food, and soda, with 8- to 12-year-olds seeing the most food advertisements. This market, the "tweens," is especially important to advertisers because it encompasses the ages at which youngsters typically begin to make some of their own buying decisions. According to Dr. Susan Linn of the Campaign for a Commercial-Free Childhood (CCFC): "We know that marketing is a factor in the childhood obesity epidemic. It is unconscionable that 8–12-year-olds see, on average, more than 7,600 food commercials a year—the vast majority for candy, snacks, cereals, and fast food."[93]

We understand that overweight is a risk factor for heart disease in adults, but the situation is more ominous still. Autopsy data from the conflicts in Korea[94] and Vietnam,[95] the Bogalusa study,[96] and the PDAY Study[97] all testify to the ubiquitous nature of the disease in young Americans. The 1992 Bogalusa Heart Study examined autopsies performed on children killed in accidental deaths. Researchers found the initial stages of atherosclerosis in the form of fatty plaques and streaks in most children and teenagers.[98]

DIET AND TYPE-2 DIABETES PREVENTION AND REVERSAL FOR CHILDREN

Research by Dr. Milagros G. Huerta has suggested that magnesium deficiency is related to Type-2 diabetes in obese children, who are more likely to have insulin resistance.[99] This study was performed to see if obese children get enough magnesium in their diets and if a lack of magnesium can cause insulin resistance and thus Type-2 diabetes. Researchers found that 55 percent of obese children did not get enough magnesium from the foods they ate, compared with only 27 percent of lean children. The results showed that obese children got 14.4 percent less magnesium from the foods they ate than lean children, even though obese and lean children ate about the same number of calories per day. Children with lower magnesium levels had a higher insulin resistance. Obese children typically eat more calories from fatty foods than lean children. In addition to not eating enough foods rich in magnesium, obese children seem to have problems using magnesium from the foods they eat. Extra body fat can prevent the body's cells from using magnesium to break down carbohydrates.

Characteristic signs of Type-2 diabetes in children include: overweight, early stages of heart disease, magnesium deficiency, and insulin resistance. Chlorophyll through a plant-sourced diet is high in magnesium. Chlorophyll is an amazing food that is essential for humans, and at the center of every chlorophyll molecule is the element magnesium. Plant blood (chlorophyll) and human blood (hemoglobin) are not so different, as shown in Figure 21.

Magnesium is seventeen times as prevalent in the human heart as any other tissue in the body. Famous research scientist Dr. Max Oskar Bircher-Brenner called chlorophyll "concentrated sun power" and said:

> Chlorophyll increases the functions of the heart, affects the vascular system, the intestines, the uterus, and the lungs. It raises the basic nitrogen exchange and is therefore a tonic which considering its stimulating properties cannot be compared with any other.[100]

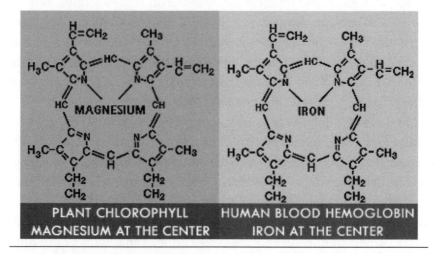

Figure 9: Plant chlorophyll and human blood hemoglobin

One of the reasons chlorophyll is so effective may be its similarity to hemin. Hemin is part of hemoglobin, the protein fraction of human blood that carries oxygen. Studies done as long ago as 1911 show that the molecules of hemin and chlorophyll are surprisingly alike, with the difference being that chlorophyll is bound by an atom of magnesium and hemin is bound by iron.[101] Experiments have shown that severely anemic rabbits make a rapid return to a normal blood count once chlorophyll is administered.[102] Although the exact chemical transaction has not been proven, the human body seems to be able to substitute iron and rebuild the blood. It is as if the anemic patient has had a transfusion.

Understanding Insulin Resistance

The diagnosis of insulin resistance is not the same as diabetes. It is associated with pre-diabetes, and exists in many Type-2 diabetics. Insulin resistance starts before diabetes and is a whole metabolic shift. About 25 to 35 percent of the population have a degree of insulin resistance and suffer from the health consequences of hyperglycemia.[103] Insulin resistance seems to be a common feature of, and possibly contributing factor to, a variety of interlinking health problems including diabetes mellitus,[104] polycystic ovarian syndrome,[105,106,107] dyslipidemia,[108] hypertension,[109,110] cardiovascular disease,[111,112,113,114,115] sleep apnea,[116] certain hormone-sensitive cancers,[117,118,119] and obesity.[120,121, 122,123] One key sign to diagnose Type-2 is called abdominal obesity, which is almost a clinical marker for this metabolic dysregulation.

Magnesium deficiency is very common in my clinical experience, and is found in about 90 percent of people with diabetes. Insulin resistance is also associated with hypertension. Experimental work with magnesium deficiency showed that giving magnesium reduces tissue sensitivity to insulin. If the diet is depleted in potassium, it can also lead to insulin resistance at post-receptor sites.[124] Zinc and chromium play a role in decreasing insulin resistance, as well as does vanadium. Biotin does appear to decrease insulin resistance according to research.[123] Vitamin

E plays a role. About 600 mg was all that was needed to make a difference in insulin resistance.

Taurine and glutathione all seem to decrease insulin resistance. CoQ10, which seems to be quite good for this, also results in improvements in blood sugar, blood pressure, and uptakes of C, E, and beta-carotene. Alpha lipoic acid is specifically good for improving insulin resistance (sensitivity). Fiber creates an improved insulin resistance. Saturated fats make the insulin resistance worse. Vegetables decrease fasting insulin. Vitamin A-rich foods decrease insulin resistance.

Stress also plays a role at the insulin resistance level. Acute stress seems to be clearly associated with severe, although reversible, insulin resistance.[126] We should pay attention to stress, and the treatment of stress.[127] A study by Nelson showed that psychosocial stress played a role in the chronic elevation of cortisol, which results in increased plasma insulin levels. A hormone called leptin is secreted by the fatty tissues. High leptin levels appear to act on the hypothalamus to decrease body fat. But as the percentage of body fat increases, even high levels of leptin are unable to stimulate the metabolic processes. So in obesity, we have a leptin resistance.[128] Leptin resistance decreases as a person becomes more sensitive to insulin.

In summary, factors that may contribute to insulin resistance and thus to diabetes include: high-fat diet; low-protein diet; deficiencies of the omega-3 and omega-6 fatty acids; a diet high in simple carbohydrates; high-glycemic meals filled with refined sugar and starches; stress; low fiber intake; deficiencies of the minerals calcium, magnesium, chromium, vanadium, potassium, and zinc; deficiency of carotenoids; low intake of vegetables; lack of exercise; watching television; and nicotine.

Gestational Diabetes

Gestational diabetes is a third major category of diabetes that needs to be addressed. It occurs in 5 to 14 percent of pregnant women. It is important to diagnose this effectively and treat it because it plays a big role in the onset of Type-2 diabetes five to ten years later. Half of women who've had gestational diabetes eventually develop Type-2.[129] It is associated with the metabolic changes that take place during a normal pregnancy. To conserve sugar for the baby, mom's placenta produces hormones that naturally increase insulin resistance, thus rerouting some of the sugar to her fetus that before pregnancy would have gone to her cells. Early in pregnancy maternal estrogen and progesterone increase and promote pancreatic beta cell hyperplasia and increased insulin release.[130]

This rise in insulin increases peripheral glucose utilization and glycogen storage and lowers glucose levels but this shifts as the pregnancy progresses. There are increased levels of human chorionic gonadatropin (HCG) which also leads to insulin resistance. Cortisol, which has the highest diabetic creating potency, peaks at twenty-six weeks. Progesterone, with anti-insulin qualities, peaks at thirty-two weeks. These two milestones, twenty-six and thirty-two weeks, encompass an important time during which the pancreas releases 1.5 to 2.5 times more insulin to respond to the resistance.[131]

THE DIABETOGENIC POTENCY OF HORMONES IN PREGNANCY

Hormone:	Peak elevation (weeks):	Diabetogenic potency:
Prolactin	10	Weak
Estradiol	26	Very weak
hCS	26	Moderate
Cortisol	26	Very strong
Progesterone	32	Strong

Figure 10: The diabetogenic potency of hormones in pregnancy

Gestational diabetes is the most common medical complication in pregnancy. Women who have it face a significantly greater risk of developing diabetes later in their life. It may be immediate or long-term, in terms of complications. Statistically associated with gestational diabetes is an increase in preeclampsia and resulting increased C-sections.

A study by Coustan and Associates showed that 6 percent were tested with irregular glucose tolerance at zero to two years post-partum; 13 percent were irregular at three to four years; 15 percent at five to six years; and 30 percent at seven to ten years post-partum.[132] Other studies have documented Type-2 diabetes at three to five years post-partum in 30 to 50 percent of the women.[133,134] Repeated insulin resistance physiologies, due to additional pregnancies, lead to an increase in the rate of developing Type-2 diabetes later. The relative risk for Type-2 diabetes was 1.95 for each 10 pounds gained during pregnancy. This is also associated with greater risk for developing hypertension, hyperlipidemia, EKG changes, and mortality.[135] Women with gestational diabetes (GDM) had higher triglycerides and fatty acids, beta hydroxy butyrate, and LDL, and lower HDL cholesterol than normals. Their offspring have an increased rate of perinatal mortality and morbidity. One study showed a fourfold increase in perinatal mortality in pregnancies complicated by improperly managed GDM.[136] Other studies have suggested an increased rate in stillbirths associated with GDM.

Maternal hyperglycemia leads to fetal hyperglycemia and fetal hyperinsulinemia with increases in fetal growth. Growth is bigger in the fatty and the liver tissues.

In studies of children of women with pre-gestational diabetes and GDM, they found that irregular glucose tolerance (IGT) was thirteen times higher than in controls. It appears that children of mothers with GDM have a higher incidence of obesity. They saw that Type-2 diabetes occurred in 8.6 percent of children with pre-diabetic mothers and 45 percent of infants with diabetic mothers.[137]

Alzheimer's Associated Diabetes

Approximately 4.5 million Americans have Alzheimer's Disease, and that figure may triple in less than fifty years, according to the Alzheimer's Association. More than 65 percent of Americans are overweight or obese, and the Centers for Disease Control and Prevention (CDC) estimates that some 54 million people are considered pre-diabetic.

Pre-diabetes and diabetes mean high blood sugar, greatly increasing the chance of developing diabetes, obesity, heart disease, and, according to new research, Alzheimer's. This link could foretell a dramatic increase in Alzheimer's cases, unless dietary and lifestyle interventions are made now.[138]

Researchers are beginning to connect Alzheimer's with diabetes, obesity, and heart disease. It is such a strong connection that Alzheimer's is being referred to by scientists at Brown Medical School as Type-3 diabetes.[139] A variety of studies have shown that people with Type-2 diabetes have about double the average incidence of Alzheimer's. One study out of the Karolinska Institute in Sweden found that even people with borderline diabetes, meaning people with high blood sugar, had a 70 percent greater risk of developing Alzheimer's.[140] Apparently the risk of dementia rises in people with high blood sugar. Speculation is that the poor brain circulation caused by diabetes is a primary factor. An eight-year study out of Kaiser Permanente tracked 22,582 patients age 50 or above with Type-2 diabetes, and found that diabetic individuals with high blood sugar experience an increased risk of dementia and Alzheimer's. Compared to those with normal glycosylated hemoglobin levels (HgbA1c less than 6), those with HgbA1c levels greater than 12 were 22 percent more likely to develop dementia, and those with HgbA1c levels above 15 were 78 percent more likely to develop dementia. As with peripheral vascular disease going to amputations, there may be a vascular dementia that is triggered by low blood flow to the brain.

New research linking diabetes and Alzheimer's suggests that the high blood sugar of diabetes can lead to the formation of advanced glycation end products, or AGEs.[141] AGEs are sugar-derived substances that form in the body through an interaction between carbohydrates and proteins, lipids, or nucleic acids such as DNA. AGEs adversely affect the structure and function of proteins and the tissues that contain proteins.[142] Recent studies have shown that both the formation and accumulation of AGEs are enhanced in diabetes.[143] According to evidence provided by Edward R. Rosick, DO:

Advanced glycation end products become even more destructive when coupled with free radicals formed during cellular energy production. These highly reactive agents produce oxidative stress that can cause cellular damage. Researchers now believe that oxidative stress may be involved in the formation of AGEs, which in turn may induce even more oxidative stress. Most AGEs that accumulate in proteins are produced under conditions of high oxidative stress. New evidence shows that oxidative stress may be an important causative factor in both insulin resistance and Type-2 diabetes.[144,145]

Brain autopsies of Alzheimer's patients find signs of significant oxidative damage by free radicals, and new research indicates that AGEs may initiate this damage.[146] It is the oxidative damage and the accumulation of AGEs in both diabetes and Alzheimer's that is the biochemical similarity between these two diseases.

We do have nutritional protection against oxidative stress of this kind. Studies show that alpha-lipoic acid (ALA) helps protect the brain against damage caused by free-radical-induced oxidative stress, which has important implications for its potential role in protecting against Alzheimer's disease.[147,148]

Other good news is that the high blood sugar of diabetes and the increased risk for Alzheimer's is related to consumption of processed high-glycemic foods, not natural foods. Juicy new research suggests that antioxidants in fruit and vegetable juices may lower the risk of Alzheimer's disease. The Kame Project, a long-term study of more than 1,800 Japanese Americans conducted in Seattle, began in 1992–1994 to study participants who had no dementia, and averaged 71 years of age. The group was followed through 2001. During that time, eighty-one cases of probable Alzheimer's were diagnosed in participants who had completed the food surveys. Those who reported drinking fruit or vegetable juices at least three times per week were 73 percent less likely to have developed Alzheimer's as those who drank juice less than once a week.[149] This is great news, as the Culture of Life anti-diabetogenic diet includes ample amounts of fresh vegetable juice.

Cancer Associations

In addition to diabetes, there is a strong link between high insulin levels and some types of cancer. In one study, ten post-menopausal women with endometrial cancer had significantly higher fasting serum insulin levels than the controls. Researchers found insulin receptors in the post-menopausal ovaries, which is a unique place to find them.[150] In a study of 752 women with endometrial cancer and with 2,606 controls, an association was confirmed between NIDDM and an increased risk of endometrial cancer.[151] Insulin is thought to affect the development of endometrial cancer through its hormonal stimulating properties. In twenty-two endometrial cancer patients in one study, those with high hyperinsulinemia had significantly more steroid hormone receptors in the tumor area, compared with patients with low insulin anemia.[152,153] Researchers also discovered a link between colon cancer and insulin levels and it may be associated with insulin's role as a growth factor in the colon. In 102 cases of colorectal cancer researchers found that those with the highest level of fasting glucose had almost twice the increased risk of colon cancer. Those with the highest fasting insulin levels also were associated with the increased risk of colon cancer.[154]

A recent study in the *American Journal of Clinical Nutrition* has shown that people who consume a large amount of processed sugar each day are at a much higher risk for pancreatic cancer, which kills about 30,000 Americans each year. Of nearly 80,000 men and women whose diets were studied during 1997–2005, 131 developed pancreatic cancer. Those who drank carbonated or corn-syrup laden drinks even twice a day were 90 percent more likely to contract pancreatic cancer than those who never drank them. Those who added sugar to their foods or beverages at least five times daily had a 70 percent higher risk of developing pancreatic cancer than those who did not.[155] Clearly, increased insulin demand due to high sugar consumption burdens the pancreas and increases pancreatic cancer risk.

Chapter 2 Summary

In Chapter 1 overwhelming data was presented that diabetes is a world-wide pandemic. In Chapter 2 the reader can see that by living in the Culture of Death (expressed by: a diet and lifestyle of highly refined carbohydrates, dairy products, processed white flour, processed white sugar, cooked animal and other saturated fats, trans fats, nicotine, coffee, commercial foods high in agrochemicals, heavy metal toxicity, vaccinations, poor air and water quality, and high stress), we have created the pandemic of diabetes. In other words, diabetes is a *symptom* of the Culture of Death.

In addition to the Culture of Death tendencies that aggravate and pull the trigger on the loaded gun of genetic propensities, there are also economic considerations. Those people living in weaker economic conditions seemed to also be more susceptible, with the exception of China, Russia, and India, where those of greater affluence have more access to junk foods and are running higher rates of obesity, which is associated with diabetes.

In general, what we are saying is that it is a world diet and lifestyle that is a Crime Against Wisdom. The point is clear. The reader is given the option to choose the Culture of Life over the Culture of Death. Chapters 3 through 6 of this book give you the wisdom to no longer suffer the Crimes Against Wisdom in the Culture of Death. These chapters will show how to do this in a straightforward, uncomplicated way that enables you to live a life of abundance, free of diabetes.

ECONOMIC STATUS IS MUTE FOR THE DETERMINED

We want to make it perfectly clear that in Western societies, a lower-class economic status does not sentence individuals or families to a cheap, highly processed diet that brings diabetes, although it does make it harder to change the diabetic trend. Being empowered by the message of this book to eat organic, whole, live foods, of which you only need to eat half as much to get the nutrients as compared with cooked food, can prevent and reverse diabetes. I have yet to find a person, no matter how difficult their economic status, who could not switch over to this Culture of Life diet and lifestyle. And the exciting thing about this in our advanced Western culture is that we are able to acquire foods and food concentrates that are allowing us to access more powerful forms of nutrition than our ancestors ever dreamed possible. This means that we can do even better than just achieve a nondiabetic physiology, but a post-diabetic physiology in which one's health is better than it was before the diabetes, and better than most people in the world who have never developed diabetes.

Even in developing societies, where urbanization with its diet and lifestyle has increased rates of diabetes, moving back to a rural agrarian lifestyle can make accessible the indigenous diets which for centuries have protected people from having diabetes. It is useful to remind the reader that the Pima Indians, who are now running a 51 percent rate of diabetes, had only one single documented case of diabetes by 1920 when they were still living on their land and eating their indigenous diet. Their cousins, the Tarahumaras, who have stuck with a natural diet and remained on their land, have only 6 percent incidence of diabetes.

I believe that these healthy results will be repeated in all indigenous cultures who give up white flour, white sugar, cooked hydrogenated and animal fats, and return to the land and their indigenous diets and lifestyles.

CHAPTER 3 PREVIEW

In the next chapter we will be discussing a comprehensive theory of the causes of diabetes which will give you more insight into how to effectively manage your metabolism. This is a theory that explains the effectiveness of the clinical results. As a scientist, one understands, as with all theories, they must be proven. Theories give us a way to investigate what is going on. Further research is then needed to disprove or prove them. The key is that there are potentially significant results and in the next chapter we will be presenting a theory that helps us develop and understand the rationale for the 21-Day+ Program for healing diabetes, especially Type-2 and gestational, as well as providing a path for future research. To prove something is more difficult than theorizing. For example, it took more than thirty years to prove that smoking was directly linked to lung cancer. The beautiful thing is that the approach is both safe and outstanding for developing high-level wellness. It is a win/win proposition.

A Comprehensive Theory of Diabetes

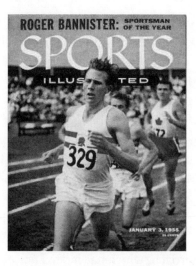

No longer conscious of my movement, I discovered a new unity with nature. I had found a new source of power and beauty, a source I never dreamt existed.

ROGER BANNISTER, ON BREAKING THE FOUR-MINUTE MILE

When Roger Bannister broke the four-minute mile in 1954, no one believed that humans had the physiological capacity to run that fast that far. Bannister clocked 3:59.4, and the glass ceiling shattered, and with it the conventional paradigm and conventional wisdom. Now it is commonplace for high school milers to run a mile in less than four minutes. *This book announces that the four-minute mile of diabetes has been broken and we have the capacity, if we so choose, to completely reverse Type-2 diabetes.*

By developing a comprehensive theory of the causative level of diabetes we become significantly empowered to develop an overall approach for the reversal of diabetes. The word *reversing* is different from ameliorating, modifying, or decreasing the amount of medication needed. I am not talking about managing Type-2 diabetes, which is the old paradigm, exemplified by a belief system stated in the *New York Times* and backed by most doctors treating diabetes: "Diabetes has no cure. It is progressive and fatal." We have the knowledge, clinical know-how, and experience to completely reverse Type-2 diabetes. The four-minute mile of diabetes has been broken. All that is needed is to let go of our belief that diabetes cannot be reversed. Then we are free to cultivate the understanding of what is possible.

Actually, doctors have been using live foods to reverse diabetes as far back as 1920 when Dr. Max Gerson healed Dr. Albert Schweitzer of diabetes with live-food nutrition. For the last twenty-five years, after turning to live foods in my own life and in using it as a baseline for all healing as a wholistic physician, this strategy has been reversing Type-2 diabetes on a regular basis. With the energy released by this understanding comes the determination to change our lifestyle, our dietary patterns, to achieve this result. The mythology supported by the allopathic treatment approach, which has indeed not been particularly successful, is that diabetes is a one-way, downhill road to death involving multiple complications. The statistics show that diabetes as currently treated will take off 10–19 years from a person's life. When we free ourselves from the lifestyle of the Culture of Death, and transition to the Culture of Life, the current pattern of irreversibility shifts to one of reversibility.

Type-2 diabetes is a disease of both a complex and simple etiology. Based on clinical experience, as well as world research, the number one culprit is the huge increase in intake of processed white sugar, white bread, and refined carbohydrates as distinct from complex natural carbohydrates such as beans and grains. The breakthrough in understanding diabetes was found in Dr. Thomas Cleave's 1975 book, *The Saccharine Disease: Conditions Caused by the Taking of Refined Carbohydrates such as Sugar and White Flour* showing that within twenty years after processed white flour and sugar are introduced into a culture, there is an "outbreak" of diabetes. His statistical analysis showed processed sugar rather than fat as the primary cause.

According to Dr. Cleave, in 1955 the primary cause of diabetes was thought to be related to fat consumption. This was because of a paper presented in 1949 by H. P. Himsworth,[1] who showed that during World War II diabetes mortality fell in direct relationship to the fall in fat consumption.

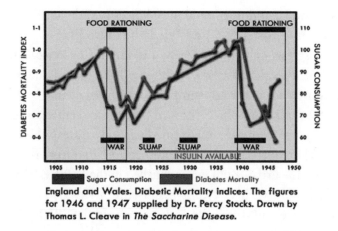

England and Wales. Diabetic Mortality indices. The figures for 1946 and 1947 supplied by Dr. Percy Stocks. Drawn by Thomas L. Cleave in *The Saccharine Disease.*

Dr. Cleave showed that when diabetes mortality was charted against the consumption of refined carbohydrates—white sugar and white flour—rather than total consumption of carbohydrates (both complex and refined), there was a much closer statistical correlation between refined carbohydrate consumption and diabetes mortality. This correlation was greater for refined carbohydrates with diabetes than for fat consumption. Dr. Cleave also showed that the increase in fat consumption from 1900 to 1960 was minor, compared with the consumption of refined carbohydrates from the 1900s when diabetes began to move from twenty-seventh in the list of causes of death to seventh by the 1960s. Only the dramatic increase in the consumption of refined carbohydrates matched the dramatic increase in diabetes mortality. This point was made clearer by the fact that in communities where refined carbohydrates were not introduced, and where a high consumption of complex carbohydrates was maintained, there was not a significant increase in diabetes.

Therefore, Dr. Cleave concluded, as we have, that the introduction of refined carbohydrates into a culture was the primary, but not sole, cause of the dramatic increase in diabetes. Other underlying causes include increased consumption of cooked animal fats and trans fats, heavy metals, agrochemicals, vitamin D deficiencies, mineral and vitamin deficiencies in general resulting from a diet of nutrient-poor processed foods, and hormonal imbalances and deficiencies such as a deficiency in testosterone. Lifestyle habits also play a role—obesity, emotional stress, inadequate sleep, and lack of exercise. Dr. Cleave's cross-cultural work, however, highlighted the main issue, which was an excess increase in the consumption of white sugar.

In 1959 G. D. Campbell[2] showed that there seemed to be a period of twenty years from the time refined carbohydrates(white sugar and white flour) are introduced into a culture and an outbreak of diabetes. Research on the urban Zulu was published in the *South African Medical Journal* in 1960.[3] This "twenty-year rule" was also confirmed by Albertson in Iceland studies. In Iceland around the 1850s, the diet was 85 percent protein and fats with no refined carbohydrate,[4] but with the introduction of refined carbohydrate, protein and fats were reduced to 45 percent, and following the twenty-year rule, there was an outbreak of diabetes.

A. M. Cohen's 1960 study of Yemenite Jews showed a low incidence of diabetes in Yemen with a general diet that was high in fat and protein, and with one of the two lowest sugar intakes in the world.[5] When these Yemenite Jews moved to Israel, there was a marked increase in white sugar consumption, and Yemenite Jews in Israel, from a culture in which diabetes was unknown, became equal for the incidence of diabetes to that of the Israeli culture.

The Canadian Eskimos also had a high raw-animal-fat diet. After refined carbohydrate was introduced into their cultures were also found twenty years later to have an increased incidence of diabetes. Dr. Cleave wrote: "With the greater availability of sugar and white flour, the consumption of the former substance amongst Canadian Eskimos has now risen to over 100 lb. per head per year and, with the expiring of the twenty-year incubation period already discussed, diabetes is now commonly occurring amongst them."

Evidence from studies in India of rural and urban groups of the same culture showed their diabetes incidence being significantly higher in the urban setting, with its much higher consumption of refined carbohydrates. It is not possible to relate it to the consumption of fats as those cultures have one-half the fat consumption that is needed for health.

In the U.S., Cherokee Indians also followed the pattern of high refined carbohydrate associated with high diabetes incidence. In the Natal Indians of the Zulu tribe, an increase in diabetes incidence was directly related to refined carbohydrate consumption, as tribal members who ate cane sugar (a complex carbohydrate) had a lower incidence of diabetes. Dr. Cleave's data suggests that there is now no country where the incidence of diabetes cannot be directly related to increased refined carbohydrate intake. Similar findings were found for all indigenous groups migrating to urban environments, such as Kurdish immigrants. Similar data has been gathered from Australian Aborigines,[6] New Guinea aboriginal groups,[7] and Polynesians in general.[8]

In summary, cross-cultural studies show the introduction of refined carbohydrates into cultures that previously had low incidences of diabetes, whether on a low-protein-and-fat and high-complex-carbohydrate diet or a high-fat and protein diet. The main environmental cause of the worldwide pandemic of Type-2 diabetes is the introduction of white sugar, white flour, and white rice into these cultures, resulting in an "outbreak" of Type-2 diabetes twenty years later. It is obvious that a successful program for healing diabetes must eliminate all refined carbohydrate from the diet.

Dr. Cleave's book synthesized and tabulated the cross-cultural studies and showed that the introduction of refined carbohydrate into the cultures with a previously low incidence of diabetes saw an outbreak of diabetes within twenty years. This indicates that the main dietary cause of diabetes is processed sugar. In my clinical experience, as in Dr. Esselstyn's discussion of the importance of avoiding oils for those with advanced heart disease, I have found that even moderate- to high-glycemic fruits in the diet raise the blood glucose levels of those with pre-diabetes and diabetes. While limited amounts of these foods may be acceptable for those not in a pre-diabetic or diabetic physiology, I do not recommend them until people are maintained in a healthy physiology (fasting blood sugar of 70–85 for at least six months to a year). At that time, it is most prudent to introduce only low-glycemic berries, cherries, and citrus to maintain a healthy physiology.

Cooked Animal Fat and Trans-Fatty Acids

The second major contributor to the onset of diabetes is a diet high in cooked animal fat trans-fatty acids. An excess of saturated animal fats and trans-fatty acids is associated with increased diabetes, cancer of the breast and prostate, immune dysfunction, and infertility. Drs. Walter Willett and Alberto Ascherio of the Harvard School of Public Health have estimated that 30,000 premature deaths each year are attributable to our consumption of trans fats.[9] Foods high in trans-fatty acids include: margarine, commercial peanut butter, and pre-packaged baked goods, cakes, pies, and cookies. Naturally occurring trans fats can also be found in some animal products such as dairy products and beef fat, since the *trans* isomer is produced by bacteria in the gastrointestinal tract of cattle and other ruminants. These naturally occurring trans fats may account for as much as 21 percent of the food sources for American adults, according to the U.S. Food and Drug Administration.[10] Trans-fatty acids disrupt cell membrane function, because they change from a *cis* fatty acid to a *trans-fatty acid*, or from a curved shape to a straight shape; their actual molecular structure is thus changed and decreases the function of the cell membrane, which some people theorize is the actual brains of the cell and certainly critical for efficient movement of glucose into the cell. The *partially hydrogenated fats* are high in trans-fatty acids and are detrimental to cell membrane function.

But let's be clear: Not all fats are harmful. The omega-3 fatty acids and monounsaturated fats improve insulin function. One study of 86,000 women followed over sixteen years, in the Nurses Health Study, found that those who consumed one ounce of nuts five times per week decreased their risk of Type-2 diabetes by 27 percent. Evidence suggests that a raw vegan diet, moderately high in walnuts, almonds, and sunflower seeds may be helpful in the prevention of diabetes and in regulating glycemic control. This may be because the omega-3 and -6 fatty acids and the monounsaturated fats act to strengthen and repair the cell membrane structure and function. The wrong types of fats in our diets create an abnormal cell membrane structure, leading to impaired action of insulin. A poorly functioning cell membrane decreases cellular viral immunity, creates low-grade inflammation, and makes us susceptible to the development of chronic disease.

ACHIEVING NORMAL BLOOD SUGAR LEVELS

On the Tree of Life 21-Day+ Program, it is common to see people shift from blood sugars of 300–400 on medication, to being taken off all medications, *including insulin,* and within one to four days achieve relatively safe or normal fasting blood sugars. Within one to three weeks many have their fasting blood sugar go down to the optimum of 85. Some people, particularly those with Syndrome X, also known as metabolic syndrome, may take three or four weeks, or even slightly longer—everyone is different. Psychological stresses, as we pointed out, create elevated cortisol, which increases inflammation and undermines our ability to control insulin and glucose. Whether it takes four days to a few weeks, or a month, or even two months isn't the point so much as that we have the capacity within us to return to a healthy physiology, with a fasting blood sugar that is consistently around 85.

Diabetes is a complicated metabolic imbalance of carbohydrates, lipids, and proteins involving inflammation, heavy metal toxicity, nutritional deficiencies, and other hormonal imbalances. Complications involve free radical damage, sorbitol buildup in the tissues and organs, and a glycosylated protein buildup. All of these greatly accelerate the aging process. Diabetes in this context can be considered a sign of accelerated aging.

Diabetes is a symptom of the Culture of Death, which now appears in the world population as a pandemic. We have the opportunity to return to a world Culture of Life and live a lifestyle that naturally protects us against diabetes, as was done by indigenous groups for thousands of years. With that in mind, we are going to take a look at the physiology of Type-1, Type-2, and gestational diabetes. Although different, there are significant overlaps. First, let us look at blood glucose levels and their impact on our health.

Blood Glucose Levels

What are conventionally considered "normal" glucose levels are actually unhealthy. It now appears that the optimal fasting blood sugar (FBS), which is one's blood glucose first thing in the morning, should be at 85. The normal range of healthy glucose is between 70 and 85. Accelerated aging occurs with an FBS of 86 or greater and with that an increased risk of premature death. We have just begun to recognize that even a high normal glucose can eventually become a serious threat to our health. The point is we need to understand the complex toxic effects that high blood sugar or hyperglycemia creates in the body. It should be clear at this point that a high blood sugar damages cells through multiple mechanisms and accelerates all elements of aging.

The following list shows the potential problems that can arise from a high-glycemic diet. Items marked with an asterisk(*) were compiled and listed by Nancy Appleton, PhD, author of *Lick the Sugar Habit,* and published in *Health Freedom News,* June 1994.

Hypoglycemia
Asthma*
Depletion and imbalancing of neurotransmitters
Migraine headaches*
Anxiety
Atherosclerosis*
Depression
Gastric or duodenal ulcers*
PMS (up to 275 percent increase)
Periodontal disease*
Increase in triglycerides
Alcoholism*
Syndrome X
Interference with the absorption of protein*
Obesity*
Acidic stomach*
Diabetes

Increased cholesterol*

Elevation of low-density lipoproteins (LDL, the "bad" cholesterol)*

Reduction of high-density lipoproteins (HDL, the "good" cholesterol)*

Insulin resistance

Arthritis*

Hypertension

Increased inflammatory prostaglandins

Cataracts*

Candida and other fungal infections

Lowered enzymes' ability to function*

Loss of teeth calcium as a result of calcium being pulled from normal blood and bone by sugar combining with it

Cancer of the breast, ovaries, intestines, prostate, and rectum*

Increase in AGEs, or glycosylated protein complexes, which accelerate aging

Increased risk of Chrohn's disease and ulcerative colitis*

Hyperactivity, anxiety, difficulty concentrating, and crankiness in children

Elevated glucose and insulin responses in oral contraceptive users*

Malabsorption in those with functional bowel disease*

Skin aging, due to changes in the structure of collagen*

Chromium deficiency

Impaired structure of DNA*

Decreased growth hormone secretion

Eczema in children*

Heart disease

Increased free radicals in the bloodstream*

Weakened immune system

Emphysema*

Appendicitis*

Hemorrhoids*

Kidney damage*
Disorganizing of the minerals in the body*
Increased fasting levels of glucose and insulin*
Interference with absorption of calcium and magnesium*
Raised adrenaline levels in children*
Varicose veins*
Gallstones*
Tooth decay*
Multiple sclerosis*
Copper deficiency*
Weakened eyesight*
Osteoporosis*
Saliva acidity*
Drowsiness and decreased activity in children*
Changed structure of protein*
Food allergies*

The key to healing diabetes is eating and living in a way that creates an FBS between 70-85. A potent means of achieving this is associated with caloric restriction. This information comes from animal studies and our clinical experience, where caloric restriction induced significant reductions in blood glucose levels.[11,12,13] The message is: The less we eat, the longer we live, and the better control we have over blood glucose. By decreasing caloric intake, our risk of age-related diseases is diminished, and a slowing of aging is activated.[14,15,16,17,18,19,20,21,22] When people eat too much in general, their blood sugar often rises. On a calorie restricted diet, their blood sugar is more likely to stay at normal levels. This observation is from my clinical experience in watching people we call the "canaries in the mine." These are people with Type-1 diabetes or sensitive Type-2s. I would ask them to try a particular food or try overeating and observe their blood glucose levels. This is not as scientifically accurate as double-blind studies, but it certainly pointed me in the right direction. With age, fasting glucose levels increase as health decreases.

To further illustrate this point, a study of 2,000 men over a twenty-year period showed that those with fasting glucose levels over 85 had a 40 percent increased risk of death from cardiovascular disease.[23] With this kind of data, one should not be surprised that the author would define an FBS above 85 as glucose toxicity. The researchers concluded that "fasting blood glucose values in upper normal range appeared to be an important independent predictor of cardiovascular death and nondiabetic middle aged men."

How did researchers decide a blood glucose of 85 was the upper limit? The pancreas is key for regulating glucose, by releasing insulin into the system. Insulin drives fat into the cells, prevents fat from being released from the cells, and makes people feel hungry. High insulin levels contribute to obesity, because insulin brings fat into the cells. Hyperinsulinemia is associated with being overweight, Type-2 diabetes, cardiovascular disease, kidney disease, and certain types of cancer. In a normal person, the pancreas stops secreting insulin when the glucose levels drop below 83 mg/dl.[24,25,26] This fact is key to our understanding of what is a healthy blood glucose. Previously we've waited until reaching an FBS of 109 before we suspected a pre-diabetic condition. Now we are looking at this in a much different way. Insulin continues to be secreted when blood glucose levels are above 83. So the body is telling us that the pancreas wants to keep the glucose levels down to a safer range than what allopaths currently consider safe or convenient. Dr. Roy Walford's work on calorie restriction showed that restricting caloric intake lowers fasting glucose by 21 percent on average from 92 to 74 in humans. Dr. Walford was the one who found that people who practiced caloric restriction also had a 42 percent reduction in fasting insulin.[27] Before the pancreas eventually gets exhausted, overweight and obese people were found to have very high insulin levels.[28,29] This research supports the teaching of "the less we eat, the longer we live." This assumption also is supported by the major long-lived human cultures averaging about 1,500 calories/day as compared to our Western culture's intake of 3,000–3,500 calories/day. My clinical observations have also been that blood sugars increase when diabetics overeat, *even if it is the overeating of healthy foods.*

This book is recommending a range of 70 to 85 as the optimal FBS. Borderline impaired fasting glucose tolerance is 86 to 99 (a precursor for pre-diabetes); and an FBS at 100 and over is considered pre-diabetes by the Tree of Life 21-Day+ standards. This is significantly different from the current assumptions. On October 24, 2003 the scientific committee of the American Diabetes Association actually did create a new and better definition of pre-diabetic or impaired glucose tolerance of a blood glucose of 100 or greater. They lowered the breakpoint from 109 to 100 mg/dl, which now means that the value of 100 or more would lead to a diagnosis of impaired fasting glucose or pre-diabetes. According to the general scientific literature, those who fall into the pre-diabetic range would probably develop diabetes within ten years.

Glycemic Index and Insulin Index

Another approach that helps lower blood glucose is decreasing the intake of high-glycemic-index foods, and high-insulin-index foods. The glycemic index (GI) is a measure of what happens to your blood sugar when you consume particular foods. GI numbers show how much one helping (50 grams) of a particular food raises your blood sugar.

Although useful, the GI does not provide a complete and accurate understanding of the full range of foods and their effect on glucose metabolism. In some instances a food has a low glycemic index rating but a high insulin index rating. Another vantage point at understanding how diet affects insulin levels has been proposed by Susanne H. A. Holt, Janette C. Brand Miller, and Peter Petocz.[30] They state that the GI concept does not consider insulin responses to particular foods. Their research proposes a method for obtaining a more accurate assessment of dietary factors to insulin response, based on a more realistic isoenergetic basis. The insulin index is based upon the insulin response to various foods, and certain foods (such as lean meats or proteins) seem to cause an increased insulin response despite there being no carbohydrates present. Additionally, other foods seem to cause a disproportionate insulin reaction for the carbohydrate load. Holt and her colleagues have noted that glucose and insulin scores are mostly highly correlated, but high-protein foods and bakery products (rich in fat and refined carbohydrates) "elicit insulin responses that were disproportionately higher than their glycemic responses."

A number of factors other than carbohydrate content mediate in stimulation of insulin secretion. For example, protein-rich foods or the addition of protein to a carbohydrate-rich meal can stimulate a modest rise in insulin secretion, without increasing blood glucose concentration. Similarly, adding fat to a carbohydrate-rich meal also increases insulin secretion even though plasma glucose response is reduced.

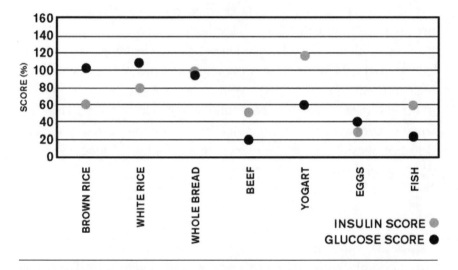

Figure 1: Insulin and glucose scores of selected foods (Source: Holt, Miller, and Petocz, "An insulin index of foods: the insulin demand generated by 1000-kJ portions of common foods." *Am J Clin Nutr,* 1997, 66:1264–1276)

From the above data, we can theorize, at least, that some complex carbohydrates do not produce insulin responses much greater than protein-rich foods such as beef or fish. Perhaps surprisingly, the insulin scores (IS) for beef and fish are greater than their glucose scores (GS), and the GS for yogurt is higher than the IS or GS of carbohydrate-rich foods such as brown rice, white rice, and bread. This will lay rest to the myth that protein-rich animal foods are somehow insulin safe when compared to carbohydrate-rich foods.

Satiety Index

The satiety index (SI) is a relatively new concept[31] that measures how full or satiated people feel after consuming a given calorie load from a variety of foods. It is measured by asking people to rate how satiated they feel after a meal and by how much food they eat after a two-hour delay after consuming the test food. Thus, a high-SI food would leave people more satisfied after eating a set amount of calories and they would also eat less two hours later when given something else to eat, presumably because they are still less hungry. It seems likely that a diet made up of higher-SI foods would likely lead to less hunger and a lower calorie intake. High-fructose corn syrup is a concern because it brings high amounts of sugar into the system, but does not activate a feeling of being satiated; thus people are more likely to keep eating. The high-fructose corn syrup sweeteners that have been implicated in the epidemic of obesity is an interesting example of a low-SI food, as it does not turn on the natural satiety response.

Glycation

Associated with a high blood sugar is the destructive effect of the glucose as it links with protein in a process called *glycation*. The higher the blood glucose, the more severe the glycation process. When the glucose non-enzymatically links with protein molecules, it results in the formation of nonfunctioning protein structures in the body. This results in poorly functioning enzymes, poorly functioning cell membranes, and cross-linkages of proteins in all tissues. Two extracellular proteins, collagen and elastin, are particularly affected, and we see it in the skin as wrinkles. The formation of AGEs throughout the body is an accelerated aging process, hence the apt abbreviation of glycosylation or glycation as AGE. AGE-related changes to collagen and elastin are believed to contribute to the stiffness of blood vessels and the urinary bladder, as well as impaired functioning of the kidneys, heart, retinas, and other organs and tissues. Moreover, damaging glycation reactions trigger inflammatory signaling, which scientists believe could provoke tissue damage and cancers.[32] As we will learn shortly, inflammation is the fourth of the Seven Stages of Disease, and it is followed by ulceration (Stage 5) and fungation (Stage 7, cancer). In diabetes, the rapid formation and accumulation of AGEs contribute to complications of disease, including injury to small blood vessels (microangiopathy) that impairs kidney and eye health.

In addition to those formed in the body, AGEs can also be introduced by external sources. For example, tobacco smoke contains precursors to advanced glycation end products, which increase AGE levels in the body. Foods that have been subjected to processing and heat also act as sources of AGEs.[33] The author concurs with Julian Whitaker, MD, that fructose is a "highly reactive molecule that readily attaches to proteins, changing their structure and interfering with normal activity. Studies show that fructose accelerates glycosylation, damaging proteins to a significantly greater degree than sucrose or glucose."[34] Our most prominent source of this damaging sugar is high-fructose corn syrup in soft drinks, which, according to the USDA Economic Research Service, comprised more than 25 percent of the beverages consumed by Americans in 1997. A 2005 study found that the low AGE content of a low-fat vegan diet could benefit diabetics.[35] The Culture of Life anti-diabetogenic diet I employ is unprocessed, unheated, plant-source-only foods, and low-glycemic, meaning that the AGEs issue is rendered moot. It is thus optimal for reducing and eliminating diabetes and its complications.

Oxidative Stress

A higher blood glucose creates an oxidative stress as well. Research has clearly shown that the antioxidants vitamin C and E inhibit the formation of AGEs,[36] and have been shown to reduce protein glycosylation both *in vivo* and *in vitro*,[37,38] with beneficial results in the treatment of Type-2 diabetes. Vitamins C and E also act as scavengers of free radicals generated by the glycosylated proteins.[39] Davie, et al. supplemented twelve nondiabetic subjects with 1 gram daily of vitamin C and demonstrated significant decreases of glycosylated hemoglobin of 18 percent and glycosylated albumin of 33 percent over a three-month period.[40] Jain, et al. found a significant reduction in glycosylated hemoglobin as well as a lowering of triglycerides in thirty-five Type-1 diabetics supplemented with 100 IU d-alpha tocopherol for three months.[41] The use of these incredible antioxidants will be discussed at greater length in Chapter 4.

Fasting Blood Sugar: Under 85

Glycosylation and oxidative stress are major reasons for why keeping an FBS of 85 and below is so important. Any FBS above 85 suggests that there is a metabolic disturbance, which is what we are describing that diabetes is. This metabolic disturbance leads to general degeneration. So, as we look at this process in terms of the carbohydrates we can understand full well all carbohydrates are not all the same. Simple carbohydrates—anything with white sugar, white bread, or high-fructose corn syrup—are very different from complex carbohydrates. Complex carbohydrates such as beans, grains, and vegetables are actually valuable in the healing of diabetes. An interesting cultural study conducted fifty years ago that makes this point is that of the O'Odham people of Southern Arizona, historically known as the River Pima and Papago, who had almost no diabetes. Now they have one of the highest levels of diabetes in the world—about 51 percent. Before the introduction of a processed diet, they were involved in desert farming and wild food gathering, which included complex carbohydrates and insulin-laden foods that protected them. Such foods had lower glycemic indexes, including lima beans, velvet mesquite pods, and non-bitter emery oak acorns. These foods had significantly lower glycemic ratings. Their diet was historically based on legumes and some corn. Some of these foods were actually high in insulin as well, and also high in gum pectins and complex carbohydrates. These desert plants used to capture and store life-giving water. are the same agent that makes beans, mesquite, plantago, belotas, chia seeds, nopalitos, and prickly pear fruit effective regulators of blood sugar. Because of their interface with Western culture and diet, and certain shifts that limited their access to anti-diabetogenic foods, they shifted to a high-refined-sugar and cooked-animal-fat diet.

Most foods high on the glycemic and insulin indexes greatly accelerate the metabolic imbalance. If you have a blood sugar that is 200 mg/dl after eating, or actually any time of day, that is considered diagnostic of diabetes. If your fasting blood sugar is 126 or higher on two separate occasions it supports a presumptive diagnosis of diabetes and merits further testing.

The glucose tolerance test (GTT) is a very sensitive test for diabetes. The classic amount is 75 grams of glucose dissolved in 300 ml of water, and if your blood glucose value is 190 to 200 or above two hours later, it is diagnostic of diabetes. Two hours after drinking the glucose, the normal value should be less than 140; anything between 140 and 180 is pre-diabetes. Levels above 180 in the first hour or 200 at the end of the first hour indicate diabetes. Levels above 140 could also indicate hypoglycemia, depending on the pattern of a full five-hour test. At the Tree of Life, we only use 40 grams of glucose in a five-hour test because the sugar is such a stress on the system. We find clinically that our results have been highly sensitive and accurate at this amount. Another test for diabetes is the glycosylated hemoglobin (HgbA1c), which is not as specific or sensitive as the glucose tolerance test, but a lot easier to do. A value of 6.0 suggests there is no diabetes. The glycosylated hemoglobin test has to do with how much protein hemoglobin in the red blood cells is glycosylated. One can use it to monitor the diabetic process every three to four months.

There is also the fructosamine test, which can be done on a monthly basis. We like to test both glycolylated hemoglobin and fructosamine. These tests can be thrown off by any occasion that creates an impaired glucose tolerance, including use of medications such as diuretics, glucocorticoids, nicotinic acid, and phenoytin. You are going to have more accuracy in monitoring the healing of diabetes by using two tests rather than one.

Dietary Fat and Diabetes

The role of high fat intake in diabetes has been suspected since the early twentieth century. As far back as the 1920s, Dr. S. Sweeney produced reversible diabetes in all of his medical school students by feeding them a high–vegetable-oil diet for forty-eight hours. None of the students had previously been diabetic.[42] Recently, this role of fat in diabetes has been highlighted by Neal Barnard, in his newest book, *Dr. Neal Barnard's Program for Reversing Diabetes*. As a vegan, he shares a certain insight about the role of animal fats as a causative factor in diabetes, and the process of reversing diabetes to an extent. His research contrasts in a positive way with the results of the American Diabetic Association diet. He has observed, as we have also observed, that a high-animal-fat diet is associated with increased incidence of Type-2 diabetes.

Dr. Barnard noted that in Japan, Thailand, other Asian countries, and Africa people on the traditional diet had a low incidence of diabetes. As soon as people from these cultures moved away from their complex-carbohydrate diet of rice, starchy vegetables, beans, and noodles they immediately began to develop high rates of diabetes. With this understanding, we have to be conscious when we use the word *carbohydrate*. Complex carbohydrates do not cause diabetes. They, plus a high-fiber diet, which these foods have, give us a slow rate of breakdown of glucose into the system and therefore do not significantly tax or stress the system. These foods have a low- to moderate-glycemic index, and a low insulin index. When people from these indigenous cultures hit the Western diet, rates of Type-2 diabetes soar. Dr. Barnard's work emphasizes that a diet high in fat, especially cooked animal fat (saturated fat), will increase the rate of diabetes.

Dr. Barnard's insight is certainly something I support as a live-food vegan: that the junk fats, trans-fatty acids, and cooked saturated animal fats tend to block and disorganize the cell membranes in a way that disrupts the insulin receptors in the cells. This clinical experience gives us an insight into fat metabolism, that we should be getting these specific fats—animal fats and trans fats—off our plate as much as possible.

Dr. Barnard's landmark twelve-week study showed that the average person on a low-fat, high-complex-carbohydrate, moderate- and low-protein diet lost 16 pounds, with fasting blood sugar dropping 28 percent. Two-thirds of the participants who were taking diabetic medications were able to discontinue or reduce them.[43] This study was interesting because there were no limits on calories or amounts of food carbohydrates, and there was no change in exercise regime. The next study he did was one that included women who were moderately or severely overweight but didn't have the diagnosis of diabetes. They were put on a diet that was zero in animal fat and low in vegetable oils. A control group was on a cholesterol-lowering diet. The vegetarian group lost about a pound per week, and the control group lost about 8 pounds in total per person.[44] The study group's body cells became more and more sensitive to insulin; at fourteen weeks their insulin sensitivity had improved by 24 percent. From these results he theorized that a low-fat diet activated the natural ability to open the insulin receptors in the cells to allow glucose into the system. In another study, he observed ninety-nine people over twenty-two weeks. Forty-nine were on a vegan low-fat diet with no animal products and no limits on complex carbohydrates. The remaining fifty people were on the basic American Diabetes Association diet. The ADA diet reduced glycosylated hemoglobin by 0.4 percent. The vegan diet was three times more effective, reducing the HgbA1c by 1.2 percentage points (one point is considered 1 percent). So the average value of gylcosylated hemoglobin fell from 8 percent to 6.8 percent during the twenty-two weeks. This is very significant. A diabetes study in the UK showed that a one-point drop in glycosylated hemoglobin with Type-2 diabetes reduces the risk of kidney or eye complications by 37 percent.[45] This vegan diet is mimicked a little bit by that designed by Dr. Dean Ornish in his famous work in 1990. His diet contained no animal products, no cholesterol, and very low fat (a 10 percent fat intake). After about one year, the angiograms showed that 82 percent of the people who started with significantly blocked coronary arteries were starting to open up their arteries. In addition people exercised, meditated, and had no smoking.[46]

A study[47] reported in the February 2004 *New England Journal of Medicine* tested young people whose parents or grandparents had Type-2 diabetes. These were healthy people, but were found to have a certain amount of excess fat in their cells, called intramyocellular fat; their intramyocellular fat was up to 80 percent higher than normal. In some cases, the excess fat was beginning to block insulin function. It is interesting that one newer theory of cell function, developed by Dr. Bruce Lipton and described in his book *The Biology of Belief,* considers the cell membrane the brain of the cell. The cell membrane is greatly affected by extracellular signaling, and insulin and glucose are extracellular signalers; consequently, both influence intracellular signaling by their action on the cell membrane. These genetically predisposed people had a much higher level of intramyocellular lipids, which seems to be significant. Intramyocellular fat accumulates to a certain extent, and tends to interfere with insulin's intracellular signaling process. The mitochondria, which burn fat and produce energy for the cells, were unable to keep up with metabolizing the accumulated fat. The study showed that limiting the fat intake enabled reversing the trend toward worsening insulin resistance. The researchers also saw that those people with Type-2 diabetes appeared to have far too much fat in their cells, and less than normal amounts of mitochondria. In other words, people with diabetes have far too few mitochondria than needed to burn up the accumulated fat. Another study[48] was done on people following a vegan diet and they found that the intramyocellular lipid in each participant's calf for vegans was 30 percent lower than in the omnivores. This makes the point that a vegan diet makes one less susceptible to activating the diabetic genes. In the case of fat, the accumulation of fat in the cells shuts off intracellular signaling of insulin.

Researchers at the Pennington biomedical research center in Baton Rouge, Louisiana, studied ten young men who were in reasonably good health, putting them on a high-fat diet. What they found is that in only three days the men accumulated significantly more intramyocellular fat. The first point this makes is it's really easy to build up intramyocellular fat on a high-fat diet. But more important, they tested the genes associated with the mitochondria and their energy production and found that the fatty foods these volunteers ate actually turned off the genes that affected the cells' ability to burn fat. The genes that produce mitochondria were in fact disabled. The implication fits with our larger theory that fat interferes with the normal workings of the cells, including the ability to adequately respond to the intracellular signaling of insulin. With the fat accumulation, the glucose is not able to be properly metabolized. Whether it is because it can't move from glycogen to glucose and therefore creates a glucose backup, or because glucose cannot get into the cell, the detrimental fatty foods seem to either disable the genes so they are not able to produce more mitochondria or eliminate the fat. Most likely, both mechanisms occur. Theoretically, the point is that a high-saturated-cooked-animal-fat, high-trans-fatty-acid, high-refined-carbohydrate diet decreases the healthy anti-diabetes gene expression and precipitates the onset of Type-2 diabetes. Fatty foods seem to disable the genes, meaning that our DNA goes to a lower phenotypic expression, and so they are not able to produce more mitochondria or eliminate the fat. The basic point is that what we eat speaks to our genes—and a high fat intake, especially of animal fat and trans-fatty acids, gives a negative message to the genes, activating increased insulin resistance and a diabetic process. Based on these theoretical understandings, the key to diabetes reversal is to activate an upgrade of the anti-diabetic phenotypic gene expression.

Just as Dr. Neal Barnard had a particularly insightful perception as a cooked-food vegan, after working with diabetes since 1973, and as a live-food vegan since 1983, I have gained certain insights about what is a healthy fat and the role of healthy fats in creating health. I have observed different things in relationship to different amounts of fat. One of the possible problems that I have seen in long-term use of a 10-percent-fat diet is the possibility of omega-3 deficiencies. Omega-3 deficiency means less effective cell membrane function, less effective nerve transmission, less effective serotonin and other neurotransmitter production, transmission, and neuroreceptor site function in the cells. Ten percent or less fat in the diet also creates the possibility of omega-6 deficiencies.

The nature of the fat is far more important than the amount of fat, although both are important. Studies by Dr. Edward Howell on the Eskimos showed that when they ate high amounts of raw blubber they did not develop heart disease, high blood pressure, or any significant morbidity. When they began cooking their blubber, they began to develop heart disease and high blood pressure. Specific data on diabetes before and after the change from raw blubber to cooked is not available, but since the switch to the Western cooked-animal-fat diet, as well as white sugar and white flour, there certainly has been an increase in Type-2 diabetes. The additional message here is that cooking destroys enzymes and alters the structure of the fat. When you cook or fry saturated fat it becomes unhealthy. In addition, the processing of fats through hydrogenation changes them from a cis- structure to a trans- structure. There is actually a physical change in the structure.

Unfortunately, there is not as much data on the subject as we would like. At temperatures of 320–428°, depending on the oil being cooked, the production of trans-fatty acids as well as more immediately harm-

CIS- STRUCTURE

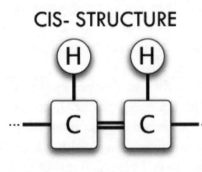

TRANS- STRUCTURE

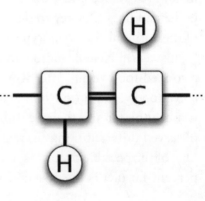

ful free-radical products starts deleterious chain reactions in the fat molecules. The antioxidants in the oil, such as beta-carotene and vitamin E, are used up as well. Also, the lipases that come in the raw blubber, needed for healthy fat metabolism, are destroyed. The hydrogenation process used to turn oils into semi-solid or solid fats requires 428° temperature for several hours. This produces high amounts of trans-fatty acids, which are more solid than cis fatty acids. In the process of physically changing its structure to a trans-fatty acid, every single cell membrane in the body is negatively affected. The defense system of the cell membranes are minimized, the immune system of the cell is lowered, and the ability of the cell membrane to do cell signaling is indeed compromised. The cell membrane can no longer act effectively as the brain of the cell.

At the Tree of Life Rejuvenation Center we have found dramatic positive results in healing diabetes by putting people on live foods with a live-moderate-fat diet. We recommend 15–20 percent uncooked fat, depending on a person's constitution. This is still moderately low. Plant source food has no cholesterol, so all blood lipid levels tend to go to normal. Because of this, we are not convinced that it is fat only that is the problem so much as whether the fat is cooked (or animal-based), in which the actual structures have changed, and therefore the cell membrane has changed with a consequent compromise in cell signaling. Plant-source-only live-food fats, such as those in almonds and walnuts, have actually been shown to lower cholesterol and help with the healing of diabetes. For example, the people in our study experienced a 44 percent average decrease in their LDL cholesterol in 21–30 days. Most of these people went to an LDL of approximately 80, which is the minimal cut-off point for the prevention of heart disease.

Cross-cultural ethnographic studies suggest that the ancient people, even 3.2 million years ago, had a relatively low-fat diet. They ate basically a plant-source diet (a chimpanzee diet) and their fat intake was less than 30 percent.

The polyunsaturated fatty acids also require a certain balance. The significance we have hypothesized about the kinds of fats, between cis being transferred to trans, appears in some research[49,50,51] that shows there are abnormal membrane phospholipid profiles in cooked fat, which is of major significance in both Type-1 and Type-2 diabetes. Insulin stimulates and glucagon inhibits a particular enzyme, which influences the availability of polyunsaturated fats for membrane incorporation. This is another aspect of the effect of insulin on the fat metabolism and how the fatty acid composition of the membrane lipids affects the function of insulin. Research shows that increasing membrane fluidity by taking in higher levels of dietary polyunsaturated fatty acids, especially the omega-3s, actually increases the number of insulin receptors, therefore increasing insulin activity.

Research[52,53] suggests that in Type-2, we have hyperinsulinemia and insulin resistance in approximately 75 percent of Type-2 diabetics in the initial phases. The elevated levels of insulin happen because insulin function is not working.[54] Later on, there is more of an inflammatory burnout of the overworked pancreatic beta cells and hence insulin production goes down. The inability of Type-2 diabetic cell membranes to process insulin is not necessarily a result only of insulin and glucagon influences, but, as we pointed out earlier, is due to high concentrations of insulin which, because of its biphasic nature, can actually turn off receptor function at high concentrations. It also suggests, and again, this is theory, that the diabetic onset of Type-2 can result from cell membrane abnormalities. One study comparing 575 diabetics with 319 normals showed there was a problem incorporating polyunsaturated fatty acids into the cell membrane.[55] All the diabetic red blood cell membranes were lower in polyunsaturated fatty acids. Plasma phospholipids, triglycerides, and cholesterol esters were also impaired, suggesting there is an impairment of polyunsaturated fatty acid metabolism in diabetes. This suggests that in non-insulin-dependent diabetes impaired insulin activity may be both a cause and an effect of membrane polyunsaturated fatty acid composition. It is complicated, but the point is to show that Type-2 diabetes is associated with dysfunctional fat metabolism.

Research has also shown that the omega-6 to omega-3 ratios are generally not in balance in Type-2, being too high in omega-6. This imbalance is made worse with the intake of approximately 13.3 grams per person per day of trans-fatty acids, as documented in the United States.[56] Research has shown that diets relatively high in saturated fat and trans-fatty acids, such as we see with flesh foods and hydrogenated fats, can significantly affect insulin efficiency and glucose response. When we increase the percentage of omega-3 fatty acids in the diet, insulin resistance can be improved or prevented.[57,58,59] It is highly suggestible that polyunsaturated fatty metabolism has some role in NIDDM.

Research does show that when you increase the ratio of polyunsaturated fatty acids to saturated fatty acids, there is an improved insulin binding.[60] Rats fed high-fat diets became insulin resistant. Saturated fatty acids caused the most deterioration. Linolenic acid (LA) caused the least problem. The use of omega-3 from flaxseed oil normalized insulin function in the saturated fatty acid group. Research has also shown that the higher the amount of saturated fatty acids in the cell membrane, the more insulin resistance there is.[61,62]

In individuals with abdominal obesity, it is worth suspecting hyperinsulinism. People with hyperinsulinism may have a diminished ability to utilize glucose peripherally; they may also have increased circulating free fatty acids, affecting glucose metabolism and creating a decline in insulin receptors.[63] The South Asian Indians and the Pima Indians have a genetic predisposition to NIDDM, but it didn't really manifest until they switched in the 1940s to a Western diet. The epidemic of NIDDM in these groups seems to be directly related to the dramatic increase in total calories of refined carbohydrates, total fat, and in the unbalanced omega-6 versus omega-3 ratios.

In summary, trans-fatty acids are indeed also a problem, as well as an increase in omega-6 versus omega-3 ratio of fatty acids. This evidence suggests that a diet that is relatively low in fat, relatively high in raw omega-3 fatty acids, and free of high-density refined carbohydrates would be very helpful to the indigenous people worldwide, and to everyone, in preventing and reversing NIDDM.

Type-1 Diabetes (IDDM)

The cause of Type-1 diabetes is somewhat different than Type-2. Its genetic component is not as direct, but transmission is believed to be an autosomal dominant, recessive, or mixed chromosome, although no mechanism is proven. The genetic research does suggest that if a first-degree relative has IDDM, a child has a 5–10 percent chance of developing it.[64]

Research has been pretty detailed on the diabetes genes for Type-2. It is believed that the susceptibility gene resides in the sixth chromosome and the major alleles that suggest risk are HLA-DR3, HLA-DW3, HLA-DR4, HLA-DW4, HLA-B8, and HLA-B15. The genes do play a role. The onset of Type-1 seems to be linked with an environmental insult, an allergen, or a virus that initiates this process in genetically susceptible people.

These insults create an inflammation response, called insulinitis. What happens is that the activated T-lymphocytes infiltrate the islet cells in the pancreas. Macrophages and T-cells appear to be involved in the destructive cycle as they release cytokines that create free radical damage. This free-radical induced islet beta cell death involves breaks

PATHOGENESIS OF TYPE-1 DIABETES MELLITUS

EVENT	AGENT OR RESPONSE
Genetic susceptibility ↓	HLA-DR3, DR4, DW3, DW4, B8, B15
Environmental Event ↓	Virus, Cow's milk protein ingested by mother *or child*
Insulitis ↓	Infiltration of activated T lymphocytes
Activation of autoimmunity ↓	Self ⟶ non-self transition
Immune attack on pancreatic beta cells ↓	Islet cell antibodies, cell mediated immunity
Diabetes Mellitus Type-1	>90% of beta cells destroyed

Source: *Harrison's Principles of Internal Medicine*

in the DNA strands. The enzyme to repair the DNA free radical damage requires large amounts of NAD-plus. This creates a depletion of the intracellular NAD pools, and that leads to islet cell death.[65] Type-1 is primarily an inflammatory response from an autoimmune reaction from antibodies being made against the beta cells.

Certain viruses seem to attack and destroy the pancreatic beta cells directly, rather than through an autoimmune reaction.[66] Mumps, prior to the onset of diabetes, was found in 42.5 percent of the subjects versus 12.5 percent in the control group.[67] There are elevated levels of Coxsackie virus IGM antibodies.[68] Exposure to virus infections *in utero* or during childhood may initiate beta cell damage.[69] Rubella and chickenpox didn't seem to make any significant difference.[70] Some research suggests that routine vaccinations may be linked with inflammation of the beta cells of the pancreas, but it isn't enough data for us to make a definitive statement.

There is a significant correlation between antibodies to cow's milk protein, particularly to bovine serum albumin, in the onset of IDDM.[71,72,73,74] Some studies have suggested that somewhere between 75 and 90 percent of the cases of Type-1 have antibodies against the beta cells of the pancreas compared to 0.5 to 2 percent of normals.[75]

Cow's milk seems to be strongly linked to the onset of Type-1. Those with Type-1 diabetes were more likely to have been breastfed for less than three months and exposed to cow's milk before four months. Research has also shown that children who consumed pasteurized cow's milk before the age of 3 months were eleven times more likely to develop Type-1 diabetes.[76] In 1992, Canadian and Finnish researchers reported in the *New England Journal of Medicine* their examination of blood from 142 children, newly diagnosed with Type-1 diabetes. They found that in those children, a high percentage of them had antibodies against certain proteins in cow's milk. These antibodies cross-reacted with beta cells of the pancreas.[77] One study in Finland, Sweden, and Estonia identified 242 newborns at risk for developing Type-1 because each had a first-degree relative with the condition. They encouraged the mothers to breastfeed, and when weaning their babies, the mothers used a specifically modified baby formula in which the dairy proteins were broken up into individual amino acids. The other families were allowed to use regular cow's milk. The children who were fed the specific formula were much less likely to develop the anti-beta cell antibodies; their risk was cut by 62 percent.[78] In 2002, in a study involving families in fifteen countries, researchers found that large proteins can pass through the Peyer's patches in the small intestine and into the system, even in adults. This study suggests that even mothers who drink cow's milk could be passing on the antigen of the cow's milk to their infants. In 1991 researchers did indeed find that cow's milk's proteins ingested by a nursing mother end up in her breast milk.[79] In 1994, the American Academy of Pediatrics issued a report after looking into the matter of antibodies to cow's milk protein in association with the onset of Type-1 diabetes in children. Based on more than ninety studies, the American Academy of Pediatrics agreed that indeed, the risk of diabetes could likely be reduced if infants are not exposed to cow's milk protein early in life.[80]

So if we really want to protect our kids, we must not expose them to cow's diary directly by drinking or through mothers drinking cow's milk. The good news here is multifold: Mother's breast milk is best; and we can also feed our children nut and seed milks made at home to provide superior nutrition *at no risk to their health*. These milks, found in the recipe section of this book, are desirable for the mother as well, before, during, and after pregnancy to support her nutritional needs.

Type-2 Diabetes (NIDDM)

In Type-2 diabetes, also called non-insulin-dependent diabetes mellitus (NIDDM), obese people in the early diabetic stages secrete an average of 114 units of insulin, which is more than three times the normal 31 units of insulin, and lean Type-2 individuals produce between 14 and 31 units daily. The great variation for Type-2s is determined by the stage of the disease. Again, this is relative as there seem to be two major stages in Type-2 diabetes. First, we have a hyperinsulin stage for the majority, and then as the beta cells of the pancreas begin to inflame, they get exhausted, scar, and create a shift from hyperinsulinemia to a state of insulin dependence. Therefore, it is very important to maintain an FBS of 85 or lower to keep pancreatic cells from wearing out and creating a hypoinsulin stage. Individuals with Type-1 secrete 0 to 4 units.

Chronic Complications

And we have made of ourselves living cesspools, and driven doctors to invent names for our diseases.

PLATO

The chronic complications of diabetes take us into another level of understanding about the seriousness of diabetes, and we first are going to focus on Type-1, then the long-term complications that apply to Type-1 and Type-2. In Type-1 you may accidentally get excess insulin, which may cause insulin shock. You have the issue of diabetic ketoacidosis, which is primarily a Type-1 diabetic problem, where fat is broken down for energy and ketones create acidity. You also have what is called non-ketogenic hyperosmolar syndrome, with rapid dehydration because you have so much sugar that your body is attempting to get rid of excess sugar and you lose large amounts of water through the urine, which is called polyuria. The hyperosmolar syndrome can be a serious problem. It can also be activated by medical problems such as pneumonia, burns, stroke, and use of certain drugs such as glucocorticoids and diuretics.

Chronic complications in both Type-1 and Type-2 diabetes are similar. They emerge from the same causal pathways. They include two main metabolic problems: the glycosylated protein and the intracellular accumulation of sorbitol. The glycosylated proteins lead to changes in the structure and function of almost all the protein systems in the body, significantly affecting the protein metabolism system, the enzyme function throughout the body, and virtually all the tissues in the body. An example of problems caused by glycosylation would be glycosylated low-density lipoproteins (LDL). LDL is usually at high levels in diabetics. The glycosylated LDL molecules don't bind to the LDL receptors and are thus unable to shut off the endogenous cholesterol synthesis. The result: You tend to get more cholesterol than your body needs. Excessive glycosylation also occurs in red blood cells, in the lenses of the eye, and in the myelin sheath of the nerves. This glycosylation creates deactivation of enzymes, inhibition of regulatory molecule binding, cross-linking of glycosylated proteins, trapping of soluble proteins by the glycosylated extracellular matrix, abnormalities in nucleic acid function, altered molecular recognition, and increased immunogenicity.[81] All this accelerates the aging process.

Sorbitol buildup inside the cells is another major serious metabolic problem. Sorbitol is a byproduct of glucose metabolism that takes place in the cells with the action of the enzyme aldose reductase. In a normal physiology, once the sorbitol is formed, it is metabolized by polyol dehydrogenase to fructose. This conversion to fructose allows it to be excreted from the cell. In the diabetic with high blood sugars, the sorbitol accumulates and plays a major role in the development of secondary complications. The sorbitol is involved in a variety of ways, but the basic mechanism can be seen in cataracts, as an example. High blood sugar, either from an inability to metabolize the sugar or by eating too much sugar foods, results in the shunting of glucose to the sorbitol pathway, which is a secondary pathway. But since the lens of the eye is impermeable to sorbitol, the lack of the polyol dehydrogenase enzyme occurs from excess demand, and the sorbitol accumulates to high concentrations. It persists even if glucose levels go to normal. This accumulation creates an osmotic gradient that draws water into the cells to maintain the osmotic balance in the eye cells. Associated with this osmotic process, the cells release small molecules such as inositol, glutathione, niacin, vitamin C, magnesium, and potassium to maintain the osmotic balance. These compounds are needed to protect the lens from damage, but are being lost because of the excess sorbitol; the loss makes the lens cells susceptible to further damage. The result: The delicate protein fibers in the lens become opaque.

This intracellular accumulation of the sorbitol is a major factor in many complications of diabetes. It is found in the lens of the eye, the

Schwan cells of the peripheral nerves, the papillae of the kidney, the Islets of Langerhans in the pancreas, and the Murel cells of the blood vessels. This tells us it seems to be associated with almost every tissue, and though its exact function is not clear, it is associated with these complications.

CARDIOVASCULAR DISEASE

People who have diabetes are two to four times more likely than non-diabetics to develop heart disease or have a stroke, and three-fourths of all diabetics (77,000 annually) ultimately die from heart disease.[82] Deaths from heart disease in women with diabetes have *increased* 23 percent over the past thirty years, compared to a 27 percent *decrease* in women without diabetes. Deaths from heart disease in men with diabetes have decreased by only 13 percent, compared to a 36 percent decrease in men without diabetes.[83] Diabetics with renal disease have a cardiovascular disease risk that is sevenfold higher than diabetics without renal disease.

Mainly, it is our Culture of Death diet and lifestyle that create cardiovascular disease. This has been proven by Dr. Caldwell B. Esselstyn of the Cleveland Clinic. Dr. Esselstyn's study, published in the *Journal of Family Practice*,[84] showed the reversal of cardiovascular disease with a 100 percent success rate among eighteen patients who followed a vegan diet with *no cooked oil*.[85] If you, or a friend or loved ones, have cardiovascular disease, the next two figures below may be the most important things you see in your life, and are resounding evidence of the need for a diet of plant foods.

The second figure supporting the case for diet as the underlying cause or prevention for heart disease is found in *Eat to Live* by Dr. Joel Fuhrman, based on data from the World Health Organization and the Food and Agriculture Organization of the United Nations.[86]

Populations with low death rates from the major killer diseases are populations that almost never have overweight members and that consume more than 75 percent of their calories from unrefined plant foods. This is at least ten times more unrefined plant source foods than the average American consumes.[87]

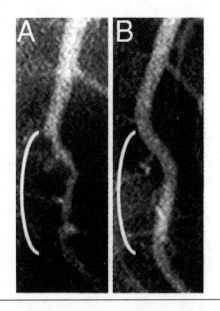

Figure 2: Coronary angiograms of the distal left anterior descending artery before (A) and after (B) thirty-two months of a plant-based diet without cholesterol-lowering medication, showing profound improvement

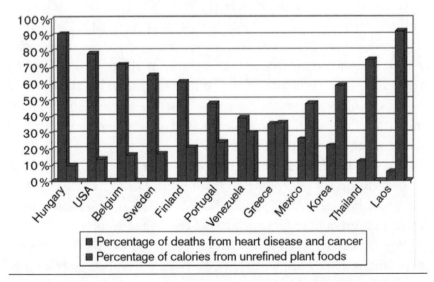

Figure 3: Unrefined plant food consumption and the killer diseases, heart disease and cancer

Even having diabetic parents can increase your risk of developing heart disease. A new study reported in the June 20, 2006, issue of the *Journal of the American College of Cardiology* showed that the blood vessels of people whose parents both have Type-2 diabetes, even if they do not have diabetes themselves, do not respond as well to changes in blood flow as those of people without a family history of diabetes. None of the thirty-eight adults (in their mid- to late-thirties) in this study had diabetes, but half of them were the offspring of two diabetic parents. The scientists restricted blood flow in the arms of the participants using a blood pressure cuff. Then, using ultrasound, they compared how blood vessels in the arms of participants responded to the surge in blood flow when the cuff was released. Blood vessel responsiveness was impaired in all nineteen participants (nine men and ten women) whose parents had diabetes. Allison B. Goldfine, MD, from the Joslin Diabetes Center and Brigham and Women's Hospital in Boston, Massachusetts, said:

> Persons whose parents both have Type-2 diabetes have endothelial dysfunction. This predisposition to atherosclerosis is present even when the offspring do not have diabetes themselves. Insulin resistance has been suggested to be important to both the development of diabetes and cardiovascular disease in large populations. However, in this high-risk group, even the most insulin sensitive offspring had diminished endothelial function.[88]

HYPERTENSION

We are looking at a target blood pressure of 130/80. According to the CDC, about 73 percent of adults with diabetes have blood pressure greater than or equal to 130/80 mm Hg or use prescription medications for hypertension.

DENTAL DISEASE

Periodontal (gum) disease is more common among people with diabetes. Among young adults, those with diabetes have about twice the risk of those without diabetes. Almost one-third of people with diabetes have severe periodontal diseases with loss of attachment of the gums to the teeth measuring 5 millimeters or more. Improving your dental health can also help with glycemic control. Researchers at the State University of New York, Buffalo, treated a group of 113 Pima Indians for periodontal disease and measured their glycemic control three months later. They found improved glycemic control along with a reduction in the bacteria that cause periodontal disease.[89]

DIABETIC NEUROPATHY AND FOOT ULCERS

Neuropathy is associated with decreased sensory and nerve conduction velocities. Diabetic neuropathy also seems to be associated with sorbitol accumulation.[90,91] Sorbitol accumulation leads to myoinositol loss. Inositol helps create healthy nerve conduction. Typically, this peripheral neuropathy is associated with parasthesias, hyperesthesias, and pain. On the neurological exam, almost every diabetic I see has a poor vibratory sense, altered pain and temperature sense, and poor deep tendon reflexes. Often on this program, these symptoms are reversed, and recent research using a vegan diet supports our results. Researchers in California studied twenty-one people with Type-2 diabetes and neuropathy, and using a low-fat vegan diet combined with exercise found that in only two weeks, seventeen of the twenty-one reported a complete cessation of symptoms, and the final four had noticeable improvement.[92]

Diabetic foot complications are the most common cause of non-trauma-based lower-extremity amputations in the industrialized world. Neuropathy, a major etiologic component of most diabetic ulcerations, is present in more than 82 percent of diabetic patients with foot wounds.[93] The incidence of gangrene is twenty times higher as compared to nondiabetics, and the risk of lower-extremity amputation is fifteen to forty-six times higher in diabetics than in those who do not have diabetes mellitus.[94,95] Each year, more than 82,000 amputations are performed among people with diabetes. Furthermore, foot complications are the most frequent reason for hospitalization in patients with diabetes, accounting for up to 25 percent of all diabetic admissions in the United States and Great Britain. With ulcers one must stop all smoking, because nicotine causes arterial constriction, and this further decreases peripheral circulation.

DIABETIC RETINOPATHY

Diabetic retinopathy is another serious complication and is the leading cause of blindness. In diabetic retinopathy the retinal vessels in the eye weaken and develop microaneurisms that leak blood plasma out of the capillaries. This results in scarring in the eye, which leads to gradual blindness. As the figure shows, it is related to the glycosalated hemoglobin, and seems to increase when the gylcosalated hemoglobin goes above 6.0.

This National Health and Nutrition Examination Survey (NHANES) III data was derived from looking at retinopathy and against fasting,

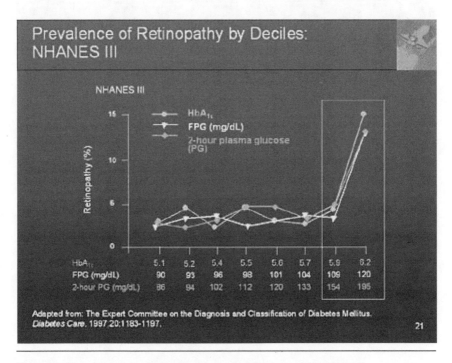

Figure 4: Prevalence of retinopathy by deciles (Source: NHANES III)

two hours postprandial, and HgbA1c. If you look at retinopathy, every-thing's fine, until one point where the rate starts to increase, and that is a HgbA1c of 6 percent, a fasting blood sugar of 110 mg/dL, and a 2-hour value of 154 mg/dL. Is this unique to the NHANES data? Well, if you look at Pima Indians and Egyptian studies you see the exact same thing. When your HgbA1c goes above the normal range, you start to develop complications.

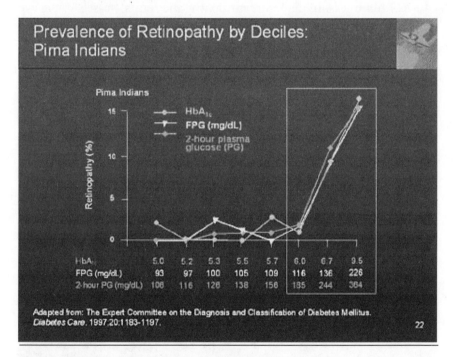

Figure 5: Prevalence of retinopathy by deciles: Pima Indians

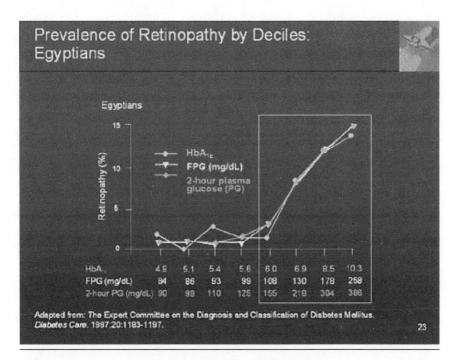

Figure 6: Prevalence of retinopathy by deciles: Egyptians

This is important data, because it puts a finer point on why we are encouraging an HgbA1c level of less than 6, and not 6.5 or 7.0.

DIABETIC NEPHROPATHY

Diabetic nephropathy, another serious complication, is the most common cause of chronic kidney failure and end-stage kidney disease in the United States. It is a common cause of high rates of dialysis and death. Once people begin kidney dialysis, they usually die within five years. The diabetic process affects the kidneys in a few ways: glomerulosclerosis, an arteriosclerosis of the entering and leaving renal arteries; arteriosclerosis of the renal artery and its interrenal branches; and deposits of glycogen, fat, and glycopolysaccharides around the tubules. Early on, nephropathy has no symptoms, but as it advances we see edema (swelling, particularly around the eyes), nausea, fatigue, headache, and generalized itching. This also has the potential to be slowly reversed on this program.

The following table summarizes the complications associated with diabetes.

THE SPECTRUM OF GLUCOSE TOXICITY	
Eyes	Retinopathy (microaneurysms, hemorrhages, exudates, neovascularization)
Kidneys	Nephropathy (albuminuria, nephrotic syndrome, hyporeninemic hypoaldosteronism, end-stage renal disease)
Nerves	Neuropathy (distal sensory ± motor neuropathy, mononeuritis multiplex, autonomic neuropathy, amyotrophy, chronic demyelinating immune polyneuropathy)
Skin and mucous membranes	Microvascular lesions, necrobiosis lipoidica diabeticorum, staphylococcus/streptococcus infection/cellulitis, fungal infections
Fetus	Macrosomia, congenital anomalies (neural tube defects), shoulder dystocia
Pancreas	Endocrine (decreased insulin secretion, ß-cell failure), exocrine (decreased digestive enzyme synthesis and secretion)
Insulin target tissues	Insulin resistance symptoms in fat deposits especially in lower abdomen, muscle, and liver
Vascular system	Atherosclerosis, endothelial cell dysfunction (decreased vasodilatation), restenosis

Subtle Insulin Physiology

The physiology of insulin as a hormone is something worth considering. It is interesting to understand that insulin is biphasic. Hyperinsulinemia results in a biphasic glucose response to epinephrine, first at low levels, then at high levels. Our emotions play an important role in insulin sensitivity or insulin resistance. Part of our treatment includes the use of homeopathic insulin to moderate the communication between the pancreas and the nervous system.

In the 1950s, scientists used the term "insulin-dependent" to mean that muscles and fat require insulin to take in glucose. Newer research tends to suggest a slightly different physiology. Glucose is transferred into the cells *with or without insulin to some extent.* There are enough GLUT-4 transporters in cell membranes to guarantee adequate glucose uptake to meet the demands of cellular respiration, even without insulin. For example, insulin is not necessary for glucose to enter the cells of the brain or kidneys. Red blood cells are also able to utilize sugar without the assistance of insulin. Furthermore, when you are exercising, the muscle cells can extract glucose from the blood without insulin, using special proteins called GLUT-4 transporters.[96] Although this may be true, Type-1 diabetics who do not receive insulin usually die, so the picture is more complicated. It also has been shown that adipose sites cannot take glucose without insulin.[97] It is interesting that in our limbic system, the area of the brain that affects our memory, sense of safety, survival instincts, eating, appetite drives, and learning contains a high density of insulin receptors.[98,99] As a homeopath, I have explored the use of homeopathic insulin, and there seem to be positive effects using it, including psychological improvement, perceptual calmness, lower blood glucose, improved elimination and metabolism, reduced metabolic wasting, and reduced development of diabetic complications. This suggests a function of insulin as a signaling molecule.

There is also a relationship between growth hormone and insulin, which is counter-regulatory. If one is high in concentration, then the other is low. Muscle protein synthesis is regulated by human growth hormone and insulin acts to prevent muscle breakdown. Insulin physiology is not exactly the way we have previously conceptualized it. Insulin is a signaling protein. It both stimulates and inhibits activities in a nonlinear curve.[100] Too much insulin can actually inhibit glucose uptake. The relationship between insulin concentration and protein synthesis suggests that most of insulin's stimulatory effect occurs at low concentrations, while high insulin concentrations may have an opposite effect. Insulin has been shown to mediate lipid, protein, and carbohydrate metabolism, converting nutrients into energy and maintaining cellular identity and replication. Insulin has been found to stimulate DNA, RNA, and protein synthesis. Yet, it inhibits these same biological functions at concentrations that are too high, which gives us another insight into the problem of hyperinsulinemia. High concentrations of insulin can result in central nervous system and circulatory depression from its inhibitory affects on glucose metabolism.

Lindsay Berkson writes in *Hormone Deception* that natural hormones are so potent they can produce very dramatic changes in cell activity with very small amounts, parts per billion or parts per trillion—a figure so minute that only extremely sensitive tests can measure them. Hormones like insulin are measured at the parts-per-trillion (ppt) level, the equivalent of putting one drop of water into a six-mile-long train with 660 tank cars. This should place the introduction of large amounts of insulin into the body in proper perspective. We have used insulin *homeopathically* (very small amounts) in a variety of ways. It does seem to help, although we have not conducted a long-term study. We use homeopathic insulin because it works on the energetic level and signaling level. Insulin may be toxic at high levels such as in hyperinsulinemia. Insulin works on many levels with complex feedback loops. Each of insulin's chemical reactions depend on bioelectric signals arising from insulin growth factor regulator (IGF-1), hormonal control, human growth hormone (HGH), and enzymatic reactions. Signaling activity begins with the insulin receptor insulin interface on the outside surface of the cell membrane. IGF-1 or anything that activates insulin receptor substrates will activate glucose uptake. This can actually happen with homeopathic insulin or IGF-1. The insulin molecule targets specific muscle fibers, fat tissues, and brain regions. Glucose metabolism is facilitated into the cell by glucose transporters and does not necessarily require insulin. Every cell in the body takes in glucose to some degree, yet every cell does not possess an insulin receptor. The insulin receptor family regulates nutritional metabolic pathways. IGF-1 receptors are in every cell in the body, and signal similar to insulin. Insulin receptor substrates transport glucose and stimulate metabolism.

Homeopathic insulin can also activate liver function. The liver is the first target of insulin and serves to increase storage of glucose as glycogen. Insulin upgrades the liver to a full state of glycogen and stimulates glyconeolysis, the breaking down of glycogen to sugar. Insulin also uses magnesium as a second messenger. Insulin helps to stabilize intracellular magnesium levels. Insulin also promotes triglyceride synthesis and mineral uptake of phosphates and potassium. So homeopathic insulin has the capacity to stimulate many functions through cell signaling. The important point here is that insulin is a hormone and affects the whole hormonal system as a signaling protein. Insulin, as we pointed out before, inhibits the breakdown of muscle fibers. IGF-1 can stimulate protein synthesis in fatty tissue and is influenced by insulin uptake of free fatty acids.

This is an immensely complex system. Type-2 diabetes and insulin resistance seem to be affected hormonally. This gives us a definite insight into the physiology. Insulin is released in response to elevated serum glucose and hyperinsulinemia and an increased insulin response to glucose are the first measurable responses. It's possible that one of the underlying causal physiology of insulin resistance is a defect in the utilization of glycogen within the cell. Some 80 percent of glucose is stored in the muscles, and 20 percent is stored in the liver. So this is a defect that could permanently affect glycogen utilization within the muscle and prevents the muscle from using glycogen stores. When you have increased glycogen storage buildup, there is a possible backup of the transport of glucose across the cell membrane for storage within the cell. There is no more room in the cell for glucose utilization and storage. This results in hyperglycemia as part of the response to the backup. Hyperglycemia then causes an increase in the release of insulin. In small doses, insulin is an anabolic steroid that optimizes lean body mass and energy utilization. In excess, however, insulin impairs cyclic adenosine monophosphate (cAMP) and inhibits the release of anabolic steroids. Therefore, it increases catabolic processes and decreases the energy available to the organism.

We are looking now at a new way of understanding this process, and this is still at a theoretical level. But as we know, endocrinologists successfully treat diseases of hormone insufficiency such as hypothyroidism and hypoadrenalism, both of which the author has seen very consistently in diabetes, as well as hypogonadism and somatotrophic deficiency of growth hormone treated by supplementing with hormones. In diseases of hypersecretion, we try to block the hormones. Thus treating hyperinsulinemia with more insulin doesn't have a lot of logic to it.

Hormone Disruption

Hormone disruptors may be another contributing factor in diabetes. For example, Vietnam veterans exposed to endocrine disruptors such as Agent Orange (a potent mixture of several hormone-disrupting pesticides such as dioxins) have a higher incidence of diabetes, as well as abnormal glucose and insulin levels.[101] Women are even more strongly affected. A follow-up study on the dioxin accident in Seveso, Italy, examined blood from 31,000 people within months of the accident and followed the exposed people for more than twenty years. They found an increased incidence of diabetes, but only in females.[102] Berkson suggests that women are more greatly affected by chemical exposures than men, probably because they have a higher ratio of body fat and different metabolic and elimination rates than men.

ARSENIC IN TAP WATER

Arsenic is another commonly found hormone disruptor suspected of playing a role in diabetes. Arsenic interferes with the action of glucocorticoid hormones, which belong to the same family of steroid hormones as estrogen and progesterone. Glucocorticoids turn on many genes that help regulate blood sugar and even ward off cancer. Repeatedly drinking water containing certain amounts of arsenic has been linked to increased rates of cancer and diabetes. The underlying mechanism is now thought to be hormone disruption.[103]

TESTOSTERONE CHANGES

Another fascinating aspect of hormonal physiology is the role of testosterone in diabetes. In the 1960s, J. Moller and other European clinicians used testosterone to treat men who had diabetes.[104] Some research suggests that testosterone can actually bring the glycosylated hemoglobin back to normal and lower insulin levels in men. The logic goes like this: Sex hormone binding globule (SHBG) binds testosterone, dihydrotestosterone, and estradiol to the cell wall. Without SHBG, no gonadal hormone can enter into the cell and generate the release of messenger RNA (mRNA) to activate gene expression. Men tend to have a lot less SHBG than women because SHBG is actually an estrogen amplifier. What we see is higher SHBG and estradiol are found in men with central obesity, gynecomastia, and Type-2 diabetes. That is a very important piece in this whole hormonal imbalance. Healthy men have more free testosterone than free estradiol only when there is adequate testosterone, and SHBG is less than 15 picomoles.[105] An increase in SHBG preferentially binds testosterone over estradiol, shifting the ratio to more free estradiol over testosterone, which isn't really great for men. By adding testosterone to the system, it's possible to create the shift away from estradiol dominance, increasing testosterone levels and lowering SHBG. Low levels of testosterone are found in diabetic men.[106,107] The absence of testosterone or low testosterone seem to be connected to insulin resistance, showing up as a diminished insulin sensitive glycogen synthetase enzyme activity.[108,109] It's possible that in men, a low secretion of testosterone might be a primary event precipitating insulin resistance. Preliminary research shows that building testosterone to normal values reduces insulin resistance.[110] When we add testosterone, it lowers SHBG; and that lowers insulin levels. Lower SHBG improves the testosterone and estrogen ratio. Testosterone also lowers insulin and decreases obesity. So we have a whole other mechanism. Perhaps this is telling us how little we know about the whole hyperinsulinism syndrome, but it gives us a clue. There is not much research about testosterone and women in this system, so there is little we can say about it.

We can take this back to understanding Syndrome X, which has the underlying physiology and symptoms of hyperinsulinemia, impaired glucose tolerance, Type-2 diabetes, obesity, hypertension, dyslipidemia, heart disease, and the inability to lose weight. N. M. Kaplan has observed that hyperinsulinemia precedes these disease states, which is a very important thing to understand in this whole process.[111] The risk of ischemic heart disease is 4.5 times greater with elevated insulin. Other researchers have found that a decrease in an endogenous testosterone is associated with an increase in triglycerides and a decrease in HDL cholesterol. So it could be that in men, it is a decreased testosterone that is associated with hyperinsulinemia and syndrome X.[112,113] We can reasonably hypothesize that in men with Type-2 diabetes there is often a state of relative hypogonadism, which leads us to hyperinsulinemia. Increasing the testosterone may be an appropriate gender-specific treatment. There does seem to be a significant correlation between insulin sensitivity and SHBG levels in men with Type-2 diabetes.[114] Research suggests that increased testosterone and DHEA seems to be associated with lowered insulin in men, which leaves us open to the idea that adding testosterone to men with Syndrome X or Type-2 diabetes, or obese middle-aged men, which is a tipoff of Syndrome X, may improve insulin sensitivity.[115,116]

Living Enzymes

Enzymes are substances that make life possible. No mineral, vitamin, or hormone can do any work without enzymes. They are the manual workers that build the body from proteins, carbohydrates, and fats. The body may have the raw building materials, but without the workers, it cannot begin.

EDWARD HOWELL, MD

Included in the Culture of Life anti-diabetogenic diet is a significant benefit we derive from the living enzymes present in uncooked foods. In research at George Washington University Hospital and Hygienic Laboratory, Drs. Rosenthal and Ziegler found that when 50 grams of raw starch was administered to patients their blood sugar rose only 1 mg and then decreased, but when the starch was cooked, there was a dramatic increase of 56 mg in one-half hour, 51 mg in 1 hour, and 11 mg in 2 hours after the meal. Researchers also gave raw starch to diabetics to whom no insulin had been given for several days. Average increase in blood sugar in these diabetics from eating the raw starch was just 6 mg in one-half hour, then a *decrease* of 9 mg in 1 hour, and a decrease of 14 mg in 2.5 hours after the raw starch meal.[117] This significant difference in raw versus cooked foods in terms of blood sugar regulation implies that the enzymes in the raw starch might be important. Also, heating activates the breakdown of complex carbohydrates to simple sugars more rapidly, thus raising the glycemic index of the food. My clinical experience over some thirty-five years has been that a raw-food, low-fat diet with the use of food enzymes and supplemental digestive enzymes has been very effective in the treatment of adult Type-2 diabetes. Cooking affects weight gain as well. Research has found that if raw potatoes are fed to hogs they won't gain weight, but when fed cooked potatoes they gain weight.

In his book *Food Enzymes for Health and Longevity,* Dr. Howell describes a study at Tufts School of Medicine related to weight gain and inadequate enzymes. They examined eleven overweight individuals and found lipase deficiency (lipase is needed to digest fats) in their fatty tissues as well as fatty tumors.[118] The lipase content of the adipose tissues of obese individuals and in lipomas was below the population norm.[119] Generally speaking, the amount of amylase (needed to digest carbohydrates) in diabetics is about 50 percent of normal. It has been shown that the amylase content of liver and spleen was raised from two to seventeen times over the original when digestive enzymes containing amylase were given.[120] There is some suggestion that the external excretion of the pancreas becomes deficient in enzymes in diabetes, and that oral administration of enzymes had a beneficial effect.[121] Dr. Bassler reported a deficiency in amylase in the duodenum in more than 86 percent of cases of diabetes he studied. Drs. Harrison and Laurent, in twenty-nine cases of Type-2, reported fourteen cases with a significantly lower blood amylase and thirteen cases with values from the low to lowest limits of the normal range.[122,123] We need again to distinguish between cooked, saturated, and animal fats, versus raw fats with their natural high lipase content, such as we see in the indigenous Eskimo diet, along with cold-pressed unrefined olive oil, avocado, as well as predigested raw nuts and seeds soaked overnight, and even sprouted grains, which are healthy sources of fat. Even raw animal fat did not seem as strongly associated with the onset of chronic disease, but eating the same diet cooked and without enzymes because they were destroyed with cooking could be associated with the enzyme deficiency that cooking creates. It could also be explained by changing fats from cis to trans. More likely it is both. A low lipase enzyme level in the body is also connected to increased obesity. Enzyme research summarized by Miehlke and colleagues showed that artery obstruction was successfully treated and improved through high enzyme intake between meals, and it didn't seem to matter whether it was through the enzymes in the food, or taken exogenously through supplementation.[124] Dr. Edward Howell's work with the Eskimos showed that they lived a disease-free life with a high-enzyme diet, rich with raw flesh foods (particularly blubber). Diabetes and degenerative diseases only became common when Eskimos began cooking their food and consuming depleted, refined carbohydrates and processed foods, both effected by encroachment of Western culture. The cooking destroys enzymes in the raw fat and in the raw meat. According to Dr. Howell in *Food Enzymes for Health and Longevity,* through the introduction of cooking, the Eskimos have become one of the most unhealthy cultures. According to one study,[125] as of the late eighties, these were the top ten foods eaten by Alaskan natives, ranked by frequency of consumption:

1. Coffee and tea
2. Sugar
3. White bread, rolls, and crackers
4. Fish
5. Margarine
6. White rice

7. Tang and Kool-aid
8. Butter
9. Regular soft drinks
10. Milk (whole and evaporated)

Notice that the only native food in the top ten is fish, and that it is outranked in consumption by coffee, tea, sugar, and white bread. According to one study[126] by the Alaska Area Native Health Service in Anchorage, comparisons with past data indicate that the prevalence of diabetes in Eskimos has increased from 1.7 percent in 1962 to 4.7 percent in 1992, a nearly threefold increase.

Proteolytic Enzymes

Our program uses proteolytic enzymes, lipases, and general combinations of proteolytic lipase and amylase. Proteolytic enzymes seem to be associated with a tendency to clotting, appear to help decrease the inflammation effect of the disease process in Type-1 and Type-2, and seem to help unclog arteries. Two cases of Type-1 diabetes were reported by Dr. William Wong in a personal communication in which they were only given proteolytic enzymes. One was an 86-year-old with fifty years of Type-1 diabetes. She had a below-knee amputation on the right and was about to lose her left foot. She had paresthesia in her fingers and forearm, scar tissue in her eyes, a gray pallor, and dry skin, and was on four injections of insulin a day. She was given the proteolytic enzymes over three months. As scar tissue in her eyes cleared, her vision became 20/10, and her left foot had a full correction. An ultrasound done after three months found no blockage whatsoever. Her skin in general and in her extremities especially became pink, her glycosylated hemoglobin went from 9 to 6, and she stopped taking insulin.

Another Type-1 diabetic was from the Flathead tribe in Montana. He was in his mid-thirties, had acquired Type-1 in his mid-twenties, and was receiving three to four injections of insulin a day. Toes in both feet had been amputated, he was suffering neurological degeneration in the legs, paresthesia in arms and hands, he had received one kidney transplant and the other one was beginning to fail. He took proteolytic enzymes for six months. Circulation improved and the regimen saved his toes and foot from amputation. His need for insulin dropped to none. His neuropathy disappeared, which I hypothesize is secondary to fibrosis in the nerve trunks, or poor circulation due to inflammation. His kidneys began to function again. We hypothesize that the inflammation and subsequent scarring in the kidneys decreased through use of the proteolytic enzymes as his only new supplement. His creatinine, an indicator of kidney function, went to normal.

These two cases suggest an interesting theoretical way to understand the disease process in Type-1 and Type-2 diabetes. A first step in the degenerative process is inflammation, termed insulinitis in Type-1, either due to antibody attack on the beta cells of the pancreas from cow's milk antibodies or against certain viruses. The inflammation progresses to scarring. In Type-2 there is a progression from hyperinsulinism and its inflammation, in which the beta cells are stressed through overproduction and free radical production. The inflammation leads to a chronic scarring, which either blocks the flow of insulin from the beta cells, inactivates the beta cells, or perhaps blocks the circulation to the beta cells. The recovery, in one case from more than fifty years of Type-1 diabetes, theoretically suggests that the beta cell function is not destroyed, but is only blocked by the scarring. This may lead to a new way to understand the intermediary degenerative process in diabetes and it gives us a new way to supplement the treatment approach by using high-potency proteolytic enzymes both for opening up general capillary, arterial, and major artery circulation and reestablishing the blocked, but not destroyed, function of the beta cells of the pancreas.

A third case was a person who developed Type-1 diabetes in his teens, starting with a rapid onset of diabetes with possible insulinitis and then scarring. He was hospitalized with an FBS of 1,200 and diagnosed as Type-1. One way to explain his rapid response to the Tree of Life program is to claim he was misdiagnosed, but that ignores the typical rapid onset and acute transition to a potentially life threatening blood sugar of 1,200. In a previously healthy person, Type-2 is classically known to have a slow, gradual onset. Since his teens he had been on approximately 20 units of insulin per day. In four days on the Tree of Life 21-Day+ Program, he was off all insulin and in two weeks, his blood sugar was below 85. All symptoms disappeared, and he is in perfect health and diabetes-free two years later. As of nearly two years later, his HgbA1c is 6.0, down from his intitial HgbA1c of 11.8.

These three cases of Type-1 diabetes experienced what is considered medically impossible. With two of them, only proteolytic enzymes were used, and the third benefited from the full Tree of Life 21-Day+ Program, which includes the use of proteolytic enzymes as well as the low-glycemic and low-insulin-index live-food diet that in itself has an anti-inflammatory effect.

To summarize the author's theory behind all this: At one level, Type-1 and late-stage Type-2 involve a chronic inflammation and scarring of the beta cells of the pancreas. In Type-2, there is a constant overstimulation of the beta cells of the pancreas, eventually moving to hyperinsulinemia, inflammation, and fibrosis. The fibrosis blocks the ducts of the pancreas and appears to kill the beta cells of the pancreas. There is also inflammation and fibrosis in the glomeruli of the kidneys and fibrin, causing atherosclerosis. The proteolytic enzymes create a lysis of the fibrin plugs in the microcirculation, in the matrix of the plaque. What we see is a significant opening of peripheral circulation and therefore a decrease in the secondary degenerative symptoms. This, of course, is a theoretical explanation for why we feel the proteolytic enzymes work to reverse the diabetic degenerative process. We don't have explicit evidence to prove this theory beyond the three examples.

We have explored most causes, except the mineral deficiencies, vitamin deficiencies, and metabolic toxins, which are the subject in Chapter 4. Minerals play a very important role, and we see specific deficiencies of magnesium, manganese, zinc, chromium, vanadium, and potassium in diabetic patients. These deficiencies could be a result of the blood hyperosmolality and the minerals being lost with excessive urination, in an attempt to get the sugar out of the system. There may be other reasons as well.

A Unifying Theoretical Approach to Healing Diabetes

In summary, there is a degenerative metabolic process that arises from a diet high in sugar, cooked animal fat, and trans-fatty acids, and low in fiber, combined with a lifestyle of stress, lack of exercise, and general toxicity that interfaces with and activates the diabetes-producing genes in both Type-1 and Type-2. We need a theory that includes these genetic realities. Genes play a more predominant role in Type-2. Diabetes affects the metabolism on many levels of fat metabolism, protein metabolism, and glucose carbohydrate metabolism. The theory must also include hormone balance and enzyme levels, as the degenerative metabolic process affects the hormone flow and is affected by it. In addition, it is affected by our enzyme levels and function, as diabetics have significantly less lipase, amylase, and proteases. The theory needs to include the process of inflammation advancing to fibrosis, which seems to be somewhat reversed by proteolytic enzymes, which also minimize and reverse the degenerative process of heart disease, kidney disease, retinopathy, and neuropathy that are the long-term complications of diabetes.

We are looking for a comprehensive understanding that can cut through the complexity of diabetes. The unifying theory and healing approach of the Tree of Life 21-Day+ Program is based on the following principle:

> What we eat and how we live speaks to our genes. We, by what we eat and how we live, can either degrade our phenotypic expression and activate the diabetic process or improve our phenotypic expression for the prevention and reversal of diabetes.

Genotype means the actual genes that were given genetically. In essence, genotype is analogous to a computer's hard drive. *Phenotype* is the way the genes express themselves, which can vary according to the signaling systems that we give them through our diet and lifestyle. Phenotypic expression is analogous to our software programs. Put a healthy program in, and we get a healthy response.

Since 1922, when Frederick Banting and Charles H. Best discovered insulin, which was a great contribution and saved many lives, we have taken a more medical or drug-based approach to the treatment of diabetes. The cross-cultural studies show that diabetes is not a natural occurrence. It is caused by a Crime Against Wisdom—eating and living in a way that downgrades our phenotypic expression so that the diabetic process is activated. Genes are polymorphic (slightly variable), and they can have multiple activators. Diet is a primary activator and exercise and lifestyle are secondary activators. Our diabetes-creating diet is a Crime Against Wisdom that brings increasing amounts of death and misery through the disease of diabetes to millions of people. We have already said that the research shows that a high-saturated-fat diet tends to shut down healthy gene expression. We have, through high intake of cooked animal fat, saturated fat, high omega-6 versus low omega-3 fats, glucose from junk food, and refined carbohydrates, created a genetic downgrade that deregulates our phenotypic expression to one that sets off the diabetic process. The Tree of Life diet—which starts out initially as a 100 percent live-food, high-complex-carbohydrate, low-glycemic and insulin-index, 15–20-percent-plant-source fat (depending on our individual constitution), and low-calorie diet—is specifically designed to upgrade the phenotypic gene expression. It results in turning off the phenotypic diabetic expression and turning on the anti-diabetogenic phenotypic expression.

Calories with Purpose

A key piece of research that supports this wholistic theory was done in 2001 by Dr. Stephen Spindler. He underfed rats by 40 percent. Within a month they had a 400 percent increase in the expression of the anti-aging genes, and an increase in the anti-inflammation genes, antioxidant genes, and anti-cancer genes. Why a live-food diet is so successful is that it turns on anti-aging genes, anti-inflammatory genes, and theoretically the anti-diabetic genes. This is because a live-food diet is a natural form of calorie restriction. When you cook your food, according to the Max Planck Institute, you coagulate 50 percent of your protein, 70–90 percent of your vitamins and minerals, and up to 100 percent of your phytonutrients. One of the phytonutrients, for example, called resveratrol, plays a very important role in activating the anti-aging genes. It is gaining growing recognition in fighting age-related diseases ranging from dementia to diabetes. On a live-food diet properly eaten, we actually eat 50 percent fewer calories as compared to a Standard American Diet (SAD), but maintain a very high level of nutrition. The reason for this is that we are consuming *nutrient-dense foods,* not just calorie-dense foods such as those offered in restaurants and fast-food dispensaries all over the Westernized world. We are becoming nations of overfed, undernourished individuals. Our bodies are rebelling through the metabolic degeneration process called diabetes. They are asking us for nutrients that are not provided through our cooked, processed diet typically found in the Culture of Death.

When we say "calorie restriction," in the Tree of Life context, which is a plant-source-only, live, organic diet, it should not be misunderstood that we are denying ourselves the fuel we need. Nor are we in a cycle of deprivation. On the Tree of Life Rainbow Green and anti-diabetic Live-Food Cuisine we are eating a delicious, filling, natural, appropriate amount of calories that are nutrient-dense enough to activate an *aliesthetic taste change.* The aliesthetic change is experienced as when we feel pleasurably satisfied from eating. It is also known as the "stop eating" signal we get from our body. This taste change most commonly happens when eating raw food. Think about it: It is not usual to overeat a salad. Eating a processed, cooked diet laden with excitotoxins (such as MSG) provides the double insult of low nutrient density combined with the supersensory stimuli of artificial flavorings, driving body and mind to continue to ask for food long after our calorie needs would have been satisfied by a tasty nutrient-dense meal. You would think that by eating a lower-calorie diet that a feeling of restriction or deprivation would result, but when your body receives all the minerals, phytonutrients, vitamins, enzymes, protein, essential fats, complex carbohydrates, and water it requires through a plant-source-only meal, a feeling of deep satisfaction is experienced right down to the cellular level. We are satiated by these foods that are high on the satiety index. A completely new sense of abundance is realized as we begin to seek quality over quantity in our food. When we eat in such a way that everything we consume has purpose, we are living in the Culture of Life. Instead of accelerating the chronic disease/aging process, we turn on the anti-aging genes and remove the underlying causes of almost every preventable chronic disease process we are now witnessing in the Westernized world.

This is the key concept: A properly eaten live-food diet turns on the anti-aging and anti-diabetic genes. On a live-food, plant-only diet people naturally tend to go to their optimal weight. Because of this you automatically lose weight on our program if you are overweight. The people in the movie had an average weight loss (with the exception of the two Type-1 diabetics who were very thin to begin with) of 25 pounds in the first month. Often we see people who are obese lose 100-plus pounds in a year on a live-food diet without doing anything but eating live foods. Since up to 90 percent of diabetics are overweight, and diabetes is related to obesity, the natural weight loss down to optimal weight on a live-food diet in this context is a powerful plus. A live-food diet creates just the opposite effect of the high-refined-sugar, high-cooked-animal-fat, low-fiber diet that is creating the pandemic today. The pandemic gets worse as we go more into industrialized foods. A 100 percent live-food Phase 1.0 diet combined with green juice fasting is the most powerful way to upgrade the phenotypic expression and turn off the diabetic genes. A Phase 1.0 diet as described in *Rainbow Green Live-Food Cuisine* is a low-glycemic, green diet with no fruits. This is the diet that a person stays on for the first three months until FBS has stabilized at around 85, and the glycosylated hemoglobin (HgbA1c) reaches 6.0 or less. Once we have stabilized into a healthy nondiabetic physiology, then we add low-glycemic fruits found in Phase 1.5, and give people the option of shifting to a diet of 80 percent live foods, which is the minimum definition of being on live foods according to the 2006 International Summit on Live Foods.

On this diet, there are some variations, but a general pattern is needed to activate healing. The general pattern, according to Ayurvedic principles is that diabetes is a *kapha* disorder, although it can happen in any of the three *doshas*. The corrective diet for a kapha disorder is a low-fat, low-sugar diet with more of a focus on bitter, pungent, and astringent foods. Kapha imbalances are made worse by a high amount of oil, a high amount of sugar, and low exercise. Kaphas tend to have constipation, and they are made better by a high-fiber diet. This has been a mode of treatment for several thousand years. The treatment program in this book is based on not only current research, but on thousands of years of effective treatment and understanding. We have simply added a unified theory that enables a very rapid approach to healing, for reversing diabetes naturally. The rapid moving to normal blood sugar levels without any medications encourages people to stay with the program because they get immediate tangible results. Therefore, even in ancient times we already had the answer: an anti-kapha diet, low in sugar, low in fat, high in complex carbohydrates, plant-only and live-food based, and naturally high in fiber. As long as we stay on this diet, we will be diabetes free.

This is an ongoing protective diet, no matter what your genetic predisposition is. *This is the breakthrough.* We are not talking about simply decreasing medication; we are talking about Type-2 people coming off all their insulin and oral medications within four days. We're not talking about twelve weeks, or two years, or anything like that. We are talking about very rapid effects. We are talking about the average person we see in our program coming in with unregulated FBS of 300 while on insulin and/or oral hypogyclemics, and in an average of two to three weeks often having an FBS of approximately 85. If a person has Syndrome X, or what we call metabolic syndrome, then it may take several weeks longer to reset the phenotypic expression and move out of the Syndrome X expression.

The Seven Stages of Disease

The Seven Stages of Disease, formulated by Dr. John Tilden more than 100 years ago, gives us another perspective in how to understand the degenerative process of diabetes and how to reverse the process. "Health is what you consistently do," and the same can be said of ill health. Disease is an acquired state that is earned over the years with identifiable stages that lead to the manifestation of symptoms, and even death, if we are not prudent enough to reverse the disease process and go backward through the seven stages. Even an acute viral-based Type-1 onset requires a disturbed terrain that allowed a weakened immune state that produced susceptibility to a viral infection, resulting in insulinitis and a rapid onset of Type-1 diabetes. Diabetes is a disease process with stages that we can progressively degenerate along, advancing the disease condition and creating complications—or we can reverse the disease process. It depends on whether we are aware of what is required to live a healthy life. Herbert Shelton called this understanding the laws of life. If you understand and follow these laws you'll be healthy. If you break them you will get sick. This is the meaning of Crimes Against Wisdom. Shelton wrote:

> The laws of life are not something imposed upon the organization of man. They are imbedded in the very structure of our being, in our tissues, our nerve and muscle cells, our bloodstream, into the total organism. . . . Since these laws are fundamental parts of us, we cannot revolt against them without revolting against ourselves. . . . We cannot run away from the laws of being without running away from ourselves.[127]

In the Tree of Life program we teach what these natural ways are, and empower you to live by them. Let's look now at the Seven Stages of Disease.

STAGE 1: ENERVATION

Enervation is the reduction of nerve energy, by which the body's normal maintenance and eliminative functions are impaired, especially in terms of the elimination of *endogenous* and *exogenous* toxins, those created from within (through normal metabolic processes) and from without (in modern times including the 65,000 human-made toxins in our environment, and the excitotoxins, food additives, and toxins created by the cooking and processing of food). A person who is enervated is generally inactive, living in a toxic environment and consuming toxins that are not being released from the body in a timely manner.

Enervation is also created by stress, which uses up the vital energy in the body that would be applied to maintenance and elimination. Constipation occurs in the bowel, lymph, and tissues of the body. This is the diabetogenic diet and lifestyle we have been illustrating throughout this book.

STAGE 2: TOXEMIA

The stagnation of Stage 1 leads to a buildup of toxins in the body, and these substances begin to saturate the blood, lymph, and cells. Stage 2 is typified by sluggish energy, and in the case of diabetes, we already have cells that are developing the preconditions for being insensitive to the signaling of insulin due to their toxic state. John Tilden writes in the chapter "Toxemia" in Herbert Shelton's *The History of Natural Hygiene:*

> The toxin theory of the healing art is grounded on the truth that toxemia is the basic source of all diseases. So sure and certain is this truth that I do not hesitate to say that it is by far the most satisfactory theory that has been advanced in all the history of medicine. It is a scientific system that covers the whole field of cause and effect—a system that synthesizes with all knowledge, hence a true philosophy.
>
> When this truth first began to force itself upon me, years ago, I was not sure but that there was something wrong with my reasoning. I saw that it would bring me very largely in opposition to every established medical treatment. I held back, and argued with myself. ... I fought to suppress giving open utterance to a belief that would, in all probability, cause me to be hissed at—subject me to the jeers

and gibes of the better class of people, both lay and professional.

Little by little I have proved the truth of my theory. I have tried it out daily for the past twenty years. I myself have personally stood the brunt of my experimenting, and have willingly suffered because of it. Every day this trying-out of the theory has convinced me more and more that toxemia is the universal cause of disease.

As has been stated continuously in my writings for the past dozen years, the habits of overeating, overclothing, and excesses of all kinds use up nerve energy. When the nerve supply is not equal to the demands of the body, organic functioning is impaired, resulting in the retention of waste products. This produces toxemia.[128]

Common sources of toxemia include various exogenous and endogenous toxins, which will now be recognizable as the diabetogenic preconditions for diabetes.

Endogenous toxins include:
- Metabolic waste, ongoing, toxic byproducts on the cellular level
- Spent debris from cellular activity
- Dead cells
- Emotional and mental distress and excess
- Physical fatigue, distress, and excess

Exogenous toxins include:
- Unnatural food and drink
- Natural foods deranged by cooking, refining, and preserving
- Improper food combinations that result in endogenous toxins
- Medical, pharmaceutical, herbal, and supplemental drugging
- Tobacco, alcohol, and all forms of recreational drugging
- Environmental, commercial, and industrial pollutants
- Impure air and water

STAGE 3: IRRITATION

The body becomes irritated by the toxic buildup in the blood, lymph, and tissues, and the interstitial space between the cells begins to resemble a toxic waste dump. The cells and tissues where buildup occurs are irritated by the toxic nature of the waste, resulting in inflammation. The waste products interfere with the proper oxygenation and feeding of the cells as well as causing the accumulation of excess water in the tissues. Pain signals coming from the tissues have at least three causes: lack of oxygen, lack of nutrition (cellular food), and pressure. The cells, subjected to the lack of oxygen, the lack of food, and the increased pressure from the retained water, begin to send out pain signals. The cells are hence *irritated*. The conventional answer is either to ignore the pain and discomfort, or to take a "pain" pill, adding more to the toxic burden as the sufferer continues living in the same manner. The toxic sufferer can feel exhausted, queasy, irritable, itchy, even irrational and hostile. This leads to the next stage of disease and body degeneration, inflammation.

STAGE 4: INFLAMMATION

The enervated body is now suffering the results of toxemia. The cells have initially become irritated. The next step of cellular changes and body degeneration is *inflammation*. The inflammation process produces the common "-itis." With the skin it is dermatitis. In the throat it may be tonsillitis and, further on, esophagitis. In the stomach we find gastritis. In the small intestine, ileitis. In the colon, colitis. The heart may have carditis. With the liver it is hepatitis. You can have an inflammation (an -itis) anywhere in the body.

The medical community has named many of the 20,000 distinctly different diseases. Allopathic practice tends to name a disease after the site where the toxins have accumulated and precipitated their symptoms. Once the set of symptoms is named, doctors usually prescribe pharmaceuticals at Stage 4, which do not remove the underlying causes that we are now familiar with. With diabetes and its complications, we see this stage of disease in the heart, kidneys, pancreas, liver, and nervous system. By allowing the accumulation of toxemia to advance, the body will continue to decline in energy and vitality. Further cellular changes will be found. Left unchecked and unheeded, the next stage of disease is ulceration.

STAGE 5: ULCERATION

An ulcer can be viewed as a consequence of body degeneration. *Ulceration* can occur with any body tissue, but the usual connotation of ulcers has to do with the skin. Tissues are destroyed. The body ulcerates, forming an outlet for the poisonous buildup. The toxic sufferer experiences a multiplication and worsening of symptoms while the pain intensifies.

Modern medical practice is usually to continue drugging, and often commence with surgery and other forms of treatment at this stage. Remember, diabetic foot complications are the most common cause of nontrauma-based lower extremity amputations in the industrialized world. Neuropathy, a major etiologic component of most diabetic ulcerations, is present in more than 82 percent of diabetic patients with foot wounds.[129] The incidence of gangrene is twenty times higher as compared to nondiabetics, and the risk of lower extremity amputation is fifteen to forty-six times higher in diabetics than in people who do not have diabetes mellitus.[130,131]

STAGE 6: INDURATION

Induration means a hardening or scarring of tissues. Induration is the result of long-standing, chronic inflammation with bouts of acute inflammation interspersed. The chronic inflammation causes an impairment or sluggishness of circulation, and as some cells succumb, they are replaced with scar tissue. This is the way we lose good, normal-functioning cells—by chronic inflammation and death of cells.

We also see low oxygen in the cells coming from induration in the blood vessels as they are glycosolated. Atherosclerosis is a form of induration. With low or no circulation, toxic buildup, and low oxygen we have the conditions for the seventh stage of disease: fungation, or cancer.

STAGE 7: FUNGATION

When the internal conditions have deteriorated to the extent that normal aerobic, oxidative processes are no longer possible, the cells can revert to a more primordial means of surviving. Biochemical and morphological changes from the depositing of endogenous and exogenous toxins bring about degenerations and death at the cellular level. The cells can carry on their life processes by anaerobic processes, the same processes that many bacteria use. When the cells have changed in form and function to this extent, this is when an oncologist will tell you that you have cancer.

TRACKING BACK THROUGH THE SEVEN STAGES TO HEALTH

The root causes of diabetes and its complications must be eliminated to be totally successful. In the language of the seven stages, the most important stages to address in reversing the diabetogenic process are toxemia and inflammation. This is another way to understand the diabetogenic degenerative process and how to reverse it. The means for reversal of toxemia and deficiency are topics we are going to investigate for the remainder of the book. When a person supplies the body with superior building materials, begins to lower the level of toxemia, and increases vitality, the body will begin to repair and rebuild. Previous complaints may surface once again as the body "retraces" and heals. The true test of any theory of disease is how well it can affect the chronic diseases such as diabetes.

Chapter 3 Summary

Diabetes is a complex metabolic dysregulation that emerges as a symptom of the Culture of Death. The lifestyle and diet of the Culture of Life is the antidote.

Although we have shared a wholistic theory, results based on the application of this wholistic theory are what are most important. Our results are very good: 100 percent of Type-2 participants being off medications in four days and many having an FBS of 85 in a few weeks. The average FBS among the participants highlighted in Chapter 4 began at 260 on medications, and ended at an average 86.6, with everyone off all medications. LDL cholesterol dropped an average of 67 points, or 44 percent, with an ending average level of 82. The rapid reversal of the seven stages is accelerated by green juice fasting and natural supplements (discussed in next chapter) of herbs, minerals, high-protease enzymes, and digestive enzymes with our food to build up the amylase, and liquid zeolite (Natural Cellular Defense, or NCD) when combined with the green juice fasting to help pull out the heavy metals and 65,000 environmental toxins. We have also found that the NCD seemed to help in decreasing the FBS. With this integrated approach the results of the Tree of Life 21-Day+ Program are so rapid and consistent. The quicker the healing, the more encouragement people have and the happier they are.

This approach, based on my clinical experience over thirty-five years and guided by a unifying theory of turning on the anti-diabetes genes and turning off the diabetes-producing genes with green juice fasting and live foods, has helped us to break the four-minute mile of diabetes. It is supported by a lifestyle that creates life and not death. The Tree of Life program we describe in the next chapter is a complete wholistic approach with the Culture of Life plant-source only live-food cuisine and lifestyle as its foundation.

CHAPTER 4

The Tree of Life
21-Day+ Program

It is a part of the cure to wish to be cured.

SENECA, PHILOSOPHER, LEGAL SCHOLAR, AND PLAYWRIGHT (TRAGEDIES)

A truly good physician first finds out the cause of the illness, and having found that, first tries to cure it by food. Only when food fails does he prescribe medication.

SUN SSU-MO, TANG DYNASTY TAOIST PHYSICIAN, IN *PRECIOUS RECIPES*

Let nothing which can be treated by diet be treated by other means.

MAIMONIDES, JEWISH RABBI, PHILOSOPHER AND
MASTER WHOLISTIC PHYSICIAN TO EGYPTIAN SULTAN

The first principle of the Tree of Life 21-Day+ Program to heal diabetes naturally is a prudent diet that we call the Culture of Life antidiabetogenic diet: organic, plant-source only, live (raw) food, relatively high complex carbohydrate, 15-20 percent (low to moderate) plant-based fats, moderate protein, low glycemic index, low insulin index, high minerals, no refined carbohydrate (especially white flour and white sugar), high fiber, moderate caloric intake, and prepared with love.

This Culture of Life diet, updated with the concept of individualization as explained in detail in *Conscious Eating,* is best known as the Genesis 1:29 Garden of Eden diet. Some people need more protein (plant-sourced), and others need a diet higher in complex carbohydrates, depending on one's constitution. Regardless of your constitution, however, this diet is high in vegetables and phytonutrients. A high-phytonutrient diet naturally includes a variety of antioxidants such as carotenes, vitamin E, vitamin C, phenol compounds, and resveratrol. You know you are getting these when there is a full rainbow of colors in your vegetables, fruits, and grains, as colors are actually the pigments containing phytonutrients, which turn on the anti-aging, anti-cancer, and anti-inflammatory genes. Most important, these phytonutrients turn off the diabetes-causing genes and turn on the anti-diabetic genes. In *Genetic Nutritioneering,* Jeffrey Bland, PhD, explains how the hormone insulin indirectly speaks to the genes and alters gene expression. Insulin also influences the other hormones in the body. A healthy flow of insulin in the body not only helps us control blood sugar, but is linked to a healthy balance of many other hormones, including insulin-like growth factor, human growth hormone, cortisol, somatostatin, serotonin, noradrenalin, and leptin.[1] Our control of hormones is found through our diet, stress, exercise patterns, and, of course, the food we take into our body. Emerging research confirms that the type of carbohydrates we eat also influences the expression of our genes through their effect on the secretion of insulin, glucagons, and other cell signaling hormones. So when we eat, we need to consciously consider that what we eat speaks to our genes, and therefore positively or negatively affects our gene expression.

Our genes carry messages that describe how sensitive we are to insulin and blood sugar. In other words, we have free choice to modify the expression of these genetic messages, by what we eat, how we exercise, how we create stress in our life, and the toxins (such as drugs, alcohol, cigarettes, and heavy metals) that we bring into our system. The point is that whether or not there is an onset of insulin resistance depends on our food and lifestyle. Insulin is a major regulator of the diabetic genes. When our insulin levels are not in homeostasis, our genes that favor the diabetic process are activated.

Studies have found that when individuals consume animal-protein-rich foods their insulin output is greater. This research done with the insulin index, as discussed in Chapter 2, shows that meat, dairy, and fish can create an excess release of insulin—that is, they have a high insulin index and therefore imbalance the system. Research by Gene Stiller, PhD, found that a protein-enhanced diet often increases insulin resistance.[2] Research generally shows that diets containing whole and natural vegetable protein have a lower insulin response than refined high-fat foods. It has been found that the amino acid mix in vegetable protein, although complete, is slightly different than, and offers certain advantages over, animal protein. Specifically for diabetes, vegetable protein positively affects many aspects of our metabolism, including the improvement of insulin sensitivity and the reduction of toxic reactions.[3] Simply changing the excess of calories in the diet and improving the ratio of protein to carbohydrates and fat according to your constitution can actually improve the regulation of blood sugar levels.[4]

Phytonutrients

One of the most potent components of food that affects gene expression on the molecular level is phytonutrients. Research on phytonutrients supports the general findings we've summarized; for example, 82 percent of 156 different published dietary studies found that fruit and vegetable consumption helped protect against cancer.[5] People who eat more fruits and vegetables have about one-half the risk of cancer mortality than those people who are not plant eaters. Plant-sourced diets are very high in phytonutrients, which include a variety of antioxidants, carotenes, vitamin E, vitamin C, phenolic compounds, and terpenoids. We get more than twice the phytonutrients from the same amount of calories on the nutrient-dense live-food diet, which also is a *natural* calorie-restricted diet. The Tree of Life World Cuisine naturally stimulates and reactivates the anti-aging, anti-inflammatory, anti-cancer, and anti-diabetic genes, and turns off the diabetes-causing genes with the aid of the rainbow menu of phytonutrients. These phytonutrients include: the *allyl sulfides* in garlic and onions, potent stimulators of improved phenotypic expression for diabetes and aids in controlling blood sugar with their sulfur components important for insulin function; *phytates* in grains and legumes, with anti-cancer effects; *glucarates* in citrus, grains, and tomatoes, improving the gene expression of detoxification; *lignans* in flax, improving the metabolism of estrogen and testosterone; *indoles, isothiocyanates,* and *hydroxybutene* in cruciferous vegetables, improving detoxification against carcinogens; *ellagic acid* in grapes, raspberries, strawberries, and nuts, improving antioxidant function; and *bioflavonoids, carotenoids,* and *terpenoids,* reducing inflammation and improving immunity. Inflammation is definitely affected by our gene expression. My favorite anti-inflammatory food is ginger; it has active phytochemicals called gingerols, which have been shown to be quite effective in the treatment of arthritis and other inflammation problems. Used in conjunction with curcumin, these two have been shown to improve gene expression in regard to the anti-inflammatory response.[6] One popular flavonoid is quercetin. Found in apples, onions, and garlic, quercetin helps improve gene expression related to allergy and arthritis, and helps maintain the integrity of vascular tissue for improved circulation. Bioflavonoids, of which quercetin is one, are among the most important modifiers of gene expression, in addition to being antioxidants.

Once we understand this first principle about eating a Culture of Life anti-diabetogenic diet, we start to understand that what we take into our body has very important healing effects. In a October 1997 article in *Science* by Dr. Caleb Finch, a professor at the Andrus Gerontology Center at the University of Southern California, Finch clearly makes the point that heredity plays a minor role in determining life span.[7] One of the most important roles in longevity is connected to lifestyle.This principle applies to the tendency to be diabetic. If we do not activate the diabetes-producing genes, with poor diet and lifestyle, then diabetes will not manifest.

Anti-Aging: Caloric Restriction and Resveratrol

To further make the point of the main theoretical principle of the Tree of Life 21-Day+ Program, *Life Extension* 2004 reports that a phytonutrient, resveratrol, has been found by Harvard medical school researchers to activate a longevity gene in yeast that extends life by 70 percent. In an interview, leading resveratrol researcher Dr. Xi Zhao-Wilson told *Life Extension:* "There has been a great deal of attention focused on resveratrol in the past few years, following a study showing that resveratrol activates molecular pathways involved in life-span extension, now demonstrated in yeast, worms, flies, fish, and mice, and which possibly bear a relationship to mechanisms underlying caloric restriction."[8] The tremendous amount of scientific evidence of the effect of caloric restriction on upgrading our gene expression supports the link of caloric restriction and longevity. In humans, the preliminary evidence is very promising: Consuming a low-calorie diet is associated with several possible markers of greater longevity, such as lower insulin levels and reduced body temperatures, along with less of the chromosomal damage that typically accompanies aging.[9] This research supports one of the main points of our program—that diabetes is an accelerated aging process, and youthing through eating restricted but nutrient-dense foods reverses the accelerated aging associated with a diabetogenic diet and lifestyle.

RESEARCH HISTORY ON CALORIC RESTRICTION

Research on caloric restriction goes back to the 1930s when Dr. Clive McKay of Cornell University found that the life span of rats doubled when their food intake was halved. Not only did the calorie-restricted rats live longer, but they were more healthy and youthful, when compared to the control rats. He found that his control rats, allowed to eat as much as they wanted, became weak and feeble, as they lived their normal life span. Calorie-restricted rats, at the time when the control rats were dying out, were still alive, youthful, and vigorous. One of the rats lived to the equivalent of 150 human years. This research was repeated in the 1960s with calorie-restricted rats at the Morris H. Ross Institute, where the rats lived up to 1,800 days, or approximately 180 human years. In the 1970s breakthrough research was done by Dr. Roy Walford and Dr. Richard Weindruch at the UCLA medical center where they found that even gradual restriction of calorie intake in middle-age rats extended life span as much as 60 percent. Research by Professor Huxley extended the life span of worms by a factor of nineteen times by periodically underfeeding them.[10] Research has also shown that undereating increases life span in fruit flies, water fleas, and trout.[11] The research by Walford and Weindruch suggested that it doesn't matter what age you start—you can still turn on a healthy gene expression. That's good news for a lot of people.

The next breakthrough began in the 1990s with Dr. Richard Weindruch and Dr. Thomas Prolla at the University of Wisconsin. Using microchip technology, they measured the expression of thousands of genes in mice, rats, monkeys, and humans. Weindruch and Prolla studied gene profiles in the muscles in normal and calorie-restricted mice and found major differences in gene expression between the two groups. In this first study of gene expression, the scientists found that gene expression was significantly positively altered by caloric restriction in a way that seemed to show a slowing of the aging process.[12] Following this significant breakthrough was work done by Dr. Stephen Spindler, professor of biochemistry at the University of California-Riverside. Using gene technologies, Spindler studied the expression of 11,000 genes in the livers of young normally fed and calorie-restricted mice, and found that 60 percent of the age-related changes in gene expression from calorie-restricted mice occurred within a few weeks after they started the calorie-restricted diet. The full effects of caloric restriction on the genetic profile for anti-aging develop quickly. Spindler found that caloric restriction results in a specifically produced genetic anti-aging profile and resulted in reversal of the majority of age related degenerative changes that showed up in the gene expression. As diabetes is an age-related degenerative process, so it follows that a general anti-aging effect should have an anti-diabetogenic effect. Spindler found a fourfold increase in the expression of the anti-aging genes in short-term caloric restrictions, and a 2.5-fold increase in the expression of youthing genes in long-term caloric restriction. He was able to reproduce this with a 95 percent success rate.

Spindler noted that caloric restriction not only prevented deterioration or genetic change gradually over the life span of the animal, but actually reversed most of the aging changes in a short period of time. His research lasted only a month with the rats. In another study, he found that the most rapid change from a genetic aging profile to an anti-aging profile occurred in older animals as well as young and middle-age ones, thus making the point that it doesn't matter at what age you begin. Caloric restriction does appear to turn on the expression of the anti-aging genes and turn off the expression of the aging genes, and most likely turns off the expression of diabetic genes. We have a full memory of all our gene expression in our chromosomes; all we have to do is push the right dietary button to get a healthy expression.

CULTURAL EVIDENCE SUPPORTING CALORIC RESTRICTION

Human cross-cultural studies reveal the same results. Dr. Kenneth Pelletier, in his research on longevity, found that cultures in which people lived the longest, healthiest lives—the natives of the Vilcabamba region of Ecuador, the Hunza of West Pakistan, the Tarahumara Indians of northern Mexico, and the Abkhasians of the Georgia region of Russia—ate low-protein, high-natural-carbohydrate diets that contained approximately one-half the amount of protein Americans eat and only 50–60 percent of the total calories.[13] Paavo Airola makes the point in *How to Get Well* that one never sees an obese centenarian.

Returning to Spindler, an important part of his research is that the short-term caloric restriction can turn on the majority of the anti-aging genes. He found that weight loss from caloric restriction improves insulin sensitivity, improves blood glucose values, decreases blood insulin levels, decreases heart rate, and improves blood pressure. In summary, Spindler's results, published in the proceedings of the National Academy of Sciences, showed:

- No matter what age you are you still get an anti-aging effect with calorie restriction
- Anti-aging effects can happen quickly on a low-calorie diet
- Caloric restriction of only four weeks in mice seems to partially restore the liver's ability for metabolizing drugs and for detoxification
- Caloric restriction seems to quickly decrease the amount of inflammation and stress even in older animals.[14] We see these same positive results in our one-week green juice fasting retreats at the Tree of Life in the U.S. and Israel.

What we eat feeds our genes as well as what we do not eat. It is our choice. This is the key to understanding the diet for reversing diabetes. We will take it one step further, so it is very clear. The Tree of Life 21-Day+ Program starts with green juice fasting for seven days, because that is the most powerful form of caloric restriction, and therefore has the most potential effect on balancing the insulin messages to our genes to turn off the diabetogenic process. We begin to see positive effects within four to seven days. This is one of the reasons we are able to get people off all their medications, including insulin, in such a short time. When there is a great deal of genetic upgrading needed, as with Syndrome X, it may take three to four weeks. Considering that most people still believe diabetes is not reversible, this is not very long.

The Culture of Life anti-diabetogenic world cuisine, besides its other qualities, is also high in enzymes, high in electron energy, and high in bio-photon energy. These areas are all discussed in depth in my book *Spiritual Nutrition.* Organic live food provides the highest-quality nutrient concentrates, the highest-quality phytonutrients, vitamins, minerals, and bioelectrical energy, which is quite important for healing and building the vital life force. It is not only activating and energizing the system and repairing it on that level, but repeating the activity in a very simple way. When we cut through the metabolic complexities of diabetes, and we simply see it as an accelerated form of aging, which it is, then we can apply an approach that gets to the core of reversing the diabetic process—turning on the anti-aging genes and the anti-diabetic genes through the Culture of Life anti-diabetogenic world cuisine.

This is the essence and the breakthrough of our program. Is this a new idea? It most certainly isn't. Genesis 1:29 says very specifically: *"Behold, I have given you every plant yielding seed that is upon the face of all the earth, and every tree with seed in its fruit; you shall have them for food."* In other words, we have already been given the optimal diet for a healthy lifestyle. But that doesn't mean that everyone chooses to follow it. The pandemic of diabetes has given us a chance to reconsider that this is advice worth following. Choosing to heal oneself from diabetes is a major diet and lifestyle choice. As it says in Devarim (Deuteronomy), one of the five books of the Torah, you can choose life or death. Which culture do you choose to live in?

Aside from pancreas problems with diabetes, there is usually significant weakness in the adrenals. In my clinical experience, there are almost ten times more problems with adrenals when people are on a high-sugar diet. Hypothyroidism is also a common tendency. Hypogonadism, i.e., low testosterone, in men is not unusual and there are herbs to improve that condition. Additional herbal and nutritional support is given for these issues according to the individualized needs of the client.

CLIENT RESULTS

You have read the theory, formulated out of thirty-five years of clinical experience. It is time to present the clinical data from the first eleven people on whom we have formally collected data. It is the author's intent to make a study that is significantly larger than this "pilot study" in the future.

It might have made sense to write this book five years from now with the results of at least 100 people. But the results have been so dramatic, and the lives of millions are so dear to us, and the preservation of life possible through this approach is so important, that I wanted to get this information out as soon as possible.

I would like to do a clinical trial of 100-200 people, and we hope to receive funding to do so. I feel the results you are about to see merit such attention, and I am actively working to receive the proper funding.

Explanation of the Data

FASTING BLOOD SUGAR (FBS)

This blood glucose level is taken with a monitor each morning before food is eaten, as well as three other times during the day. A range of 70 to 85 is the optimal FBS. Borderline (or early pre-diabetes) impaired fasting glucose tolerance is 86 to 99, an FBS of 100 and higher is considered pre-diabetes, and above 126 is diabetes by the Tree of Life 21-Day+ standards. Below is a summary of the FBS results that we achieved for our eleven participants, all off their oral hypoglycemics or insulin. The initial fasting blood sugar results were achieved with all on oral hypoglycemics and insulin. Everyone was off these medications within four days of beginning the program.

CLIENT	INITIAL FBS	ENDING FBS	FBS POINT DROP	% CHANGE
Client 1	293	88	205	70%
Client 2	287	74	213	74%
Client 3	400	85	315	79%
Client 4	400	109	291	73%
Client 5	248	83	165	67%
Client 6	130	82	48	37%
Client 7	111	87	24	22%
Client 8	300	70	230	77%
Client 9	144	82	62	43%
Client 10	120	65	55	46%
Client 11	279	126	153	55%
AVERAGES	247	86	161	65%

GLYCOSYLATED PROTEIN (HGBA1C)

The HgbA1c test measures the percentage of hemoglobin that is non-enzymatically linked to glucose, also known as glycosylated hemoglobin. The life span of red blood cells is about four months, so the HgbA1c test gives a three- to four-month view on blood glucose control. People with diabetes have high blood sugar levels, and thus more glucose is glycosylated to the hemoglobin. An HgbA1c test result above 6.0 is considered diabetic.

Research shows, as we saw with the Pima Indians data on retinopathy, that HgbA1c levels of 6.0 or less is where complications are minimized and eliminated most significantly. It is estimated that for every 1 percent drop in HgbA1c levels, the reduced risk of long-term diabetic complications is as much as 37 percent.

FRUCTOSAMINE

While the HgbA1c test measures blood glucose over the last three or four months, the fructosamine test gives an indication of glucose control over the past month. Fructosamine is a term referring to the linking of blood sugar onto protein molecules in the bloodstream. This is a useful test to use when changing protocols in a specific person because changes in diabetic control can be detected earlier than with the HgbA1c test.

LDL/HDL CHOLESTEROL

According to Dr. Caldwell B. Esselstyn, who has reversed cardiovascular disease with a 100 percent success rate using a vegan diet,[15] we do not see heart disease in people who have a total cholesterol of lower than 150 or an LDL of less than 80. In our results, you will notice that the low-density lipoproteins (LDL) went close to normal range, with an average drop of 67 points, or 44 percent, to an average LDL of 82 over a period of 21–30 days. LDL is known as "bad" cholesterol because a high reading is associated with increased risk of heart disease. Many authorities are now encouraging LDL levels at less than 80 for those with diabetes, because the number one cause of death among diabetics is heart disease. Although an LDL of less than 80 is relatively safe, your risk of heart problems drops as LDL decreases, until it reaches a level of approximately 40 mg/dl.[16] HDL (high-density lipoprotein) is called "good" cholesterol because it carries cholesterol out of the body. Optimum target levels for HDL are above 45 mg/dl for men, and 55 mg/dl for women. HDL can also be interpreted in relation to total cholesterol. A favorable HDL would be at least one-third of total cholesterol, so if 150 is our goal, then a healthy HDL would be 50 and over.

TRIGLYCERIDES

These are fat particles traveling in the bloodstream. Normal concentration is less than 150 mg/dl. Lowering triglycerides is another important way to reduce the risk of heart disease. This is easily accomplished on a Culture of Life anti-diabetogenic diet and lifestyle. Our clients routinely see their triglycerides going to normal after one month on live foods.

C-REACTIVE PROTEIN (CRP)

CRP is a pro-inflammatory cytokine that is a cardiovascular disease risk factor. The C-reactive protein reading indicates a degree of inflammation; it is determined by measuring the amount of a specific protein in the blood. Recent research suggests that patients with elevated levels of CRP are at increased risk for diabetes,[17] hypertension, and cardiovascular disease. A study of more than 700 nurses showed that those in the highest quartile of trans fat consumption had blood levels of C-reactive protein that were 73 percent higher than those in the lowest quartile.[18]

As we now know, inflammation is the fourth stage of disease, so we can use this test to first determine how far along someone is in the disease process and, even more important, to mark one's progression back through the seven stages to a healthy physiology. Inflammation contributes to complications that are further along than the fourth stage of disease, such as ulceration (Stage 5), so seeing this marker come down is a significant sign of improvement in health. We measured an average CRP decrease of 70 percent, after one month on the program.

WEIGHT

The results summarized in the success stories that follow are occurring in people who are dramatically overweight. We are not operating a weight loss clinic, but our observation is that 82 percent of people will come into a normal weight within two years of adopting a Culture of Life anti-diabetogenic cuisine and lifestyle. In all cases people felt stronger and healthier. At the end of the movie made at Tree of Life, the five people felt so much better by all their indicators that they were able to climb Red Mountain, a 1,000-foot plus climb over difficult terrain. For many diabetics, even those in a post-diabetes physiology, weight loss may need to continue to further reduce the risk of the complications of overweight, including increased insulin resistance and the temptation to return to a diabetogenic lifestyle. The average weight loss after one month was 25 pounds for those who were overweight at the beginning of the program.

Eleven Success Stories

CLIENT 1

This 59-year-old male had a health history of Type-2 diabetes for ten

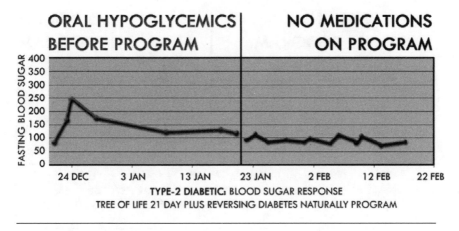

Figure 1: FBS for Client 1

years, and an FBS near 300 before starting the program. Additional chronic conditions included heart disease with pacemaker, hypertension, obesity, and stroke.

This client came to the Tree of Life with a history of blood sugar levels near 500, and at the start of the program his blood sugar before lunch on the 14th of January was 330. Within a few days of officially beginning the program, on the 22nd of January, his FBS had already dropped to 123, and by the 27th, just five days later, he reached an FBS of 88, close to a normal, nondiabetic FBS. When he began the program, his weight was 288; one month later he was down to 256. His fructosamine levels dropped into normal range, from 313 at the start to 262 after one month. C-reactive protein went from 8.8 to 3.8. Total cholesterol dropped from 147 to 107, and triglyceride levels held steady at 113.

CLIENT 2

This 25-year-old male had a medical history of hospital-diagnosed Type-1 diabetes for more than five years. His medications included Lantis 15U, and Glucophage 500 mg twice/day.

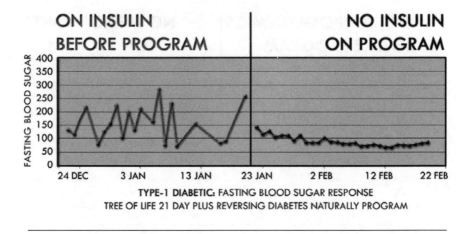

TYPE-1 DIABETIC: FASTING BLOOD SUGAR RESPONSE
TREE OF LIFE 21 DAY PLUS REVERSING DIABETES NATURALLY PROGRAM

Figure 2: FBS for Client 2

After just four days on the program, Client 2 was off his insulin completely, with an FBS of 88. By two weeks his FBS was consistently below 83 and remains there two years later. His fructosamine dropped from 480 to 340, within normal range, in three weeks. His glycosylated hemoglobin HgbA1c has returned to 6.0 from 11.8. Total cholesterol went from 216 to 150, and LDL cholesterol from 142 to 88, essentially eliminating him from the pool of people who tend to develop heart disease. His triglyceride level fell from 65 to 53. Weight loss was not a serious need for this client; he lost 6 pounds in twenty days, and then gained back 3 pounds. To resolve the question of whether this patient was Type-1, the patient on his own went to his local MD for further tests to determine whether he was Type-1 or Type-2. His beta cell antibody titers were significantly high at 8.9 (normal is 0–1.5), strongly suggesting that he is indeed a Type-1 diabetic. His clinical history, which was a rapid and fulminating onset of diabetes, causing him to be hospitalized with a blood sugar of 1,200, is consistent with a medical history of Type-1 diabetes, as contrasted with Type-2, which is characterized by a slow onset of symptoms. It is interesting, and perhaps historic in the field of diabetes research, to note that in a one-year follow-up his serum C-peptide, which is associated with a precursor to insulin, was originally less than 0.5, and is now 0.7. This suggests that the program is actually beginning to rebuild or reactivate the beta cells of the pancreas.

CLIENT 3

This client began the program on March 27th. Before she arrived, her blood sugar had hit levels as high as 465 just three weeks before the program.

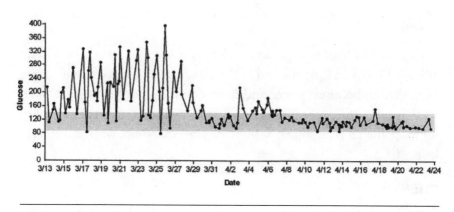

Figure 3: FBS for Client 3

By her twenty-first day on the program, her FBS had reached 85, and weight loss was 25 pounds.

CLIENT 4

This diabetic was 39 years old with Type-2 for five years, and a medical history of hypertension and obesity—in my estimation, a classic example of Syndrome X. At the start of the program her FBS was 400 ahd her weight was 352 pounds. After one month her FBS dropped as low as 109 and her weight dropped to 329 pounds. Her CRP dropped from 37.8 to 8.6. Her total cholesterol dropped from 237 to 171 and trigycerides dropped from 225 to 123 in one month.

CLIENT 5

This client was a 55-year-old Type-2 diabetic for ten years and manifested a Syndrome X pattern. He started with an FBS of 248 and within eighteen days on the program his FBS reached 83, off all medications.

CLIENT 6

This Type-2 diabetic started with an FBS of 130 on oral diabetic medications. In one week while off all medications, her FBS dropped to 82. She also lost 13 pounds in three weeks. Her total cholesterol dropped from 217 to 140 and LDL went from 148 to 46.

CLIENT 7

A 61-year-old female Type-2 diabetic for ten years, this client had an average FBS of 111. By the end of the program her thinking, which had been slower, became clearer and more connected to the environment. By the end of the program her FBS was 87 and has remained in the 80s for more than a year, shown at our one-year follow-up, with an HgbA1c level of 5.5.

CLIENT 8

Type-2 diabetes was diagnosed for this 55-year-old two months after her last baby was born, thirty-five years ago. She came to us with an average FBS of 300, and was using four doses of oral hypoglycemic medications each day. On day one, she eliminated her use of oral hypoglycemics, and achieved an FBS of 105. Days two through four, her FBS was 50, and then rose to 77, 84, and 70 for days five, six, and seven, respectively. Several weeks after her green juice fast she continued to remain with an FBS of around 70 with one spike up to 170 when she ate something sweet. This spike helped convince her not to succumb to the idea of "moderation" in the Culture of Death.

CLIENT 9

This client had Type-2 diabetes for ten years, with a history on metformin and glucorite for the past three years. On day one, she stopped the use of medications. Her FBS was 144 on day one, 129 on day two, and by day seven was 102. On day eight, she achieved a nondiabetic FBS of 82.

CLIENT 10

This Type-2 diabetic started the fasting program with an average FBS of 110–120. By day two, the FBS was 98, and by day seven, 65.

CLIENT 11

This is an interesting case because it shows that healing does not necessarily occur completely in three to four weeks. During her one-month program, she lost 26 pounds, went from using 35 units of insulin a day to 0 units, discontinued the use of the pharmaceuticals Lantis, Byetta, Neurontin, and Monopril within four days, saw a decrease in her C-reactive protein levels from 8.4 to 2.6, lowered her total cholesterol from 210 to 136 (with LDL dropping from 142 to 85 and HDL rising from 25 to 29), and lowered her FBS from 279 to 126 for a 55 percent drop without any medications. This particular client was well on her way to a healthy reversal when she returned home.

Foods, Juices, Herbs, Vitamins, and Minerals– An Eloquent Healing Message

The results summarized above were achieved by a very conscious choice of foods and their juices, herbs, vitamins, amino acids, minerals, and enzymes. The incredible resolutions of the diabetic physiology to a nondiabetic physiology have as much to do with what we did include, as what we *removed* from the diet and lifestyle. You are now aware that we have eliminated processed sugar, white flour, cooked carbohydrates, processed foods, excitotoxins such as artificial flavorings and colorings, animal fats, trans fats, cooked fats, smoking, and television. Before we discuss the nutritional and lifestyle elements that we do include in the program, it is important to mention that there are some plant-source foods that are typically eaten, and even recommended by medical professionals as part of diabetes-amelioration programs, that we do not use.

WHEAT

Wheat, according to Ayurvedic principles, is kaphagenic (heavy and sweet), and therefore not recommended for diabetics. We do not include wheat, specifically white bread, also due to its *alloxan* content. Alloxan is the chemical that makes white flour look clean, white, and beautiful. A remarkable discovery that a single injection of alloxan can produce diabetes mellitus in laboratory animals was made in 1942, in Glasgow, by John Shaw Dunn and Norman McLetchie.[19] Scientists and FDA officials have known about this connection for years. Alloxan causes diabetes by creating free radical damage to the DNA in the beta cells of the pancreas. The *Textbook of Natural Medicine* calls alloxan a "potent beta cell toxin." It is unfortunate that the FDA still allows companies to use it to process foods we eat. Research also shows that we are able to reverse the effects of alloxan with vitamin E. According to Dr. Gary Null's *Clinicians' Handbook of Natural Healing*, vitamin E effectively protected lab rats from the harmful effects of administered alloxan.

In support of that, researchers have found that among rats that are genetically susceptible to IDDM, feeding wheat gluten will cause 40 percent of the subjects to develop IDDM. Several other groups of rats with the same genetic inclination to develop IDDM were fed gluten-free diets, and only 10–15 percent developed IDDM. Further, the rate and severity of diabetes could be manipulated by varying the amount of gluten in the diet. Others have shown that delaying introduction of dietary gluten in animals delays or prevents diabetes. Most authorities in this area of diabetes research conclude that gluten is a major factor in causing the development of IDDM in genetically predisposed animals.[20]

SOY

Soy is also a diabetogenic and kaphagenic food. It is a low-mineral food that robs the body of minerals. About 90 percent of all soy is genetically modified (GMO). Soy is also one of the top seven allergens, and is widely known to cause immediate hypersensitivity reactions. While in the last forty years soy has occupied an important place in the transition from an unhealthy meat-based diet to vegetarian and vegan cuisine, it is time for us to upgrade our food choice to one having more benefits, and fewer negative possibilities. In 1986, Stuart Berger, MD, placed soy among the seven top allergens—one of the "sinister seven."[21] At the time, most experts listed soy around tenth or eleventh. Bad enough, but way behind peanuts, tree nuts, milk, eggs, shellfish, fin fish, and wheat.[22] Scientists are not completely certain which components of soy cause allergic reactions. They have found at least sixteen allergenic proteins, and some researchers pinpoint as many as thirty.[23]

Kaayla T. Daniel writes in *The Whole Soy Story:*

> Allergic reactions occur not only when soy is eaten but when soybean flour or dust is inhaled. Among epidemiologists, soybean dust is known as an "epidemic asthma agent." From 1981 [to] 1987, soy dust from grain silo unloading in the harbor caused 26 epidemics of asthma in Barcelona, seriously affecting 687 people and leading to 1,155 hospitalizations. No further epidemics occurred after filters were installed, but a minor outbreak in 1994 established the need for monitoring of preventive measures. Reports of the epidemic in Barcelona led epidemiologists in New Orleans to investigate cases of epidemic asthma that occurred from 1957 [to] 1968, when more than 200 people sought treatment at a Charity Hospital. Investigations of weather patterns and cargo data from the New Orleans harbor identified soy dust from ships carrying soybeans as the probable cause. No association was found between asthma-epidemic days and the presence of wheat or corn in ships in the harbor. The researchers concluded: "The results of this analysis provide further evidence that ambient soy dust is very asthmogenic

and that asthma morbidity in a community can be influenced by exposures in the ambient atmosphere."

Soy contains built-in insecticides called *isoflavones* (genistein and daidzein). Isoflavones are estrogen-like substances that have the same effect in the body as estrogen, and eating soy can make a person estrogenic, contributing to problems such as cancer, irritability and mood swings, fat gain from the waist down, fibrocystic breast disease, and uterine fibroids.[24,25,26] Isoflavones decrease thyroid hormone production. This can stunt children's growth. Hypothyroid is associated with raised serum cholesterol and tends to create fatigue and obesity.[x27,28,29] This further encourages and enhances a diabetogenic reality. Isoflavones decrease the good cholesterol (HDL), thus contributing to heart disease, the number one killer of diabetics.[30,31]

Soy may also be connected with Alzheimer's disease, now thought to be a complication of hyperglycemia and diabetes. In a major ongoing study involving 3,734 elderly Japanese American men, those who ate the most tofu during midlife had up to 2.4 times the risk of later developing Alzheimer's disease. As part of the three-decade-long Honolulu-Asia Aging Study, twenty-seven foods and drinks were correlated with participants' health. Men who consumed tofu at least twice weekly had more cognitive impairment than those who rarely or never ate the soybean curd.[32,33] Going further, higher midlife tofu consumption was also associated with low brain weight. Brain atrophy was assessed in 574 men using MRI results and in 290 men using autopsy information. Shrinkage occurs naturally with age, but for the men who had consumed more tofu, lead researcher Dr. Lon R. White from the Hawaii Center for Health Research said, "Their brains seemed to be showing an exaggeration of the usual patterns we see in aging."

In men, eating soy isoflavones can significantly reduce testicular function and lower luteinizing hormone (LH) production, which is what signals the testicles to work. A high soy intake and potentially lower level of LH increases the probability of estrogen dominance in men, contributing to hair loss, swollen and cancerous prostates,[34,35] and insulin resistance. Dorris Rapp, MD, a leading pediatric allergist, asserts that environmental and food estrogens are responsible for the worldwide reduction in male fertility.[36]

For women, female children fed the estrogens in soy formula and products hit puberty early, sometimes as young as age 6 to 8.[37] Eating soy products during pregnancy may affect the sexual differentiation of the fetus toward feminization; studies even show malformations of the reproductive tract or offspring born with both male and female sexual organs.[38] Kaayla T. Daniel writes:

> Ingrid Malmheden Yman, PhD, of the Swedish National Food Administration, wrote to the Ministry of Health in New Zealand informing the agency that children with severe allergy to peanut should avoid intake of soy protein. To be on the safe side she further advised parents to make an effort to "avoid sensitization" by limiting both peanuts and soybeans during the third trimester of pregnancy, during breast feeding, and by avoiding the use of soy formula. Controversy has raged since the 1920s as to whether or not babies could be sensitized to allergens while still *in utero*. In 1976, researchers learned that the fetus is capable of producing IgE antibodies against soy protein during early gestation and newborns can be sensitized through the breast milk of the mother and later react to foods they've "never eaten." As Dr. Stefano Guandalini, Department of Pediatrics, University of Chicago, writes, "A significant number of children with cow's milk protein intolerance develop soy protein intolerance when soy milk is used in dietary management." Interestingly enough, researchers recently detected and identified a soy protein component that cross reacts with caseins from cow's milk. Cross reactions occur when foods are chemically related to each other.
>
> Matthias Besler of Hamburg, Germany, and an international team of allergy specialists report on the website www.allergens.de that adverse reactions caused by soybean formulas occur in at least 14 to 35 percent of infants allergic to cow's milk. On another valuable

allergy website www.medicine.com Dr. Guandalini reports the results of an unpublished study of 2108 infants and toddlers in Italy, of which 53 percent of the babies under three-months old who had reacted poorly to dairy formula also reacted to soy formula.[39]

"The amount of phytoestrogens that are in a day's worth of soy infant formula equals 5 birth control pills," says Mike Fitzpatrick, a New Zealand toxicologist.[40] A study reported in *The Lancet*[41] found that the "daily exposure of infants to isoflavones in soy infant-formulas is 6–11-fold higher on a bodyweight basis than the dose that has hormonal effects in adults consuming soy foods." This dose, equivalent to two glasses of soy milk per day, was enough to change menstrual patterns in women.[42] In the blood of infants tested, concentrations of isoflavones were 13,000 to 22,000 times higher than natural estrogen concentrations in early life.

Soy is a mineral-deficient food and, adding insult to injury, contains phytin, which chelates essential minerals such as iron, zinc, and magnesium out of the body before they can be absorbed.

In 2003, a study[43] was done comparing the bodily IGF-1 increase promoted by 40 grams of soy (the amount in one soy candy bar and a soy shake, or four soy patties) versus 40 grams of milk protein. Soy was found to be almost twice as powerful as milk protein in increasing IGF-1 levels (36 percent for milk, 69 percent for soy). This new IGF-1 data potentially places soy in the category of a powerful cancer promoter of the breast, prostate, lung, and colon.[44] The implications are, first, that this establishes soy as a very kaphagenic food, as IGF-1 is the end product of growth hormone stimulation. Although it is controversial, there are many in the medical world who feel that excessive IGF-1 could stimulate the aforementioned cancers if they are already present. This is why Canada does not allow rBGH milk from the U.S. because it is so much higher in IGF-1. In essence, this is still at the level of theoretical speculation but we feel it merits a preventive attention. Our sense is that one should have at best a minimum of soy in the diet if including any cooked food as part of an 80-percent-live, 20-percent-cooked food cuisine. The following chart shows how pervasive soy is in our so-called health foods. The 40-gram level of IGF-1-creating soy protein from the study, as you will see in the chart, is easy to achieve.

EATING PROCESSED SOY EASILY ADDS 40 GRAMS OF HARMFUL PROTEIN CONCENTRATE TO YOUR DIET		
ITEM	**SERVING**	**GRAMS OF PROTEIN**
Desserts and Snacks:		
Cliff® Builder's Bar	1 bar	20
Cliff® Bar (Oatmeal, Raisin Walnut)	1 bar	10
Revival Soy Bars®	1 bar	17
Atkins Nutrition Bars®	1 bar	21
ZonePerfect Nutrition Bars®	1 bar	15
Revival Soy Shakes® Splenda®	1 shake	20
Meats:		
Morningstar Farms® Sausage Patties	1 patty	10
Boca© Breakfast Links	1 link	8
Gardenburger® Chik'n Grill	1 patty	13
Boca Burger® Original	1 burger	13
Boca® Ground Burger	2 ounces	13
Boca® Chicken Patties	1 patty	11
Smart Dogs®	1 dog	9
Boca® Chili	1 serving	20
Cheeses:		
Veggie Shreds® (Cheese)	2 ounces	6
Boca® Pizza	1 slice	13
Tofu with Added Isolates:		
Lite Tofu®	3 ounces	5
Flour:		
Benesoy® High Protein Soy Flour	1 ounce	15

John McDougall, *The McDougall Newsletter,* April 2005, 4(4),
www.drmcdougall.com.

Eliminating soy from your diet can be tough if you are just eating processed vegetarian or vegan. Many pre-packaged and prepared foods contain soy as an ingredient, but it may be listed as "textured vegetable protein" (TVP), "textured plant protein," "hydrolyzed vegetable protein" (HVP), "vegetable oil," or "MSG" (monosodium glutamate). You may also find "lecithin," "vegetable broth," "bouillon," "natural flavor," or "mono-diglyceride" ingredients that are often soy products. We suggest eating a live, plant-sourced diet that is not processed or cooked, and to avoid restaurants that serve foods with soy products in them. The recipe section of this book will provide you with ample foods that are nutrient-dense, non-allergenic, delicious, and filling, and that will have you wondering why you ever ate processed soy-containing meals.

Excitotoxins

Excitotoxins represent another health disaster associated with the better-living-through-chemistry paradigm of the Culture of Death. In an attempt to avoid dealing with the problems associated with the craving for the sweet taste of sugar, and instead of facing our sweet taste issues which are more of an acquired taste at the level of excess that is practiced in the world today, we have invented artificial sweeteners and excitotoxins. The negative health consequence of this has become more and more significant. Russell Blaylock, author of *Excitotoxins: The Taste That Kills,* writes:

> There are a growing number of clinicians and basic scientists who are convinced that a group of compounds called excitotoxins play a critical role in the development of several neurological disorders including migraines, seizures, infections, abnormal neural development, certain endocrine disorders, neuropsychiatric disorders, learning disorders in children, AIDS, dementia, episodic violence, lyme borreliosis, hepatic encephalopathy, specific types of obesity, and especially the neurodegenerative diseases, such as ALS, Parkinson's disease, Alzheimer's disease, Huntington's disease, and olivoponto-cerebellar degeneration.[45,46]

An enormous amount of both clinical and experimental evidence has accumulated over the past decade supporting this basic premise.[47] These excitotoxins are food additives such as MSG, hydrolyzed vegetable protein, and aspartame. This excitotoxins increase our cravings for the junk foods they are added to and thus make people more vulnerable to the problems associated with junk foods and diabetogenic foods because the excitotoxins stimulate the appetite rather than activate the satiety response. In this context, excitotoxins are great for building the wealth of the food companies and excellent for destroying the health of the population. For example, since 1948 the amount of MSG added to foods has doubled every decade. By 1972, 262,000 metric tons were being added to foods each year. More than 800 million pounds of aspartame have been consumed in various products since it was first approved. Ironically, these food additives have nothing to do with preserving food or protecting its integrity. They are used to alter or "enhance" the taste of food.

MONOSODIUM GLUTAMATE (MSG)

When one cooks soy, evidence suggests that MSG is a naturally created by-product. Many people in the live-food movement thought that the creators of Bragg's Liquid Aminos were adding MSG to the product, because people were having MSG reactions to it. They were not adding MSG. Patricia Bragg would never do that. Instead, what was happening was that people were reacting to the normal MSG created by the heating of the soy in their recipe.

Ingesting MSG creates an excess of glutamate, which the body has trouble converting. MSG causes a very large insulin response after it is ingested, because there are glutamate receptors in the pancreas which are activated by the glutamate increased by the MSG and which then cause a release of insulin. MSG also opens calcium channels, thus constricting blood vessels—this may put diabetics with high blood pressure at risk by negating calcium channel blocker medication.

Conventional wisdom has been that MSG does not result in a corresponding increase in blood levels of free glutamic acid, but according to research done in Canada, MSG does result in higher plasma concentrations of free glutamic acid, aspartate and higher insulin levels as well as insulin. In addition, plasma insulin concentration almost triples in response to MSG ingestion. This increase in plasma insulin can exacerbate hypoglycemia.[48] This is especially important in diabetics since prolonged elevation of the blood sugar produces a down-regulation of the glucose transporter and a concomitant "brain hypoglycemia" that is exacerbated by repeated spells of peripheral hypoglycemia common to Type-1 diabetics.

MSG has also been associated with damage to the hypothalamus and concomittant resulting obesity. In 1968, John W. Olney, MD, a respected researcher at Washington University Medical School, St. Louis, Missouri, and member of the National Academy of Science, found that mice in his laboratory in which the administration of MSG had resulted in retinal damage, had become grotesquely obese. Since 1969, many scientists have confirmed Dr. Olney's findings of damage to the hypothalamus from MSG with resulting obesity. There is abundant literature demonstrating that MSG and aspartic acid cause hypothalamic lesions, which, in turn, can cause gross obesity. Although there are a number of causes for obesity, there is no question that one of the contributing causes for the obesity epidemic is the ever increasing use of MSG and aspartame. The damage to the hypothalamus is even worse in the womb and the first two years of life, when the young child is developing. The use of MSG during this critical developmental time may create severe endocrine problems later in life including decreased thyroid function, increased tendency toward diabetes, and higher cortisone levels than normal. A child consuming a soup containing MSG plus a drink with NutraSweet will have a blood level of excitotoxins six times the blood level that destroys hypothalamus neurons in baby mice.[49]

ASPARTAME

Aspartame, commonly thought to be a benefit to diabetics as a sweetener because it is low glycemic and low caloric, has actually been linked to the activation of diabetes. According to research conducted by Dr.

H. J. Roberts, a diabetes specialist, a member of the ADA, and an authority on artificial sweeteners, aspartame leads to the creation of clinical diabetes, causes poorer diabetic control in diabetics on insulin or oral drugs, causes convulsions, and leads to the aggravation of diabetic complications such as retinopathy, cataracts, neuropathy, and gastroparesis. Dr. Roberts found ". . . the loss of diabetic control, the intensification of hypoglycemia, the occurrence of presumed 'insulin reactions' (including convulsions) that proved to be aspartame reactions, and the precipitation, aggravation or simulation of diabetic complications (especially impaired vision and neuropathy) while using these products."[59] Russell Blaylock, MD, author of *Health and Nutrition Secrets,* writes: "Diabetics who drink large amounts of aspartame-sweetened drinks are more likely to go blind. Aspartame is composed of the excitotoxin aspartic acid; phenylalanine; and methanol, a known eye toxin."

General Anti-Diabetogenic Diet

The following charts show low-glycemic, low-insulin-score Rainbow Green food for Phases 1.0 and 1.5 of the Tree of Life cuisine program.

RAINBOW GREEN CUISINE, PHASE 1.0
All vegetables except cooked carrots and cooked beets
All sea vegetables
Non-sweet fruits: tomatoes, avocados, cucumber, red pepper, lemons, limes
Fats and oils: flax oil, hemp oil, sesame oil, walnut, almond, sunflower, and avocado, coconut (not more than 1 tablespoon per day)
Nuts and seeds (except cashews), coconut pulp
Superfoods: Klamath Lake blue-green algaes (E-3Live is the most active), spirulina, chlorella, Green Superfood powder mixes
Sweeteners: stevia, cardamom, cinnamon
Salt: Himalayan and Celtic sea salt

RAINBOW GREEN CUISINE, PHASE 1.5
(ADDITIONS TO PHASE 1.0)

All vegetables: carrots (raw), beets (raw), squash (raw)

Fruits: low-glycemic fruits—blueberries, raspberries, cherries, fresh and unsweetened cranberries, pomegranate, goji berries, grapefruit, lemons, limes

Condiments and sweeteners: mesquite, cacao, carob

Bee pollen granules

Grains: quinoa, buckwheat, millet, amaranth, spelt

Fermented and cultured foods: apple cider vinegar, miso (non-soy), sauerkraut, probiotic drinks

Notes:

Phase 1: no grains, not sweet or fermented

Phase 1.5: grains stored less than 90 days, low-sweet fruits, and fermented food

Phase 1.5: A small amount of Phase 2 fruits and veggies in a large salad

DIABETIC TRANSITION CHART
(TRANSITIONING TO A LOW-GLYCEMIC,
LOW INSULIN-INDEX CULTURE OF LIFE CUISINE)

Conventional Diabetic Culture of Death Foods	Organic Plant-Source only Antidiabetogenic Culture of Life Foods
Meat:	**High-Protein Plant Foods:**
Beef, pork, lamb, chicken, turkey, tuna, and all fish	Nuts and seeds; nut and seed pâtés and cheeses; high-protein superfoods—spirulina, blue-green algae, green superfood mixes, hemp protein, maca; beans
Eggs	Flax with omega-3 fatty acids
Dairy Products:	
Milk and cream	Nut and seed mylks
Butter, margarine, shortening, lard	Coconut oil, cold-pressed oils, cacao butter

Dairy Products (continued)

Cheeses	Nut and seed cheezes; fatty nuts— brazil, pine, macadamia, and pecan
Yogurt	Walnut yogurt; coconut cream (plain or fermented); cultured nut and seed mylks with probiotics
Sour cream	Sunflower and sesame sour cream
Ice cream	Nut-based ice creams; sorbets made in high-speed blender with frozen blueberries, raspberries
Whipped cream	Coconut cream
Milk chocolate bar	Raw chocolate bar made with cacao

Grains:

White rice, whole wheat	Amaranth, millet, quinoa, spelt, and buckwheat
Cakes and pastries	Live chocolate cakes, carrot cake, live cheese cakes
White or whole wheat bread	Flax crackers, nut and seed crackers and breads
Commercial cereals	Buckwheaties; live granola

Roasted/Salted Nuts and Seeds:

Peanuts, cashews, almonds, macadamia nuts and their butters	Raw nuts and seeds and their nut and seed butters—walnuts, flax seed, almonds, brazil nuts, sesame seed, chia seeds, pumpkin seeds, sunflower seeds

Vegetables—Cooked and Processed:

Instant foods; frozen, canned, fried, boiled, salted, and baked vegetables	Fresh vegetables, salads, soups, green smoothies, dehydrated foods

Fruit—canned and sweetened, dried and sulphered:

	Fresh, low-glycemic fruits; dehydrated fruits

Beverages:

Chlorinated, fluoridated tap water	Filtered, blessed, structured water

Beverages (contined):

Fruit juices—pasteurized	Fresh juices, preferably low-glycemic Green Vegetable Juice
Soda	Herbal noncaffeinated teas and fresh vegetable juices
Alcoholic beverages	Herbal noncaffeinated teas and fresh vegetable juices
Coffee	Cacao beverages; green tea (transitional)

Sweeteners:

White sugar, brown sugar, molasses, corn syrup, maple syrup, dextrose, sucrose, fructose, aspartame, mannitol, saccharin, sorbitol, and xylitol	Stevia, licorice root, carob, chia seed, mesquite, cardamom

Oils:

Hydrogenated vegetable oils	Cold-pressed oils: coconut, flax, hemp, sesame, almond, sunflower, avocado, olive (accompanied with high antioxidant foods or supplements)

Salt:

Iodized table salt	Himalayan crystal salt, Celtic sea salt

Particular Anti-Diabetogenic Foods

JERUSALEM ARTICHOKE

Jerusalem artichoke is an herbal medicine that contains fructose oligosaccharides (inulin) which may be helpful in diabetes. The body breaks down inulin slowly so your blood sugar doesn't rapidly increase.

CABBAGE

The protective action against oxidative stress of red cabbage (*Brassica oleracea*) extract was investigated in diabetes induced rats for sixty days.[51] Researchers found a significant increase in reduced glutathione and superoxide dismutase activity and a decrease in catalase activity and in the total antioxidant capacity of the kidneys. Daily oral ingestion of *B. oleracea* extract from cabbage for sixty days reversed the adverse effects of diabetes in rats. They found lowered blood glucose levels and restored renal function and body weight loss. In addition, the cabbage extract attenuated the adverse effect of diabetes on malondialdehyde, glutathione, and superoxide dismutase activity as well as catalase activity and total antioxidant capacity of diabetic kidneys. In conclusion, the antioxidant and anti-hyperglycemic properties of *B. oleracea* in cabbage may offer a potential therapeutic source for the treatment of diabetes.

HUCKLEBERRY

The huckleberry juice compounds may also offer significant protection against diabetic retinopathy and cataracts. Such huckleberry compound extracts are being widely used throughout Europe in the prevention of diabetic retinopathy. All of this work with huckleberry in ophthalmology actually began back in World War II when some Royal Air Force pilots in Great Britain swore that eating huckleberry jam or drinking huckleberry cordials prior to flying night missions over Germany significantly improved their visual acuity in the darkness. Such reports generated a lot of interest in the medical community in Europe, which led to a number of studies being done with the berry.

BITTER MELON

Bitter melon, also known as *Momordica charantia* or balsam pear, is a tropical fruit known throughout Asia, Africa, and South America. Its green fruit looks like an ugly cucumber. Bitter melon is made of several compounds that have anti-diabetic properties, including charantin, which has been shown to be more powerful than the hypoglycemic drug tolbutamide, and an insulin-like polypeptide called polypeptide-P, which lowers blood sugar when injected into Type-1 diabetics.[52] In one study, it decreased the glucose tolerance by 73 percent when people were given

2 ounces of the juice.[53] In another study there was a 17 percent reduction in glycosylated hemoglobin in six people. Still another study found that 15 g of the aqueous extract of this herb produced a 54 percent decrease in blood sugar after eating and a 17 percent reduction in the glycosylated hemoglobin in six patients.[54]

There are different preparations. The fresh juice is probably the strongest in terms of its effect. A variety of human clinical trials have established blood sugar lowering action of the fresh juice or abstract.[55,56] More than 100 studies have demonstrated bitter melon's ability to decrease the blood sugar, increase the uptake of glucose, and activate the pancreatic cells that manufacture insulin. The peptide it has acts like bovine insulin. So it has several effects: improved glucose tolerance without increasing insulin levels, stimulating the beta cells of the pancreas, suppressing the urge to eat sweets, and action similar to that of insulin.

Unripe bitter melon is available at Asian markets, and the fresh juice is probably the best, per the traditional use in the studies. Bitter melon is difficult to make palatable, as its name implies. The best way to use this effective plant is to juice 2 ounces, and hold your nose as you drink it with celery-cucumber juice and some lemon.

CUCUMBER

Cucumber contains a hormone needed by the beta cells of the pancreas to produce insulin. The enzyme erepsin in cucumbers is targeted toward breaking down excessive protein in the kidneys. In our program, we use a lot of cucumber juice, for drinking as well as in salads.

CELERY

Celery also has some general anti-diabetogenic affects, as well as being helpful for people with high blood pressure such as we see with Syndrome X. Celery juice has a calming effect on the nervous system, due to its high concentration of organic alkaline minerals, especially sodium. The minerals contained in celery juice make the body's use of calcium more effective, balancing the blood's pH. Celery should be the center of your green vegetable juices, and can be included in green soups and smoothies to alkalinize a system taxed by acidifying Culture of Death foods and lifestyle choices.

NOPAL CACTUS

Nopal is prickly pear cactus, widely used as a traditional food throughout Latin America. Researchers[57] gave eight fasting diabetics 500 grams of nopal. Five tests were performed on each subject, four with different cooked or raw preparations and one with water. After 180 minutes, fasting glucose was lowered 22–25 percent by nopal preparations, as compared to 6 percent by water. In a rabbit study, nopal improved tolerance of injected glucose by 33 percent (180-minute value for comparison) as compared to water.[58] Nopal researchers concur that although cooked and raw cactus are effective, preparations from commercially dehydrated nopal are not.

GARLIC AND ONION

Garlic and onions contain sulfur compounds that are believed to be responsible for their anti-diabetic qualities. S-allyl cysteine sulphoxide in garlic is one of these. It has been reported to decrease fasting blood glucose and lower cholesterol levels in diabetic rats,[59] and in one human study, onion extract was shown to reduce hyperglycemia in a dose dependent manner.[60]

GRAINS AND BEANS

The following grains and beans are high-fiber complex carbohydrates that have been found to be important for the prevention and healing of diabetes. They are part of the indigenous diets, especially of the Native Americans, that made diabetes a rarity before these cultures began to accept the Western diet in the 1940s and their rate of diabetes began to soar.

- Millet
- Brown rice
- Oats

- Buckwheat
- Amaranth
- Mung beans
- Garbanzo beans
- Pinto beans
- White tepary beans
- Green beans
- String beans
- Papago beans

NUTS AND SEEDS

Recent research suggests that regular nut consumption is an important part of a healthy diet,[61] despite the fact that in the past, nuts were considered unhealthy because of their relatively high fat content at 14–19 grams/ounce. Most of the fats in nuts are the healthier monounsaturated and polyunsaturated fats.[62] Monounsaturated fats, such as those in olive oil, almonds, and avocados, improve insulin sensitivity.[63] A Harvard study in 2002 on the benefits of nuts concluded that high dietary nut consumption decreased the risk of sudden cardiac death, a leading cause of death among diabetics. Nuts and seeds are also high in plant sterols (phytosterols), which decrease cholesterol and improve heart health.[64,65] In the intestinal lumen, phytosterols displace cholesterol and inhibit cholesterol absorption.[66]

Nuts and seeds are great for plain eating, and for making pâtés, soups, salad dressings, and nut mylks. When you see the nut mylk recipes in Chapter 6, you will wonder what you were ever doing with cow, soy, and rice milk. The anti-diabetogenic and nutritional benefits of nuts and seeds are worth knowing.

In a study presented to the American College of Cardiology March 14, 2000, Richard Vogel, MD, head of cardiology at the University of Maryland in Baltimore suggested that olive oil may be nearly as dangerous as saturated fats in clogging arteries. He found that olive oil impaired vascular function to the same extent as a Big Mac, fries, or Sara Lee Cheesecake—an arterial constriction of 34 percent. These vascular constrictions are significant because they injure the endothelium of the blood vessel and may contribute to heart disease, because it predisposes one to atherosclerotic cardiovascular disease. He also found that oils with high omega-3s, which olive oil does not have, did not cause an impairment in blood vessel function. Dr. Vogel pointed out that it is not a question of whether it is monounsaturated or polyunsaturated, but the omega-3 levels. Olive oil is very high in omega-9. This raises a more serious question, which Dr. Vogel has answered: It was not the olive oil that was key in the Lyon Diet Heart Study of the Mediterranean cuisine, but rather, it may have been the fruits, vegetables, nuts, bread, and fish that were key, in conjunction with less meat in the diet. Actually, Vogel points out, the Lyon Diet did not use olive oil.

The research suggests that olive oil is not heart-healthy, although olive oil is clearly healthier than foods saturated with trans fats. But being better than those foods is not saying much. When researchers at the University of Crete compared residents who had heart disease with those free of the disease, those with heart disease ate significantly higher quantities of olive oil and all fats in their diet. In essence, what Dr. Vogel has pointed out is that the protective elements in the Mediterranean diet are the antioxidants found in the plant sources of the cuisine. He felt that there was some protection against the direct impairment of endothelial function produced by high-fat foods, including olive oil. In another study exploring the same issue, reported in the *American Journal of Cardiology,* they also found that the constriction was worse in twelve healthy and twelve high-cholesterol subjects after consuming olive oil.

Extra Virgin olive oil does contain polyphenols that give some antioxidant protection. However, most plant foods are rich in polyphenols and provide more polyphenols per calorie than olive oil. For example, an 11–calorie serving of green leafy lettuce gives you the same amount of polyphenols (30 mg) as 120 calories of olive oil. Another group of researchers studied 200 men using three different olive oils for three weeks; one of the oils was Extra Virgin, the other two were not, and low in polyphenols. The scientists found that the Extra Virgin had better heart health effects, including higher HDL cholesterol levels and less oxidative stress. The oxidative stress is what increases inflammation in the arteries, disrupting the endothelial cells and predisposing one to plaque rupture and heart attack.

Olive oil does not lower LDL cholesterol, a potential indicator for heart disease. However, the studies have produced some confusion, as people substitute olive oil for their intake of saturated fats and trans fats, and see the LDL going downward. The point is that it is not the addition of olive oil, but the removal of harmful fats from the diet, that has decreased harmful LDL cholesterol.

Given the preponderance of evidence from these studies, we cannot say that olive oil is heart healthy. In fact, the people with the longest life expectancy and fewest heart attacks have diets low in olive oil but high in plant foods.

We do need to keep in mind that there are very few studies on the topic at this moment, so we can only make a suggestive warning rather than a definitive statement about the adverse affect of olive oil on cardiovascular health. One study reported in the March 27 issue of the *Archives of Internal Medicine* showed that eating olive oil can lower high blood pressure. In a group of twenty-three patients, Italian researchers found that after eating olive oil for six months, blood pressure medications were lowered by 48 percent, and eight participants were able to discontinue their medications altogether. Sunflower oil had no effect on their blood pressure.

In the December 1999 issue of the *American Journal of Clinical Nutrition*, Danish researchers reported that olive oil worked better than canola oil at inhibiting blood clots after a fatty meal.

Even Dr. Vogel, who found the 34 percent endothelial constriction, suggested that when olive oil is combined with the eating of antioxidant-rich fruits and vegetables, the vessel-constricting effect disappears. Therefore, on a live-food diet rich in antioxidants, or with supplements such as vitamin E (400–600 IU), Vitamin C (2000 mg), L-argninine (2,000 mg), garlic, alpha-lipoic acid (300 mg/day), and flavonoids (there are 5,000 different flavonoids—potent antioxidants found in plant foods) all improved endothelial function and blood vessel tone. Therefore, if one is healthy and on a live-food diet high in antioxidants, and uses Extra Virgin olive oil, the vascular constricting endothelial effect of olive oil should be mitigated.

We also would suggest that people with serious ASCVD follow Dr. Esselstyn's recommendation and eliminate olive oil and other saturated cooked fats, and minimize raw fats from their diet in their vegan approach to healing atherosclerosis. Likewise, those people diagnosed with diabetes for more than a year have, with nearly 100 percent certainty, a degeneration of the endothelium of the arteries, and are most prudent to avoid or minimize the use of olive oil until the diabetic physiology has been reversed completely for two years. Even though the high-antioxidant, high-omega-3 oils are a good alternative, we do also recommend that one consider creating dressings from whole pulverized nuts and seeds rather than the oils of these high-quality nuts and seeds, which only contain the fat-soluble antioxidants. In general, even though these oils are beneficial, we still recommend that one keep a relatively low fat intake (approximately 15–20 percent of total calories) in the process of healing diabetes through a live-food diet. Taken in this context, because on a live-foods cuisine you can eat half as much with the same nutritional benefit, this is actually healthier and theoretically superior to having 10–15 percent of calories from fat in a cooked food diet.

The best oils to use in salad dressings are those high in omega-3 such as walnuts, flax, and hemp, as well as sesame oil, which is very high in antioxidants. We recommend in our recipes that one can try substituting these oils for olive oil.

In our clients put on a 100-percent living and raw foods diet with 15–20 percent raw plant fat, including raw nuts, seeds, and avocado, we saw an average 44-percent drop in LDL with an average drop to an LDL of 82. We saw relief from all diabetic degenerative symptoms, including improved mental function. The improved mental function suggests an increase in blood flow to the brain. These results support the large studies cited about the beneficial use of whole raw nuts and seeds such as walnuts and almonds.

WALNUTS

Walnuts are exceptionally high in monounsaturated fat and the omega-3 fatty acid, alpha-linolenic acid. A study published in November 2004 by Kris-Etherton et al. showed that ALA reduced cholesterol and fats in the blood, and also C-reactive protein (CRP), an inflammatory marker associated with heart disease.[67] Additionally, walnuts combine these heart healthy fats with a hefty dose of the antioxidants, including at least sixteen antioxidant phenols, vitamin E, and ellagic and gallic acid. In 1993 the *New England Journal of Medicine*[68] reported that eating 8–16 walnuts per day decreased total and LDL cholesterol by 5–10 percent, and reduced incidence of stroke and clogging of arteries up to 70 percent.[69] Additional research has confirmed that when walnuts are eaten as part of a modified low-fat diet, the result is a more cardioprotective fat profile in diabetic patients than can be achieved by simply lowering the fat content of the diet. In a study published in the *Journal of the American Dietetic Association,* all fifty-five study participants with Type-2 diabetes were put on low-fat diets, but the only group to achieve a cardioprotective fat profile were those who ate walnuts (30 grams—about one ounce—per day).[70] Other studies have found similar results.[71,72,73,74] Dr. Emilio Ros of Barcelona reported in the October 17, 2006 *Journal of the American College of Cardiology* that eating walnuts could reverse the impairment of endothelial function associated with eating a fatty meal, but olive oil did not show any measurable effect. He found that eating a handful of walnuts prevented the increase in inflammation in the arteries and of endothelial dysfunction, while olive oil did prevent the increase in inflammatory molecules but did not prevent the endothelial dysfunction associated with eating fatty foods. In a previous study reported by Dr. Ros, he showed that eating walnuts over four weeks helped repair endothelial dysfunction. Dr. Ros pointed out that walnuts have several components that help in this repair function, including polyunsaturated fats, ALA, omega-3 fats, arginine, and many antioxidants. He recommends eating at least 6–8 walnuts a day.

ALMONDS

Almonds may also play a role in controlling diabetes. In a study[75] involving twenty free-living individuals, researchers examined the effect of 100 grams (about 3.5 ounces) of almonds a day. Researchers found that LDL and total cholesterol levels decreased while glycemic control did not change. In the crossover arm of this study, total and LDL cholesterol decreased 21 and 23 percent, respectively, and glycemic control was unaffected. This study shows that almonds can be incorporated into a healthful diet without negatively affecting glycemic control while also lowering cholesterol. The *Journal of Nutrition* also reported that when walnuts and almonds were added to a meal, they gave glycemic control after eating a high-carbohydrate meal. A 160-calorie handful of almonds supplies vitamin E, magnesium, and fiber. All are important in protecting against diabetes. Almonds and walnuts are the two most studied nuts in regard to diabetes and heart disease.

Sea Vegetables

People all over the world have been eating sea vegetables (known generically as seaweed) for thousands of years. Four varieties of sea vegetables have been found preserved in Japanese burial grounds that were 10,000 years old. The Australian Aborigines use three different types of sea vegetables. The Native Americans include alaria (wakame-like), nori (laver), and kelp in their traditional diets. The Atlantic coastal people of Scandinavia, France, and the British Isles also have been eating sea vegetables for centuries.

Gram for gram, they are higher in minerals and vitamins than any other class of food. They are rich in vitamins A, B, C, and E. The minerals in sea vegetables are found in similar ratios to those in the blood. Sea vegetables produce substantial amounts of proteins, complex carbohydrates, carotenes, and chlorophyll. For example, dulse and nori have 21.5 and 28.4 grams of protein, respectively, per hundred grams of sea vegetable. They have approximately 2–4.5 percent fat, and 40–45 grams of carbohydrate per hundred grams of sea vegetable. Alaria (essentially identical to the Japanese wakame) and kelp are extremely high in calcium. All of the sea vegetables seem to be high in potassium, with kelp being the highest, followed by dulse and alaria. Alaria and kelp are high in magnesium, each having three times the RDA per 100 grams. Kelp and alaria have very high amounts of iodine; 100 grams of kelp have approximately ten times the estimated RDA of iodine. One hundred grams of alaria and nori have approximately 8487 and 4266 IU of vitamin A. One hundred grams of most of the sea vegetables have about one-third the RDA of the B vitamins, one-tenth the RDA of vitamin C, and about one-third the RDA of vitamin E. As pointed out earlier, these sea vegetables also contain chelating agents that are effective for protection against the absorption of radioactive particles.

KELP

Kelp absorbs from seawater almost all the nutrients, minerals, and trace elements that are essential to life. Kelp contains more than sixty minerals and elements, twenty-one amino acids, simple and complex carbohydrates, and several essential plant growth hormones. Being rich in amino acids, vitamins, minerals, and trace elements is one of the key reasons why kelp is known as a great promoter of glandular health, especially for the pituitary, adrenal, and thyroid glands. Kelp was first used medicinally to treat enlarged thyroid glands. Physicians didn't know why kelp was effective, until it was discovered that it was exceptionally rich in iodine and that enlarged thyroids were caused by iodine deficiency. Because iodine stimulates the thyroid gland, which controls the metabolism, it was noted that those who took iodine lost weight more easily. From these observations, kelp was then used to assist in weight loss. It has been suggested that kelp's positive effects in assisting metabolism may help in lowering cholesterol. This versatile sea-vegetable is also widely used to maintain healthy skin and hair. Kelp's most dramatic application is its ability to neutralize heavy-metal pollution and radiation in the body.

Algaes

CHLORELLA AND SPIRULINA

Chlorella and spirulina are two of the most nutrient-dense foods known, and easily qualify as whole, perfect superfoods. They have a balanced complement of protein (60 percent), carbohydrate (19 percent), fat (6 percent), bio-available minerals (8 percent), and moisture (7 percent).

Chlorella gets its name from the high amount of chlorophyll in it, up to ten times that of spirulina, which is itself very high in chlorophyll. Another hallmark of this superfood is chlorella growth factor (CGF), 3 percent of the chlorella cell that is responsible for its ability to quadruple in quantity every twenty hours. CGF stimulates tissue repair, even if it has been ulcerated, as we see in advanced cases of diabetes. CGF has been proven effective against memory loss, depression, and other psychiatric diseases. It also helps boost the immune system, stimulating the production of interferon and the activity of macrophages (important defense cells in our immune system). Chlorella is the best algae for pulling heavy metals out of the system, particularly mercury, lead, cadmium, uranium, and arsenic—all known to be diabetogenic. The antiviral effects of chlorophyll and CGF have also been found beneficial in cases of blood sugar imbalances such as diabetes because chlorella's digestible protein smoothes blood sugar fluctuations. Chlorella helps diabetics by reducing AGEs, the toxic metabolites resulting from consuming refined sugars.[76]

Spirulina contains gamma linolenic acid (GLA), an essential fatty acid needed by diabetics. The Delta-6 desaturatase enzyme, which is necessary to convert linoleic acid to gamma linolenic acid (GLA), is inhibited in diabetes. And by giving GLA, an omega-6 fatty acid, researchers found that receivers of GLA did better in all sixteen parameters evaluated in one study.[77]

GLA has been found to enhance nerve conduction and blood flow in diabetic rats. These essential fatty acids seem to improve circulation, improve nerve conduction, and increase prostaglandin PG-1, which has an anti-inflammatory effect and helps ameliorate neuropathy. Spirulina is also 95 percent digestible, higher than any food known. It contains more beta-carotene than any other whole food, as well as 92 trace minerals and other nutritional elements such as vitamins, chlorophyll, glycolipids, phycocyanin, carotenoids and sulfolipids. It is also abundant in superoxide dismutase (SOD, an antioxidant), RNA, and DNA, which were identified in 1990 as essential nutrients. The high amounts of beta-carotene in spirulina have shown to be effective in fighting oral cancer in animals.[78] In India, the beta-carotene in spirulina was studied for its effectiveness and absorption in young children and found to be extremely effective.[79]

Spirulina and chlorella are excellent in juices, smoothies, on salads, and even in plain water. These are two superfoods you do not want to be without.

Sweeteners

Stevia is the only sweetener we recommend. Fifteen times sweeter than sugar, with no calories and a glycemic index of 0, the powdered leaf of *Stevia rebaudiana Bertoni* has recently become highly sought after as a supersweet, low-calorie addition to a low-glycemic diet. It gives a sweet taste, and does not raise the blood sugar as all the other natural sweeteners do. Unlike nutrient-empty synthetic sugar substitutes, stevia is loaded with vitamins and minerals, including magnesium, niacin, riboflavin, zinc, chromium, and selenium. Stevia is also one of the oldest, safest, and most highly esteemed South American herbs known, with a centuries-long history of safe use. By 1921, stevia was being hailed by American trade commissioner George Brady as a "new sugar plant with great commercial possibilities." He was so convinced that it made "an ideal and safe sugar for diabetics" that he presented it to the United States Department of Agriculture.

Several modern clinical studies suggest that stevia may have the ability to lower and balance blood sugar levels, support the pancreas and digestive system, protect the liver, and combat infectious microorganisms.[80,81,82,83,84]

Vitamins

NIACIN (B-3)

As early as 1950, researchers had discovered that niacinamide could provide protection against the development of diabetes.[85] These studies, and some performed thirty years later, sparked several human-based studies that have again demonstrated niacin's ability to not only prevent Type-1 diabetes but, if given soon enough after diagnosis, to slow the progression of and sometimes even reverse the disease, restoring pancreatic function to the point that insulin is no longer required.[86]

Niacinamide has been shown to be effective in preventing the development of diabetes in high-risk children. Researchers divided a group of high-risk children into two groups; fourteen were given niacinamide and eight were not. All eight of the untreated children eventually developed diabetes, compared to only one of the treated children.[87]

Researchers have now shown that niacinamide acts as a protective antioxidant. It also inhibits components of the immune system that target the pancreas.[88] Niacinamide also stimulates the pancreas to secrete more insulin and increases insulin sensitivity within cells.[89]

Enzymes that contain niacin play an important role in energy production and the metabolism of fat, cholesterol, and carbohydrates as a pre-hormone component in the sex and adrenal hormones, as well as a neurotransmitter precursor. Niacin is part of the glucose tolerance factor as well. Using niacinamide has had significant effects in Type-1 and Type-2 diabetes. There is some suggestion that niacinamide given within the first five years of the onset of Type-1 may help ameliorate the effect. It has also been shown to reduce total cholesterol and triglycerides, and increase HDL levels. It may turn out to be an essential part of any diabetic program.

Niacinamide has the capacity in vitro of disrupting the pathogenic mechanisms of NIDDM. Animal studies have shown significant beta cell protection from niacinamide. Many of these studies have been done since 1987 and have played a role in helping prevent the destruction of pancreatic beta cells in patients newly diagnosed with Type-1 diabetes.

Niacinamide prevents the depletion of intracellular NADH.[90,91] Low intracellular NADH levels contribute to the death of islet cells of the pancreas. Niacinamide does seem to help prevent pancreatic beta cell death, but it does not seem to intervene in the inflammatory process, which is why the live-food diet and Vitalzym X play an important role in reducing inflammation. B-3 is good for the functioning of glucose tolerance factor and it decreases lipid buildup.

Because of these interesting results, several pilot studies were designed to see if nicotinamide was a viable way to prevent Type-1 diabetes from manifesting, or after manifesting, to prevent the beta cells from further destruction or reduce the rate of destruction. In these studies seven participants were given 3 grams of niacinamide. After six months, five patients in the niacinamide group and two in the placebo group were not needing insulin. Their blood glucose levels and HgbA1c levels were normal. At twelve months, three patients in the niacinamide group and none in the placebo group remained diabetes-free.[92] Could niacinamide prevent diabetes from progressing? There have been at least ten studies attempting to answer this question of the effectiveness of niacinamide treatment for recent onset of Type-1 or cases of less than five years duration. Of these ten studies, eight were double-blind, and of the eight, four showed a positive effect compared to placebo in terms of prolonged non-insulin need or lower insulin requirements, which, in essence, is better metabolic control. They also had increased beta cell functions as determined by C-peptide secretion.[93]

Because of these tentatively positive results, two large studies were conducted, the Deutsche Nicotinamide Intervention Study and the European Nicotinamide Diabetes Intervention Trial (ENDIT); neither found significant benefit. However, in the face of some of the above studies, if my child had Type-1 diabetes, I would certainly add nicotinamide to the mix because of its minimal toxicity, and the fact that it is inexpensive. A dosage of 2,000 mg a day would cost around $7.00 a month.

Dosage: The typical dosage used is 500–1,000 mg three times a day, taken with food. Those at risk for developing Type-1 diabetes, or those who have already been diagnosed, are well advised to use niacinamide. The research has shown that it is most helpful either before or in the initial phases, i.e., during the first five years of the disease. Dosage recommendations are approximately 25 mg of niacinamide for every 2.2 pounds of body weight, so a person weighing 150 pounds would need about 1.7 grams, or 1,700 milligrams a day. Studies have shown no side effects other than one case of diarrhea, and dosages up to 3 grams daily for six months have produced no problems.

If you are taking niacinamide, it is wise to use a B-complex supplement in conjunction with it, to ensure that the larger therapeutic doses create no other B-vitamin deficiencies. Food sources of niacin are spinach and hazelnuts.

VITAMIN B-6

Vitamin B-6 is very helpful in reversing diabetic neuropathy, and protects against peripheral nerve degeneration. Diabetics with neuropathy have been shown to be deficient in B-6 and benefit from supplementation.[94] It seems to also inhibit glycosylation of proteins.[95] It also helps with magnesium metabolism.

Dosage: With regard to gestational diabetes, a study published in the *British Medical Journal* showed that women taking 100 mg of B-6 reversed the condition in twelve of the fourteen women.[96]

VITAMIN B-12

Thirty-nine percent of meat eaters are deficient in B-12 and up to 80 percent of vegans and live-food eaters are deficient in B-12 after six years. So it is absolutely essential that we supplement with this nutrient. Research has found that vitamin B-12 is also very helpful in maintaining proper function of the nervous system in individuals with Type-2 diabetes. Increased levels of B-12 were closely correlated with reduced oxidative stress in individuals with poor blood sugar control.[97] People's needs for B-12 are quite variable, and stress plays a big role in those needs. Vitamin B-12 deficiency can result in memory loss, depression, and numbness or burning feelings in the feet. We have used it along with the total program in helping to reverse diabetic neuropathy.

Dosage: We recommend a form of B-12 that is vegan, made from bacteria. It is called Nano B complex. Anyone on this diet is well advised to take it protectively. We need about 6 mcg twice a day as a minimum.

BIOTIN

Biotin is another vitamin that seems to be important for carbohydrate fat and protein metabolism. A plant-source-only diet seems to increase the intestinal bacteria in a way to enhance biotin synthesis and absorption. Biotin seems to increase insulin sensitivity, as well as activate glucokinase, which is involved in the utilization of glucose by the liver. This is important because in diabetics glucokinase concentrations are low. Biotin also helps to decrease fasting blood sugar. Biotin deficiency results in impaired utilization of glucose.[98] Blood biotin levels were significantly lower in forty-three patients with NIDDM than in nondiabetic control subjects, and lower fasting blood glucose levels were associated with higher blood biotin levels. After one month of biotin supplementation (9 mg/day), fasting blood glucose levels decreased by an average of 45 percent.[99] Reductions in blood glucose levels were also found in seven insulin-dependent diabetics after one week of supplementation with 16 mg of biotin daily.[100] Biotin has also been found to stimulate the secretion of insulin in the pancreas of rats, having the effect of lowering blood glucose.[101] An effect on cellular glucose (GLUT-4) transporters is currently under investigation.

Dosage: Biotin is appropriate for Type-1 and Type-2 diabetes. Type-2 diabetics were given 9 mg per day for one month, and compared to a placebo group; the diabetics experienced an average drop of 45 percent in their blood glucose levels.[102] Similar improvements were noted in a study of Type-1 diabetics with a daily dose of 16 mg of biotin.[103] Biotin is very safe—no side effects have been reported. Food sources include avocados, raspberries, artichokes, and cauliflower.

VITAMIN C

Vitamin C plays a very important role in the healing of diabetes and reversing complications. This antioxidant inhibits accumulation of sorbitol, reduces glycosylation of proteins, and preserves endothelial function. It inhibits aldose reductase, which creates a buildup of sorbitol, which is associated with many of the long-term complications of diabetes. One of the key gifts of vitamin C is its role in the function and manufacture of collagen, as well as maintaining the integrity of the connective tissue, which makes it important for two diabetic concerns: wound repair and maintaining healthy gums. Vitamin C seems to be important in the immune system and in the manufacture and metabolism of neurotransmitters and hormones. Insulin facilitates the transport of vitamin C into the cells, so when there is an insulin deficiency, what we actually get is a deficiency in intracellular vitamin C—thus the relative deficiency in vitamin C in many diabetics.[104] This leads to a subclinical scurvy problem, which creates an increased tendency to bleed, poor wound healing, microvascular disease, heart disease, elevation of cholesterol, and a depressed immune system.

Perhaps a most important effect of vitamin C (at doses of 2,000 mg/day) is its ability to reverse the glycosylation of proteins.[105,106] The sorbitol accumulation and cross-linking, or glycosylation, are linked to many complications, especially eye and nervous system and circulatory disorders. Vitamin C may be one of the best and safest nutrients for the inhibition of sorbitol accumulation in the cells. One study[107] showed that when researchers measured red blood cell sorbitol, then supplemented with either 100 mg or 600 mg vitamin C, then measured participants again in thirty days for their red blood cell sorbitol, the controls had nearly double the sorbitol of those who received vitamin C supplementation. This normalization of the sorbitol seemed to be independent of changes in diabetic control. The researchers concluded that the vitamin C supplementation was distinctly effective in reducing the buildup of sorbitol in the red blood cells.

Dosage: Even though the study was done with 100 or 600 milligrams of vitamin C, we suggest clinically that one should take 1,000 mg of food-sourced C three times a day because of the overall effects. Foods high in vitamin C include goji berries, grapefruit, lemons, broccoli, red peppers, Brussels sprouts, camu camu berries, and acerola berries.

VITAMIN D

Vitamin D is actually a hormone rather than, strictly speaking, a vitamin—one of the most powerful hormones in your body. It is active in quantities as small as one-trillionth of a gram.

Studies have shown vitamin D to have a protective effect against Type-1 diabetes. The results of a large pan-European trial, published in the journal *Diabetologica* in 1999, suggest that vitamin D supplements taken in infancy protect against, or arrest, the initiation of a process that can lead to insulin-dependent diabetes in later childhood. If this is the case, it seems reasonable to suggest that exposure to sunlight in early childhood may be important in preventing the onset of the disease.[108] For adults, studies have shown that the lower your vitamin D level, the higher your blood glucose.[109] One twenty-minute full-body exposure to the summer sun will result in putting 20,000 IU into the body within forty-eight hours. However, if you are older, obese, or dark-skinned, you will get far less. In fact, using sunscreen of even a low SPF rating of 8 reduces vitamin D production by 95 percent.[110] Dr. Robert Heany of Creighton University, one of the top vitamin D researchers, has stated that as many as 75 percent of the women in the U.S. are deficient.[111]

Just in case you are wondering about vitamin D levels and a raw vegan diet, researchers led by Luigi Fontana, MD, PhD, of Washington University[112] looked at eighteen men and women, ages 33 to 85, who had maintained a raw vegan lifestyle for an average of 3.6 years. They were compared with a matched group of eighteen controls who ate a standard American diet containing animal fat and processed foods. The average vitamin D levels were higher in the raw vegan group than in the control group, despite an extremely low dietary intake of vitamin D, indicative of the increased personal sun exposure.

If you live above 38 degrees north latitude (above Baltimore, St. Louis, Denver, and San Francisco), the sun is too weak from mid-fall through the following spring to stimulate significant vitamin D production. Other challenges are aging, as our skin becomes less efficient at producing vitamin D, and excessive fat layers that inhibit production. The latter is a common concern for those of us who are healing obesity and diabetes.[113] Therefore, supplementation is advised at 800 IU per day.

The benefits of sunlight or supplementation for adequate vitamin D levels do not stop with diabetes, but significantly affect the complications associated with a diabetogenic history and a Westernized diet and lifestyle. Research shows that vitamin D has a variety of important benefits besides lowering blood sugar. It seems to protect against eighteen different kinds of cancers, has a significant positive impact on the immune system in fighting colds and flus, viruses, and TB, and protects against rickets and osteoporosis.

VITAMIN E

Diabetics seem to have an increased need for vitamin E. It reduces glycosylation, improves insulin sensitivity, and inhibits platelet clumping. It regulates intracellular calcium and magnesium in the blood vessels. It helps to protect against oxidation, helps improve the action of insulin, and helps prevent many of the long-term difficulties and complications of diabetes, including neuropathy.[114] A recent study found a biochemical marker of oxidative stress to be elevated in diabetic individuals.[115] Supplementation with 600 mg of synthetic alpha-tocopherol daily (equivalent to 300 mg of natural, *RRR*-alpha-tocopherol) for fourteen days resulted in a reduction in the oxidative stress marker. One study reported improved control of blood glucose levels with supplementation of only 100 IU of synthetic alpha-tocopherol daily (equivalent to 45 mg of natural, *RRR*-alpha-tocopherol).[116]

In a human double-blind study, twenty-four hypertensive patients were given 600 mg of vitamin E per day. Those given vitamin E showed increased insulin sensitivity and improved concentrations of cellular magnesium. Magnesium is believed to protect against oxidative damage and normalize circulating glucose levels.[117] It can also play a role in preventing diabetes. One study followed 944 men, ages 42 to 60, who did not have diabetes at the beginning of the study. Forty-five men developed diabetes during the four-year follow-up. The study indicated that a low vitamin-E concentration was associated with 3.9 times greater risk of developing diabetes.[118]

It is important that one use a natural vitamin E with all the tocophenols and tocotrienals factors.

Bioflavonoids

Recent research indicates that flavonoids may be useful in treating diabetes.[119,120] Flavonoids include quercetin, which promotes insulin secretion and is a potent inhibitor of sorbitol accumulation. Quercetin has been found in vitro to inhibit sorbitol accumulation in human lenses,[121] and has been found to slow the course of cataract formation.[122,123] Other flavonoids include naringin and hespertin; both have been found to be aldose reductase inhibitors, therefore protecting against the accumulation of sorbitol.[124,125]

The nutritional benefits of flavonoids include the increase of intracellular vitamin C levels, a decrease in the leakiness and breakage of small blood vessels, the prevention of easy bruising, and immune system support—all of great benefit in diabetes.[126] Bilberry, grapeseed, and ginkgo are important plant sources of flavonoids.

Essential Fatty Acids (EFAs)

The essential fatty acids also play a very important role, which is why I am very hesitant to encourage dietary fat intake that is too low to get the benefits of EFAs.

In diabetes the essential fatty acid metabolism is impaired. The Delta-6 desaturatase enzyme, which is necessary to convert linoleic acid to gamma linolenic acid (GLA), is inhibited in diabetes. By giving GLA, which is an omega-6 fatty acid, researchers found that in a study of 111 diabetics, those who received GLA supplements did better in all sixteen parameters studied, compared to the placebo group.[127] GLA has been found to enhance nerve conduction and blood flow in diabetic rats. GLA and other essential fatty acids seem to improve circulation, improve nerve conduction, and increase prostaglandin PG-1, which has an anti-inflammatory effect and helps ameliorate neuropathy.

The omega-3 and omega-6 fatty acids are the biological precursors to a group of highly reactive, short-lived, molecular, hormone-like substances known as *prostaglandins* (PGAs). The PGAs play a role in regulating the second-by-second functioning of every part of the body. Each organ produces its own PGAs from the essential fatty acids stored in that organ. The PGAs are critical for cell membrane function because they become a part of the membrane construction themselves. PGAs help to balance and heal the immune system as well as reduce inflammatory reactions such as those seen in arthritis and allergic reactions. If there are dietary imbalances that lead to imbalances in the PGAs, then disease may arise. Although the research is not definitive, a ratio of omega-6 to omega-3 fatty acids of approximately 2/1 seems to be the best balance.

In the omega-6 series there is linoleic acid (LA), gamma linolenic acid (GLA), dihomo-gamma linolenic acid (DGLA), and arachidonic acid (AA). The omega-6 fatty acids are found in seed oils such as sunflower, safflower, corn, soy, and evening primrose. Peanut oil has some omega-6, as do olive, palm, and coconut oils. High amounts of GLA are found in mother's milk and primrose, borage, and black currant oils.

Fish are found to have high amounts of eicosapentaenoic acid (EPA) and some moderate amounts of the precursors of the omega-3 series. Fortunately, vegetarians do not have to worry about sources of omega-3 fatty acids because flax seed, hemp seed, purslane, walnuts, legumes, and sea vegetables have high concentrations. In the omega-3 series, there is alpha-linolenic acid (ALA) and the long-chain omega-3s EPA and docosahexaenoic acid (DHA).

OMEGA-3 BENEFITS

The omega-3 series should constitute approximately 10–20 percent of our fat intake. Some of the reported benefits of the omega-3s include protection against heart disease, strokes, and clots in the lungs; anti-carcinogenic activity against tumors; *protection against diabetes;* prevention and treatment of arthritis; and treatment for asthma, PMS, allergies, inflammatory diseases, water retention, rough or dry skin, and multiple sclerosis. The omega-3s are reported to increase vitality and contribute to smoother skin, shinier hair, softer hands, smoother muscle action, the normalization of blood sugar, increased cold weather resistance, and a generally improved immune system. Omega-3s are also important for visual function, development of the fetal brain, brain function in adults, adrenal function, sperm formation, and the amelioration of some psychiatric behavior disorders. It may take three to six months after starting flax seed oil supplementation to see results.

FLAX VERSUS FISH OIL: FLAX WINS

Flax seed contains 18–24 percent omega-3, compared to the low content in fish of 0–2 percent. This is significant because many people mistakenly think that they need to eat fish in order to get the omega-3-derived EPA for heart and artery protection. Abundant research on the subject indicates that this is simply not true. The vegetarian flax seed has many major advantages over fish oil. The first is that the omega-3 is a basic building block in the human body for many functions, only one of which is to make EPA. The fish oil doesn't supply omega-3; it supplies the EPA and therefore limits the body's options to make what it needs from the omega-3. Thus, the omega-3 is a better nutritional resource than the high-EPA fish oil.

Another major difference is the fiber that comes in the flax seed. Fish has no fiber and also is a highly concentrated food. Unlike many other plants, flax seed has a special fiber called lignin that our body converts to lignans, which help to build up the immune system and have specific anti-cancer, anti-fungal, and anti-viral properties. High levels of lignans are associated with reduced rates of colon and breast cancer. Just 10 grams, or about one to two teaspoons of flax seed oil per day, raises levels of the lignans significantly.

A third advantage of the flax seed oil over fish oil is that fish and fish oil are high in cholesterol. Three and one-half ounces of cod liver oil contain 570 milligrams of cholesterol, which equals the amount found in two egg yolks.

The fourth advantage of flax seed oil over fish oil is the fact that fish are often high in toxic residues because they live in polluted waters. The fifth reason flax seed is more propitious is that high levels of fish oil are rich in vitamins A and D, which can be toxic in high doses. Please note that the provitamin carotene, which is converted by the body to utilizable vitamin A, cannot be toxic like animal-sourced vitamin A.

ALPHA LIPOIC ACID (ALA)

One of the most important antioxidants, although we need a variety of them, is alpha lipoic acid. ALA helps with a variety of problems, one of which is the cardiovascular complications of diabetes having to do with small-vessel damage from inflammation. We also use a proteolytic enzyme called Vitalzym X to neutralize and reverse this inflammatory process. Vitamin E also seems to play a role at 1,200 IU per day in creating a reduction in LDL oxidation.[128]

ALA is a physiological constituent of all cell membranes, and is a very potent antioxidant both in lipid and water-soluble areas of the body. It acts within the cell membrane, reacting with and neutralizing reactive oxygen species, including super oxide radical, singlet oxygen, hydrogen radicals, peroxide radicals, and hydrochloric acid.[129] It has been used successfully in Germany for the treatment of diabetic neuropathy.[130] Lipid peroxidation, which is free radical oxidation of the lipids, is increased in diabetic neuropathy and neutralized by alpha lipoic acid.

ALA also tends to prevent protein glycosylation oxidation, because it acts as an antioxidant and stimulates glucose uptake by the cells. ALA is actually approved for the treatment of diabetes in Germany for diabetic neuropathy. A high dose, about 600 mg per day, is needed to improve diabetic neuropathy.[131] ALA's primary effect is its antioxidant reaction. In summary, ALA improves blood sugar metabolism, reduces glycosylated protein, improves blood flow to peripheral nerves, and actually stimulates the regeneration of nerve fibers.[132,133,134,135]

Research has shown that ALA increases insulin sensitivity. In one study, seventy-four patients with Type-2 diabetes were randomly assigned to receive either a placebo or 600, 1,200, or 1,800 mg a day of ALA.[136] After four weeks, those receiving ALA supplements had statistically improved insulin sensitivity, and all three dosages of ALA were effective. Other studies have supported these findings. There is some suggestion that lipoic acid reactivates vitamins C and E when they have performed their antioxidant function, and works synergistically with niacin and thiamine, as well.

GAMMA LINOLENIC ACID (GLA)

GLA reportedly can reverse nerve damage to peripheral nerves in patients with diabetic neuropathy. GLA regulates insulin, and seems to protect against diabetic heart, eye, and kidney damage. GLA has an insulin-sparing activity that allows insulin to be more effective. Diets that are relatively high in linoleic acid appear to decrease the progression of microangiopathy in diabetics.[137] Excellent sources are evening primrose oil and flax seed oil.

Amino Acids

ACETYL-CARNITINE

Another nutrient, acetyl-carnitine, has been found to improve peripheral nerve function by normalizing nerve conduction. It seems to restore myoinositol levels that are depleted by sorbitol buildup.

L-ARGININE

Arginine is another nutrient that seems to boost insulin sensitivity, as well as cardiovascular function. One study showed that insulin sensitivity was increased by 34 percent with the use of arginine, versus 4 percent for a control group. Supplementation of L-arginine can be beneficial for individuals who have increased AGEs and free-radical induced aging that accompanies poor control of blood sugar and insulin. In a clinical study done at the University of Vienna Department of Medicine, 1 gram of L-arginine was given twice daily to individuals who had oxidative stress as a consequence of poor blood sugar control. Results of the study revealed significant reduction in oxidative stress reactions, and L-arginine supplementation also reduced the amount of damage to DNA and other important cellular materials, thereby reducing the processes associated with accelerated aging.[138]

Arginine seems to increase the neurotransmitter nitric oxide. Nitric oxide also dilates the blood vessels and helps to decrease blood pressure and increase blood flow. The more blood flow there is, the more circulation and healthier your tissues can be.

Minerals

A highly mineralized body is a more disease-resistant and anti-aging body. Minerals play an important role in the treatment of diabetes. Most diabetics suffer from mineral deficiencies beyond the depletion of minerals in the soil that affects everybody eating a nonsupplemented diet, due to mineral loss through polyuria (excessive urination). The key minerals that need to be replenished are vanadium, magnesium, chromium, calcium, zinc, manganese, and potassium. The beta cells of the pancreas are high in zinc, manganese, potassium, and chromium.

Planet Earth is made of minerals and our body is made of minerals. Minerals are catalysts for enzymatic reactions in the body. They activate the vitamins and all the enzymes. They activate all the organ structures, and in fact, are the basis of all the organ and cellular structures of the body. Minerals are the builders of the system, and they act as the frequency rates in the system. They are not necessarily the energy makers, however. The human body is composed entirely of minerals and water. The water molecule is the one that acts as a powerful solvent in the human system, bringing in nutrients and washing out waste particles. Without the essential minerals and trace minerals, we could not survive.

Of a total of ninety minerals, there are approximately twenty-three key minerals, including sixteen major minerals and seven minor, or trace, minerals. All key minerals are needed for the body to function at the highest level. They need to be replenished in the system through water-soluble ionic forms. As early as 1936, the U.S. Senate declared: "99 percent of the American people are deficient in minerals, and a marked deficiency in any one of the more important minerals actually results in disease." This is one of the most intelligent things that has ever come out of the U.S. Senate, and something that was beyond even the scope of medical school. Now, many years later, we are subjected to junk foods, foods that have been pesticided and herbicided, microwaved foods, and foods harvested from increasingly mineral-deficient soils. The situation has only gotten worse. This is why most everyone needs mineral supplementation, whether they are vegan or meat eater. Dr. Linus Pauling, winner of two Nobel prizes, said, "You can trace every sickness, every disease, and every ailment, ultimately, to a mineral deficiency." Research by Dr. Maynard Murray, author of *Sea Energy Agriculture,* shows that a highly mineralized body is a more disease-resistant and anti-aging body.

For a mineral to be utilized at the intracellular level, it must be *angstrom-size* (that is, so infinitesimal it is measured in units of angstroms), and these particles must be completely water-soluble. Only the ionic form, on angstrom-size level, of minerals can enter the cells and activate the proper DNA structures to actuate the guiding frequencies for the function of the body. An angstrom (named after Johan Angstrom) is one-thousandth of a micron, and one-millionth of a meter. The significance of this information is that almost all the mineral supplements on the market are larger than micron sizes. Now, it can get a little confusing, but think about it this way: Particles that are micron in size and larger will be absorbed by the blood, but they are too large to be absorbed intracellularly and inside the nucleus. These larger forms stay in the bloodstream, and eventually become deposited in various tissue locations. Angstrom-size particles travel through the cells, and if the body doesn't need them, it will simply discharge them with no buildup of the minerals to create potential toxicity in the tissues.

We observe that the roots of the plants are designed to break down the soil and utilize and absorb mineral particles, at angstrom-size— that's what they do. With the help of fulvic acid in the humus material, plants are able to take in these minerals, and break them down into angstrom-size particles, which they use. Once we understand that, we understand that the vegetables we eat transfer angstrom-size minerals from the soil to us via the plants. They do not absorb larger-size particles, because they cannot assimilate, them. Angstrom-size minerals are key to optimal mineral absorption. *It takes about twelve years for farmland to become deficient of angstrom-size trace minerals.* For this reason, traditionally, farmers would often move every twelve years.

Minerals of micron-size or larger can cause a variety of problems. The paradox, which is hard to understand, is that while the tissues are full of minerals in a sense, the cell is lacking in the angstrom-size minerals. This is one reason why we can use salt (Himalayan or Celtic sea salt) products for our bodies with amazing results, because they are in ionic angstrom-sizes. If salt isn't in the ionic form, we simply aren't able to absorb it into our bodies. Table salt (straight sodium chloride) is not available for use in the body and can cause a toxic buildup. This may also potentially apply to salts that are sun-dried. The process of sun drying, like many other forms of heating, causes electrons not to be available and the ions to form more tight bonds that make them inaccessible for assimilation. If salt creates a savory and watery feeling in the mouth, then it is still ionic. If it dries the mouth, this suggests that it has converted to the less assimilable covalent form. Although larger mineral forms or covalently bonded salt may help us initially on one level, eventually they have the potential of building up to toxic overload.

Paradoxically, one of the most effective ways to pull out these accumulated minerals is to provide the same mineral in angstrom-size. Angstrom-size minerals act as building blocks for the more than six thousand different enzymes needed for optimal function in our bodies. If we don't have the proper minerals for those enzymes to work in the particular organs where they are needed, we do not, in a sense, have the cellular building materials for repair and regeneration of our tissues. For example, in diabetes, because of all the refined foods we eat, we have created a deficiency of chromium because chromium is pulled out of our own tissues to help metabolize the refined foods, which no longer have the chromium needed to metabolize them. The long-term result is a deficiency in chromium. So when we are taking in lots of refined carbohydrates and need chromium to help metabolize the sugar and to make the insulin work correctly, we become chromium deficient. When we eat junk foods, or food from depleted soils and synthetic fertilizers, we really aren't able to metabolize the sugars and carbohydrates properly. This adds to a diabetic condition.

In essence, minerals take us to the very formation of life. All qualities of positive or negative health can be traced back to a lack of minerals. To get adequate mineralization, as we said, the minerals need to be in angstrom-size form—0.001 micron. They need to be attached to covalent hydrogen in the water, which will pull them inside the cell. It is at the intracellular level where the action happens. When the minerals reach the nucleus and mitochondria of the cell, there's a transmutation on the cellular level that activates the DNA. The nucleus and the mitochondria are both the energy centers and the creative centers of the cell. Mitochondria also have a particular form of DNA, which is different than nuclear DNA. The minerals activate the primordial DNA. These minerals activate electromagnetic communications both intracellularly and extracellularly that organize the system and communicate about what activities must be done. Some of the DNA frequencies are received in the cell wall.

In essence, we can say that the soil in the United States, and in most of the world, is overworked and underfed—and getting worse. This soil exhaustion creates exhausted and diseased plants, exhausted and diseased animals, and exhausted and diseased human beings.

The Tree of Life 21-Day+ Program employs several routes to remineralization: fresh organic plant foods eaten, juiced, and blended (including sea vegetables); superfood powder blends; and bioavailable mineral supplementation. Our means for getting nutrient-dense plant foods will be fully discussed in the recipe section, but here let us investigate key minerals that can help support and heal the pancreatic beta cells, improve insulin sensitivity, regulate blood glucose levels, and prevent or reverse diabetic complications.

VANADIUM

Vanadium is an important trace mineral in healing diabetes naturally. It seems to keep blood sugar from rising too high. It supports the absorption of blood sugar into the muscle system and protects against elevated cholesterol, particularly a buildup of cholesterol in the central nervous system. At the Tree of Life, we use vanadium frequently to help with insulin resistivity and Type-2 diabetes. Vanadium has been found to be helpful in protecting against diabetic cataracts and neuropathy.[139] It reduces gluconeogenesis and increases the development of glycogen deposits.[140] It seems to be associated with modest improvements in fasting glucose and hepatic insulin resistance. Clinical trials have found a significant decrease in insulin requirements in patients with insulin-dependent diabetes after vanadyl sulfate therapy. They have also noted a decrease in cholesterol levels for both IDDM and NIDDM. It has also been found to stimulate glucose uptake and metabolism that leads to glucose normalization. In some cases it helps to restore insulin production in diabetic rats.

Kelp and sea vegetables are good sources of vanadium.

MAGNESIUM

Magnesium depletion is commonly associated with both insulin-dependent (IDDM) and non-insulin-dependent diabetes mellitus (NIDDM), and is one of the most important minerals to replace. Between 25 percent and 38 percent of diabetics have been found to have decreased serum levels of magnesium (hypomagnesemia),[141] and supplementation may prevent some of the complications of diabetes such as retinopathy and heart disease.[142] One cause of the depletion may be increased urinary loss of magnesium as a result of the increased excretion of glucose that accompanies poorly controlled diabetes. Magnesium deficiency has been associated with insulin resistance. Intercellular depletion of magnesium has been found to be a common feature of insulin resistance. Research has also shown that a decrease in insulin sensitivity occurs with a magnesium deficiency.[143] There seems to be a clear association between the lowest consumption of dietary magnesium and the highest amount of insulin resistance in nondiabetic subjects.[144] Other research has noted that magnesium deficiency resulted in impaired insulin secretion, and magnesium replacement restores insulin secretion. Dietary magnesium supplements (400 mg/day) were found to improve glucose tolerance in elderly individuals.[145]

In two new studies, in both men and women, those who consumed the most magnesium in their diet were least likely to develop Type-2 diabetes, according to a report in the January 2006 issue of *Diabetes Care*.[146] Until now, very few large studies have directly examined the long-term effects of dietary magnesium on diabetes. Dr. Simin Liu of the Harvard Medical School and School of Public Health in Boston, said, "Our studies provided some direct evidence that greater intake of dietary magnesium may have a long-term protective effect on lowering diabetes risk."[147]

Diabetics often have low magnesium levels in their cells and blood, and some researchers believe that they might even have a defect in the metabolism of magnesium that exacerbates the disease. Even if you're not a diabetic, you're likely to suffer from insulin resistance if you're low in magnesium. One recent study found that normal, healthy adults developed a 25 percent greater insulin resistance on a magnesium-deficient diet.[148]

Magnesium is also very alkalizing to the body, and helps counter the tendency to acidity from a diabetogenic lifestyle and physiology. Its highest concentration is in leafy green vegetables, nuts, whole grains, unpolished rice, and wheat germ. Generally high-magnesium foods include apples, apricots, avocados, beet tops, berries, black walnuts, Brazil nuts, cabbage, coconuts, comfrey leaves, figs, dulse, endive, greens, spinach, rye, walnuts, watercress, and yellow corn.

Dosage: 400 mg/day. Also, diabetics should take at least 50 mg of vitamin B-6 per day, as the level of intracellular magnesium is dependent on vitamin B-6 intake. Without B-6, it is difficult for magnesium to readily enter the cell.

CALCIUM

Calcium is an alkalinizing mineral that helps neutralize the acidity of diabetes. It has not been well studied in relation to diabetes, but following the use of calcium as a supplement, a patient of mine had decreased fasting plasma insulin levels and a significant increase in insulin sensitivity.

ZINC

Zinc seems to be important for preventing insulin resistance, as a low zinc level seems to be associated with increased insulin resistance. It seems to be involved in almost all aspects of insulin metabolism, including synthesis, secretion, and utilization. Lower levels may affect the ability of the islet cells of the pancreas to produce and secrete insulin, particularly in Type-2 diabetes.[149] Zinc seems to have a protective effect against beta cell destruction as well as anti-viral effects. Increased urinary zinc excretion appears to contribute to the marginal zinc nutritional status that has been observed in diabetics,[150] and it needs supplementation for that reason. Zinc supplementation has been shown to improve insulin levels of both Type-1 and Type-2 diabetics.[151] Zinc also helps with wound healing, a phenomenon frequently observed in diabetics. Zinc deficiencies in diabetics are associated with excess free radical activity, and the increased oxidation of fats.[152] When fats become oxidized, they become more reactive and damaging to the heart, arteries, and other integral parts of the vascular system.

Foods that contain zinc include legumes, nuts (especially almonds), and seeds (particularly pumpkin and sunflower seeds).

POTASSIUM

Potassium helps reduce insulin resistance at post-receptor sites. It seems to improve insulin sensitivity and insulin secretion. For diabetics using insulin, the use of insulin therapy causes the loss of potassium. High potassium reduces the risk of heart disease, and lowers high blood pressure. A number of studies indicate that groups with relatively high dietary potassium intakes have lower blood pressures than comparable groups with relatively low potassium intakes.[153] Data on more than 17,000 adults who participated in the Third National Health and Nutritional Examination Survey (NHANES III) indicated that higher dietary potassium intakes were associated with significantly lower blood pressures.[154] The results of the Dietary Approaches to Stop Hypertension (DASH) trial provided further support for the beneficial effects of a potassium-rich diet on blood pressure.[155] Compared to a control diet providing only 3.5 servings per day of fruits and vegetables and 1,700 mg per day of potassium, consumption of a diet that included 8.5 servings per day of fruits and vegetables and 4,100 mg per day of potassium lowered blood pressure by an average of 2.8/1.1 mm Hg (systolic BP/diastolic BP) in people with normal blood pressure and by an average of 7.2/2.8 mm Hg in people with hypertension.

There is some danger with potassium excess, especially with diabetes and kidney disease. If someone is receiving a high potassium supplementation, kidney function should be periodically evaluated. Potassium is also alkalinizing.

Good food sources of potassium are prunes, tomatoes, artichoke, spinach, sunflower seeds, and almonds.

MANGANESE

Manganese is an important co-factor in many enzyme systems that are associated with blood sugar control, energy metabolism, and thyroid hormone function.[156,157] Guinea pig research showed that a deficiency of manganese resulted in diabetes and birth of offspring that developed pancreatic abnormalities. Most diabetics have about half the manganese levels of normal individuals, and urinary manganese excretion tended to be slightly higher in 185 diabetics compared to 185 nondiabetic controls.[158] A study of functional manganese status found the activity of the antioxidant enzyme, MnSOD, to be lower in the white blood cells of diabetics than in those of nondiabetic controls.[159]

Dosage: Not more than 30 mg per day.

CHROMIUM

Chromium is an essential nutrient for sugar and fat metabolism. Because chromium appears to enhance the action of insulin and chromium deficiency results in impaired glucose tolerance, chromium insufficiency has been hypothesized to be a contributing factor to the development of Type-2 diabetes.[160,161] Individuals with Type-2 diabetes have been found to have higher rates of urinary chromium loss than healthy individuals, especially those with diabetes of more than two years duration.[162]

In twelve of fifteen controlled studies of people with impaired glucose tolerance, chromium supplementation was found to improve some measure of glucose utilization or to have beneficial effects on blood lipid profiles.[163] Chromium used synergistically with biotin seems to work to improve beta cell function and enhance glucose uptake by both liver and muscle cells and inhibit excessive glucose production in the liver. About 25–30 percent of individuals with impaired glucose tolerance eventually develop Type-2 diabetes.[164]

In 1997, the results of a placebo-controlled trial conducted in China indicated that chromium supplementation might be beneficial in the treatment of Type-2 diabetes.[165] In the study, 180 participants took either a placebo, 200 mcg/day of chromium, or 1,000 mcg/day of chromium (both of the latter groups in the form of chromium picolinate). At the end of four months, blood glucose levels were 15–19 percent lower in those who took 1,000 mcg/day compared with those who took a placebo. Blood glucose levels in those who took 200 mcg/day did not differ significantly from those who took a placebo. Insulin levels were lower in those who took either 200 mcg/day or 1,000 mcg/day. Glycosylated hemoglobin levels, a measure of long-term control of blood glucose, were also lower in both chromium-supplemented groups, but they were lowest in the group taking 1,000 mcg/day.

Women with gestational diabetes whose diets were supplemented with 4 mcg of chromium per kilogram of body weight daily as chromium picolinate for eight weeks had decreased fasting blood glucose and insulin levels, compared with those who took a placebo.[166,167]

Dosage: Niacin-bound chromium is more bioavailable than chromium picolinate. A recent study at the University of California found that chromium polynicotinate was absorbed and retained up to 311 percent better than chromium picolinate and 672 percent better than chromium chloride. Generally, chromium supplementation at doses of about 200 mcg/day, in a variety of forms for two to three months have been found in studies to be beneficial.

Herbal and Natural Teas

Caffeine elevates blood sugar by stimulating and aggravating the adrenal glucose axis, causing imbalanced and elevated blood sugars, and therefore keeps imbalancing the attempt of the healing diabetic body to achieve a normal physiology. Caffeine is also a diuretic and creates dehydration, which is a tendency in diabetes because the body is trying to rid itself of excess blood sugar by urination (diuresis).

If you have pre-diabetes or diabetes, I suggest you not use caffeinated drinks such as black tea (containing 60 mg/cup caffeine), green tea (25–30 mg/cup), or even Yerba Mate (25 mg/cup). Do not drink coffees (100mg/cup caffeine), even if they are decaffeinated. Instead, consider the herbal teas and other teas made from natural plant sources.

STRINGBEAN POD

According to Paavo Airola in *How to Get Well,* stringbean pod tea is an excellent natural substitute for insulin and therefore extremely beneficial in diabetes. The skins of the pods of green beans are very rich in silica and certain hormone substances closely related to insulin. One cup of stringbean skin tea is equal to at least one unit of insulin.[168] At the Tree of Life we juice the whole stringbean in the juice aspect of the program.

A product called Beanpod Tea is an all-natural, mild, and pleasant tasting tea that is very beneficial for diabetics. This tea is a natural detox tea, detoxifying the pancreas and related organs. Beanpod Tea is composed of the pods of kidney, white, navy, great northern, and baby lima beans. Beanpod Tea contains the amino acids tyrosine, tryptophan, and arginine, plus the B vitamin choline and the enzyme betaine. Patience is the key word in the usage of this tea. Most people will not experience instant relief with the usage of this tea. Diabetics must drink Beanpod Tea on a regular basis for approximately three months in order to help normalize their blood sugar levels.[169]

KIDNEY BEAN

According to John Heinerman, kidney bean pods are effective in lowering elevated blood sugar levels. Since almost 16 pounds of pods would have to be consumed each day to have an effect, this works best as a tea. The pods should be picked before the beans inside ripen, and *fresh* pods are more effective than dried ones by 8 to 1.

Heinerman advises to bring 3 quarts of water to a boil, toss in five handfuls or coarsely cut kidney bean pods, and simmer uncovered for 3 hours. Strain and drink three-quarters of a quart each day with meals.[170]

DANDELION

It has been said that dandelions are nature's way of giving dignity to weeds. Dandelion is well-known for its beneficial effects on liver problems, including cirrhosis, jaundice, hepatitis, gallstone removal, and liver toxicity. Dr. David Peterson, a licensed, practicing medical herbalist in Great Britain, once wrote that the high insulin content of the root may be regarded as something "to prescribe for people with diabetes mellitus."

Heinerman suggests 3 capsules of dried root each day.[171]

Herbs

GYMNEMA

Gymnema sylvestre decreases glucose absorption from the intestines; it seems to regenerate the beta cells in the pancreas and improves insulin secretion, as well as increasing the permeability of cells so that they absorb more insulin. In the November 1999 *Journal of Endrocrinology,* School of BioMedical Sciences, King's College, London, researchers

S. J. Persaud and P. M. Jones reported, "Results confirming the stimulatory effects of gymnema sylvestre on insulin release indicate that this herb acts by increasing cell permeability."

Native to India, its Hindi name *gurmar* means "sugar destroyer," and it has been used for the treatment of diabetes for more than 2,000 years in that part of the world. Research on gymnema goes back to the 1930s. In one study, a water-soluble extract of gymnema leaf was administrated to twenty-seven Type-1 diabetics at a dose of 400 mg/day for approximately a year. The subjects' insulin requirements decreased by half. Average blood glucose dropped from 230 to 152 mg per milliliter. The HgbA1c levels decreased the first six to eight months but still remained above normal. Decreases in the amounts of glycosylated proteins, cholesterol, and triglycerides were also noted.[172] In another study, gymnema extract doubled the number of islets and beta cells in the pancreas, which supports the theory that it increases the insulin secretion by creating a regeneration of the pancreas.[173]

Considered one of the most powerful herbs for improving blood sugar status, gymnema has been shown to help normalize blood sugar and triglycerides, reduce sugar cravings, and decrease insulin needs. Other research has found that this herb causes a reduction in the activities of enzymes that are normally increased in diabetes such as glycogen phosphorylase, glyconeogenic enzymes, and sorbitol dehydrogenase. The researchers also found that the glycogen depletion in the liver and lipid accumulation in diabetic animals was reversed. In another study of Type-2 diabetics, twenty-two were given this herbal extract along with their own oral hypoglycemic drugs. All of these people had an improved blood sugar control. Twenty-one of the subjects were able to reduce their drug dosage significantly. Five were able to discontinue their medication and maintained blood sugar control with this herb alone.[174]

Dosage: The average dose per day in many of these studies was 400 mg.

CURCUMIN (TURMERIC)

Curcumin is a strong antioxidant, and has been associated with treating complications in diabetes. It inhibits oxidation—an internal rusting—because it protects against free radicals that are caused by the cross linkages and high sugar. So curcumin prevents free radical damage, reduces oxidative stress associated with diabetes, and helps to clean up metabolic waste.

Curcumin is a very good herb for the liver, which is affected in diabetes.

FENUGREEK

Fenugreek has been studied in India for the treatment of Type-1 and Type-2 diabetes.[175,176,177,178] Administration of 5 grams of powdered fenugreek seed (as a 2.5-g capsule twice daily) resulted in significant lowering of blood glucose (fasting and post-prandial) in non-insulin-dependent diabetics with and without coronary artery disease (CAD). In the diabetic patients with CAD, fenugreek also significantly lowered total cholesterol and triglyceride levels.[179] In another study, defatted fenugreek seed powder was given to insulin-dependent diabetes patients at 100 g daily in two divided doses over ten days. The treated group exhibited a 54 percent decrease in twenty-four-hour urine excretion of glucose, as well as a reduction in total cholesterol.[180] Fenugreek seeds are also 55 percent fiber, so they slow down the rapid absorption of glucose. Fenugreek normalizes glucose after meals and improves insulin response in the body, and it lowers total cholesterol and triglycerides.

CINNAMON

Cinnamon is a powerful herb for blood sugar control. Dr. Richard Anderson, in a study with the U.S. Department of Agriculture's Beltsville Human Nutrition Research Center, found that cinnamon can improve glucose metabolism in fat cells by twenty-fold.[181] Of the forty-nine herbs, spices, and medicinal plant extracts they studied on glucose utilization, they found that cinnamon was the most bioactive.[182] Cinnamon has a key substance called methyl hydroxy chalcon polymer (MHCP) that stimulates glucose uptake. Scientists at Iowa State University determined the polyphenols polymers in cinnamon are able to up-regulate the expression of genes involved in activating the cell membrane's insulin receptors, thus increasing glucose uptake and lowering blood glucose levels.[183] So cinnamon improves glucose intake by the cells, increases the effectiveness of insulin, and also increases the antibacterial, antiviral, and anti-fungal processes. In a study published in *Diabetes Care,* cinnamon was found to simultaneously reduce triglyceride levels, LDL cholesterol, and total cholesterol. Participants in three groups consumed 1, 3, or 6 grams of cinnamon daily. All three levels of cinnamon reduced mean fasting serum glucose levels by 18–29 percent. The 1-gram dose also reduced triglyceride levels by 18 percent, LDL cholesterol by 7 percent, and total cholesterol by 12 percent. Higher doses of cinnamon produced even greater reductions in triglycerides, LDL, and total cholesterol.[184]

Dosage: To achieve therapeutic effects similar to those in the studies above, you will need to eat 1/4 to 1 full teaspoon of powdered cinnamon a day. This is easy to do with smoothies, teas, and nut and seed mylks.

CAYENNE

Also known as the common chili pepper, this herb contains the element capsaicin, which alleviates nerve pain (neuropathy) associated with diabetes.

HOLY BASIL

Holy basil, known as the herb of Vishnu, is considered in India to be an adaptogen, improving immunity and generally strengthening the body. A significant placebo-controlled study published in the *Journal of Clinical Pharmacy and Therapeutics* showed a 17.6-percent reduction in blood sugar. It also normalizes triglyceride levels in the blood, lowers cholesterol, and decreases blood pressure and inflammation in mild to moderate cases of diabetes.

PARSLEY

Parsley is excellent for kidney support in diabetics.

BANABA

Banaba leaf, known for its high concentration of corosolic acid, acts as a natural insulin agent. In animal studies extracts of this herb created a significant decrease in blood glucose. It balances the blood sugar, transports blood sugar into our cells, and reduces the conversion of blood sugar into fats. It helps with weight loss and to decrease triglyceride levels. This herb helps transport blood sugar into our body cells. It also helps control carbohydrate cravings.

Aside from the banaba leaf, corosolic acid is found in Queens crepe myrtle. It is a promising blood sugar regulating herb. Studies in Japan have suggested that corosolic acid is an activator of glucose transport and decreases blood sugar. In one American study with ten Type-2 diabetics, the blood sugar dropped 31.9 percent after two weeks of 480 mcg of corosolic acid per day. Nondiabetics had no change in their blood sugar. Repeated studies have found approximately the same results.

SHILAJIT

> There is hardly any curable disease which cannot be controlled or cured with the aid of Shilajit.
>
> **VAID CHARAK (FIRST CENTURY A.D.)**

Shilajit in Sanskrit means "conqueror of mountains and destroyer of weakness." The herb comes from the rocks in the lower Himalayas and is the most important natural remedy of Ayurvedic medicine. Shilajit is an ancient herbomineral extract from the Himalayas; it improves glycogen stores in the liver, and has been shown to help reduce sugar in the urine, promote regeneration of the pancreatic beta cells, and reduce oxidative stress. It is not that well known, but we have used it for mineral replacement. The active principle of shilajit is fulvic acid, which improves the bioavailability of important trace minerals, and there is some feeling that it creates regeneration in the pancreatic cells. It is known as an adaptogen and should be taken mostly during the winter.

COCCINIA INDICA

Coccinia indica seems to have a blood glucose lowering effect that operates on the same mechanism as bitter melon.[185],[186]

GINGKO BILOBA

Gingko biloba has membrane-stabilizing flavones and anthocyanides, which seem to protect against retinopathy.[187]

AMERICAN GINSENG

A team of researchers at the University of Toronto medical facility at St. Michael's Hospital in Toronto used American ginseng (*Panax quinquefolius*) in the treatment of Type-2 diabetes.[188] The authors in an earlier study showed that 3 grams of American ginseng, either with or 40 minutes before a 25-gram oral glucose challenge, significantly reduced the blood glucose levels in Type-2 diabetes.[189]

Another study was done with ten Type-2 diabetics, six men and four women who had diabetes from two to twelve years. Seven were on antidiabetic drugs and three were on diet alone. Their average age was 63. The American ginseng showed a clear benefit, reducing the total postprandial glucose by 15–20 percent over the two-hour trial. All three dose levels that they used seemed to come out the same. A 3-gram dose of American ginseng taken two hours before the glucose challenge is just as effective as a much higher dose (25 grams), so we just need 3 grams three times a day. Also, American ginseng is a very good general adaptogen.

GOAT'S RUE

In medieval Europe, goat's rue (*Galega officinalis*) was traditionally used as a treatment for diabetes. Goat's rue contains guanidine, the herbal prototype for the pharmaceutical drug Metformin, which improves insulin sensitivity and is used to treat both Type-1 and Type-2 diabetes. Metformin has been claimed to be one of the best anti-aging drugs currently available. Goat's rue causes a long-lasting reduction of blood sugar in rats and an increase in carbohydrate tolerance. In one study, goat's rue extract lowered the blood sugar of diabetic rats by 32 percent.[190] Goat's rue extracts have increased glycogen levels in the liver and myocardium of both healthy and diabetic rabbits. In addition, this potent herb lowers blood sugar in both normal and diabetic humans.[191]

PTEROCARPUS

Pterocarpus marsupium balances glucose and lowers cholesterol. It was able to reverse the damage to pancreatic beta cells in different studies. This is quite impressive. Even more so, it also helps to counter the effect of insulin resistance, maintains blood sugar levels, restores insulin release from the pancreas, and in some cases, resulted in almost complete restoration of normal insulin secretion.

BILBERRY

Bilberry (*Vaccinium myrtillus*) has a long history of being used as a treatment for diabetes. Bilberry fruit contains flavonoids known as anthocyanidins, plant pigments that have excellent antioxidant properties. They scavenge damaging particles in the body known as free radicals, helping to prevent or reverse damage to cells. Antioxidants have been shown to help prevent a number of long-term illnesses such as heart disease, cancer, and the eye disorder called macular degeneration. Bilberry also contains vitamin C, another antioxidant.

Anthocyanidins found in bilberry fruit may also be useful for people with vision problems. During World War II, British fighter pilots reported improved nighttime vision after eating bilberry jam. Bilberry has also been suggested as a treatment for retinopathy (damage to the retina) in diabetics because anthocyanodins appear to help protect the retina. Bilberry has also been suggested as treatment to prevent cataracts.

Bilberry was also able to lower glucose by 26 percent in diabetic rats, and lowered triglycerides by 39 percent.[192] Bilberry has also been found to stabilize collagen[193] and decrease capillary permeability.[194] Increased capillary permeability, resulting in retinal hemorrhage with resultant abnormal collagen repair, is an underlying cause of diabetic retinopathy. Bilberry can decrease abnormal collagen formation and capillary permeability, thus helping prevent retinopathy.[195] In another study, fifty-four diabetic patients were treated with 500–600 mg per day of an extract for eight to thirty-three months. Almost total normalization of collagen polymers was achieved, as well as a 30 percent decrease in structural glycoprotein.[196]

Dosage: Prepare bilberry tea as an infusion, using one teaspoon of dried berries in 1 cup of water. Drink one cup per day. For blood glucose control, make a tea from 2/3 cup of leaves in 2 cups of water boiled for 25 minutes, and drink 2 cups daily.

MILK THISTLE

Milk thistle has been found to be beneficial in a wide range of liver disorders. Eighty-percent silymarin extracts of milk thistle (for example, a 200-mg capsule of milk thistle will have 160 mg of silymarin) have been found to have antioxidant and glucose-regulating properties. In a study at Monfalcone Hospital in Groiza, Italy, sixty insulin-dependent diabetics took either 600 mg of silymarin or a placebo for twelve months. After the first month, in which fasting glucose levels were elevated, fasting glucose declined by 9.5 percent and average daily glucose dropped 14.9 percent among the treated group. In addition, glucosuria (sugar in the urine), glycosylated hemoglobin levels, and insulin requirements declined significantly.[197]

Additional Supplements from the Program

VITALZYM X

There is some suggestion that Vitalzym X, and other high-potency proteolytic enzymes, create a lysis, or loosening or dissolution, of the fibrin plugs in the vascular system and helps reverse the general fibrosis scarring that goes on in the body. It helps specifically to deal with the inflammation we see in diabetes, particularly Type-1 but also Type-2, where the organs are inflamed and stressed and begin to scar. I believe it also prevents cross-linking going to polymerization.

DIGESTIVE ENZYMES

Digestive enzymes, according to our theory, help slowly to overcome the general enzyme deficiencies that are documented in diabetics. They do this by helping the body use less of its own enzyme power for digesting the foods so that these enzymes, by the law of adaptive secretion of enzymes theorized by Dr. Howell, will build up the depleted levels of amylase, lipase, and proteases in the system. Sometimes diabetics suffer from gastric paresis, which is a slowing of the emptying of the stomach associated with poor digestion. The general trend is that most people older than 45–50 have a progressive weakening digestion and are therefore not able to properly assimilate the nutrition in their food. This is why we also suggest the use of HCl supplementation to assist in the digestion of protein, assimilation of minerals, and B-12. In other words, digestive enzymes on many levels provide a tonic effect on the overall healing energy and capacity of the organism.

NATURAL CELLULAR DEFENSE (NCD)

Another important component of our supplement program is the use of NCD (Natural Cellular Defense), a liquid purified form of natural zeolite that safely chelates out heavy metals. Heavy metals, pesticides, herbicides, and a total of 70,000 chemicals are used commercially in the U.S., according to the EPA. Sixty-five thousand of these chemicals are considered hazardous to our health. The Environmental Defense Council reports that more than four billion pounds of toxic chemical are released into the environment each year. Although there is not a lot of data available, it does suggest that the heavy metals, especially arsenic, mercury, cadmium and lead, interfere with the specific function of insulin and the insulin receptors. Others, like fluorine in our water and a variety of pesticides and herbicides, are metabolic poisons that may further derange the already deranged metabolism of diabetics.

Since approximately 80 percent of Type-2 diabetics are overweight and most of these toxins are stored in the fat tissues, as people begin to lose weight these toxins are released into the bloodstream and lymph in higher concentrations. In our preliminary clinical research at the Tree of Life we have been able to measure the incidence of twenty-six toxins, including heavy metals, depleted uranium, and a variety of pesticides and herbicides. Usually people have all twenty-six that we check for. University research has shown that NCD is effective for removing heavy metals; when we combine it with our green juice fasting we have found a powerful synergy that greatly accelerates the removable of toxins and thus optimizes our ability to rapidly bring diabetics back to a healthy physiology. There have been some reports that the NCD also helps to decrease elevated blood sugar by directly absorbing it in its metallic structure and carrying it out of the system.

Lifestyle Habits

EXERCISE

In the case of insulin resistant or Type-2 diabetes, exercising regularly can mean the difference between pharmaceutical dependence and drug-free blood sugar control. Diabetics who exercise experience many levels of improvement, including enhanced insulin sensitivity, and therefore have less need for injecting insulin, improved glucose tolerance, reduced total cholesterol and triglycerides with increased HDL levels, and improved weight loss. The Diabetes Prevention Program (DPP) study, conducted in the U.S. from 1997 to 2001, showed that participants who lost 5–10 percent of their body weight, kept the pounds off if they did about half an hour a day of moderate exercise, cutting their risk of developing diabetes by 58 percent.[198] Some research suggests that exercise increases the number of insulin receptors in IDDM.[199]

In Type-1 diabetics, there needs to be a little bit of attention when exercising because exercise may create an immediate release of lactic acid and glucagons, which may increase the blood sugar level, especially for those whose blood sugar levels are above 250 mg. Another danger of exercise is that if you have very low glucose while on your insulin, your body may switch to fat to get energy, and this could result in ketoacidosis. For this reason, your blood sugar level should be checked before intense exercise. Another risk could be aggravating a cardiovascular condition, as well as ocular complications. Exercise in Type-2 diabetes usually lowers the blood glucose. For this reason before intense exercise Type-2 diabetics should take less insulin or less oral hypoglycemics. Once we make these cautions, we strongly recommend moderate exercise for all diabetics.

The best exercise in general is jumping on a high-quality rebounder for up to 16 minutes a day four to five times a week. Other cardiovascular exercises would include moderately fast walking, jogging, swimming, and so on. There is no need to make exercise a complicated procedure, but to find exercise that is enjoyable and that finds you feeling positively stimulated rather than exhausted.

REBOUNDING

Jumping on a rebounder, or mini-trampoline, is possibly the best and most fun cardiovascular and lymphatic stimulating exercise, requiring the least amount of time of any exercise system. It is my favorite aerobic and lymphatic stimulating exercise.

MUSCLE BUILDING

When you consider that muscle tissue is responsible for 80 percent of blood sugar uptake following a meal, it is easy to understand why every bit of extra muscle helps. Another important benefit of muscle tissue is that, unlike fat tissue, it constantly uses energy. The more muscle tissue you have, the higher your metabolic rate will be, because while you burn a certain amount of calories during exercise, your muscle tissue will continue to burn calories hours after you exercise.[200]

MEDITATION AND PRAYER

The Tree of Life 21-Day+ Program also includes training in meditation, as stress has been distinctly related to an increase in blood sugar secondary to an increase in epinephrine and corticosteroid secretion. This leads to an increase in insulin resistance. The value of meditation and yoga have been shown in such well-known programs as that of Dr. Dean Ornish, in which they were able to reverse atherosclerosis, as well as the large body of research linking meditation to general improvement in health, vitality, and longevity. It is interesting to note that researchers at the Medical University of South Carolina found that people with diabetes who regularly attend religious services had lower levels of C-reactive protein, an inflammatory risk factor for cardiovascular disease, the leading cause of death among diabetics.[201] On a deeper level, it has been my consistent observation that those who have some sort of spiritual connection increase their ability to heal. There is never enough food for the hungry soul, and meditation and prayer feed the hungry soul.

YOGA

In addition to meditation, we also teach Kali Ray TriYoga™, which is good for decreasing physical and mental stress. Yoga in general is another form of exercise, but has many more uses than just cardiovascular exercise. It is a total system that creates a flow of energy through the body, helps to heal the body, and stimulates the pancreas and other internal organs. Although there are certain traditional poses associated with the healing of diabetes, we prefer this system because not only does it include these diabetes-healing poses but the flowing system creates an energy that has a greater overall healing effect. In general, almost all forms of yoga provide a helpful tonic for the stimulation and healing of the internal organs such as the pancreas, liver, kidneys, and adrenals. Practiced regularly, yoga can help regulate blood glucose levels, reduce stress-hormone levels, and help with weight control. Find a knowledgeable and experienced yoga teacher in your local area who feels comfortable using yoga as a means for supporting the healing of your diabetes.

SKIN CARE

The most important thing about skin care is to be very observant of the skin condition of your feet, as that is the first place where the diabetic process manifests deterioration.

Alan Dattner, MD, a wholistic dermatologist based in New York City, recommends lotions that are high in omega-6 fatty acids, essential fats that diabetics don't produce well. Avoid glycolic acid and other strong fruit acids, as they are too harsh for the skin, warns Jeanette Jacqui, MD, a wholistic dermatologist in Phoenix, Arizona. Also too strong are alcohol, iodine, mercurochrome, salicylic acid, and benzoyl peroxide.[202]

ZERO POINT PROCESS

One of the most important parts of the program is the Zero Point course, a psycho-spiritual four-day training that helps people let go of their dysfunctional eating and lifestyle habits and let go of their desire and resistance to heal from diabetes and the Culture of Death, to which many diabetics, like the rest of our society, are addicted. This course also helps the diabetic let go of the allopathic myth that Type-2 diabetes is not curable and is a slow and steady downhill death march. During the course participants open up the doors to loving themselves in a deeper way, which of course helps to facilitate healing.

This course takes place in the second week of the 21-Day+ Program. In the Zero Point process, clients receive two of the most important gifts one can receive in any healing program: first, clearing negative thought forms usually associated with the shadow of the Culture of Death, which leads to the second, allowing you to love yourself and activating the belief of your power to heal yourself.

Chapter 4 Summary

The use of herbs, nutrients, and supplements is one of the ways to support and accelerate the overall return to a normal physiology from the dysfunctional aging process of diabetes. With all of these helpful additions to the healing process we must remember that there is only one thing that counts. The foundation for reversing diabetes is turning on the anti-aging genes, and turning off the expression of the diabetogenic genes. This profoundly and positively affects the protein, lipid, and carbohydrate metabolism in diabetes. As we turn off the diabetogenic process, and activate the healthy genes with the use of the Culture of Life anti-diabetogenic world cuisine, we create the conditions for a rapid reversal of the diabetogenic process. This is the centerpiece in our program of reactivating our healthy genetics and of the success in our program to reverse diabetes naturally. By its very nature it also helps those who are overweight to naturally and easily lose weight, because eating a live-food diet enables us to eat half as much as we do on a nutrient-poor standard American diet. This live-food diet is not one of deprivation but one that is satisfying, pleasurable, and nutritionally nurturing to our senses, as well as to our body and mind. It brings in a tremendous amount of live enzymes and electrical energy that improves the functioning of all cellular activities in the system. It brings in phytonutrients that further activate the anti-aging and anti-diabetic genetic effect. Generally, it improves all aspects of health. This is the key to the program, and everything else supports this foundation.

Once we have reached a certain level of repair and have returned to a normal healthy physiology, we do not need to use all these herbs and supplements. We also will move clients from a Phase 1.0 to a Phase 1.5 and often will stop the supplements after people have returned to and sustained a normal physiology for three to six months.

The delicious Culture of Life anti-diabetogenic cuisine at Phase 1.5 is, however, what we will always need to eat in order to maintain a healthy phenotypic expression, and live a new whole way that not only prevents the onset of diabetes but also creates a healthy body, mind, and joyous spirit. The Culture of Life plant-source-only, 80-percent raw food diet is the primary foundation of the program and the herbs and supplements are secondary foundations that accelerate and support the healing.

A most important key to the success of the program is its sustainability. My clinical results with the use of live foods and green juice fasting leave no doubt that we can rapidly and safely take people off insulin and oral hypoglycemics with very rapid returns to a healthy FBS. The key question that remains is the sustainability of living in the diet and lifestyle of the Culture of Life and not be swallowed again by the shadow of the Culture of Death, which is the predominant culture in the world today. It is this shadow of the Culture of Death in which diabetes is a pandemic symptom and our primary challenge here. Global warming is a similar symptom out of the shadow of the Culture of Death. The very life of the planet is at stake, but the world has been in denial and now, even admitting the problem, the world refuses to change its high CO_2-producing lifestyle while giving lip service to how important it is to do so. To a reasonable and scientific person it is apparent that a "moderate" solution takes us deeper into the shadow because it creates the feeling that we are doing something to significantly change what is happening, while in fact we are only dipping our toes in the water.

One advantage of the 21-Day+ Program is its rapid results, which make the point clearly that something can be immediately done to reverse the diabetic physiology back to normal. The power of the immediate results is overwhelming. This is not a compromised or "moderate" approach that slows the march to diabetic death. My observation is that it takes about two years to become firmly rooted in this Culture of Life diet and lifestyle. Included in our 21-Day+ Program is a one-year follow-up with a variety of support systems. A key understanding is the teaching that what the death culture euphemistically calls "moderation" actually kills. Moderation in this context kills because it reactivates the death sentence. There is an old Chinese saying that if you do not change the way you are going you will end up in the direction you are going. Moderation in this context does not change the way you are going and has not been shown to achieve the results it would have us believe it gives the illusion of attaining. This is why the ADA and most doctors say that diabetes is not curable or reversible because they are prescribing moderation, which simply does not work by their own admission. It is actually a path of *immoderation.*

The approach we are offering is prudent and one that brings immediate results. It succeeds in changing the way you are going and saves your life. That is true moderation, acknowledging the truth of a situation and doing what is appropriate to heal the situation. It is not living in the shadow of death and denial which we euphemistically call "moderation" to give ourselves the illusionary warm, fuzzy feeling that we are acting reasonably.

We believe that the ultimate long-term success of the program depends on the support system created through the Zero Point course, the new dietary training, and the one-year follow-up. Our goal is to create an organized study with at least 200 people total from both the U.S. and Israel with our attention on the percentage of people who are able to maintain a healthy physiology over a year's time.

In the third week of the 21-Day+ Program, there is training in how to prepare Phase 1.0 plant-source-only 80-100 percent live foods. This is a five-day course in which we like to include the family. The focus is to empower people in the fundamentals of the Phase 1.0 Culture of Life live-food plant-source-only cuisine. This will be covered in depth in the recipe section of this book.

For those who need ongoing work on losing weight, we offer a Juice Feasting program that can be continued at home until a client's weight returns to a normal healthy weight. This program was developed by my research assistant David Rainoshek, MA, based on his education from colleague John Rose, and helps to establish clients in the Culture of Life diet and lifestyle. The details of this are covered in Chapter 5.

In Chapter 5, we also cover the stabilizing and sustaining part of our program—helping people to fully integrate the Culture of Life into their personal lives at home. The happy continuation of this work goes on for one year with monthly check-ins to support people in staying in and celebrating the Culture of Life. It is during this time that we get HgbA1c readings every three months, and create the time and space for people to stabilize their new-found healthy and joyous physiology. We do not really consider that a person is healed from the consciousness and physiology of diabetes until he or she has had two consecutive HgbA1c tests with results in the normal range, and has a regular FBS of 70 to 85 on a regular basis without the use of any traditional diabetic medications.

CHAPTER 5

Happy Continuation: Living in the Culture of Life and Juice Feasting

You are not what you are, rather, what you are is what you can be. The most interesting thing about life is that you can become more than you were before. You can become stronger, wiser, and healthier than you ever dreamed possible. You can achieve your true potential. You can completely re-form your physical structure, your intelligence, your emotional poise, your spiritual power. This is about how to biologically transmute the lead of life into the white gold of glory.

DAVID WOLFE, *THE SUNFOOD DIET SUCCESS SYSTEM*

Breaking the four-minute mile of diabetes by reversing diabetes completely will require continued prudent action at home, after the 21-Day+ Program. By the time your blood sugar has reached nondiabetic levels, your cholesterol, triglycerides, and C-reactive protein levels most likely will have normalized. Your weight, depending on where you started, may not yet be optimal. Returning home, you will be taking with you the gift of non-fear and an enthusiastic and deep knowing that you have the ability to succeed in the next and perhaps most crucial step in this healing process of becoming a healthy human being—stabilizing in the Culture of Life anti-diabetogenic diet and lifestyle. You recognize that life does not have to be lived in a diabetogenic wasteland, that complications can be reversed, and that you can achieve a level of health that is well beyond what you have been experiencing for yourself.

For all of us, as we move into a healthy physiology, this positive state has an ascending effect on the higher levels of our being, right up through our mind, emotions, and spirit. Healing from years of diabetes and complications means that something that has taken up such a large space in our lives is now gone. Our own life potential opens up, and we expect more of ourselves, as will others who see what a vibrant example of humanity we have become. Any attachment we had to the diabetic that we were, and the diet and lifestyle of the Culture of Death in which we lived that created it, is in the process of transformation.

After the 21-Day+ Program in a protected environment in the shade of the Tree, you return home to familiar surroundings, and the next phase of your sustained healing begins. What you are about to learn is how to live in the Culture of Life *in your old world*. An immediate challenge is how to establish a physiology (cellular memory) that does not continue to ask for the familiar foods of the old culture that helped create diabetes. You will begin to learn how to respond to the compliments, questions, skepticism, and enthusiasm of friends and co-workers. It is good to allow time for the mind to adapt to your new healthy diet of plant-source, nutrient-dense foods. You will naturally become more conscious of how living in the Culture of Life colors every aspect of your new life.

Sustainable Diet, or a Fad?

All of this is much easier to implement than it seems. The biggest hurdle is not the physiological but psychological. As Walter Bagehot once remarked, "The pain of a new idea is one of the greatest pains in human nature.... Your favorite notions may be wrong, your firmest beliefs ill founded." And your favorite foods may be the root cause of your greatest pains! It's a fact of life that people find it easier to believe a lie they've heard a thousand times than a fact they've never heard before.

DANIEL P. REID, *THE TAO OF SEX, HEALTH, AND LONGEVITY*

Let us state that these are not passing fad diets: the Tree of Life 21-Day+ Program, the Culture of Life anti-diabetogenic diet (an organic, plant-source-only, and 80-100 percent live-food diet).

The history of eating a diet of plant foods, of abstaining from meat eating, of fasting and drinking plant juices, and using herbs to heal goes back possibly further than recorded history itself. Hippocrates, the father of medicine (460–357 BC) said, "He who does not know food, how can he understand the diseases of man?" We have read Genesis 1:29 about a plant-source diet. *The Ethics of Diet* by Howard Williams outlines an entire recorded history of abstaining from flesh-eating and returning to a natural diet, citing more than fifty major Western thinkers such as Hesiod (eighth century BC), Pythagorus (570–470 BC), Plato, Ovid, Seneca, Plutarch, Thomas More, Voltaire, Rousseau, Leonardo da Vinci, Schopenhauer, and Albert Einstein. A plant-source only diet is advocated by most every major world religious tradition, as illustrated in *Food for the Gods* by Rynn Berry. This reality is also concisely stated in the chapter "Vegetarianism in the World's Religions" in my book *Conscious Eating* and in *Spiritual Nutrition,* two books containing arguably the best scientifically documented case for a life-long vegan diet of live foods. We have seen evidence that a processed diet is a diabetogenic diet, and the Culture of Death way of eating and living creates far more suffering and sickness worldwide than just diabetes. It also bears repeating that the Culture of Life anti-diabetogenic cuisine, adopted globally as our true potential, would make enough food available for the people of the world to be fed seven times over at current agricultural production levels. Again, *this is no fad;* it is rooted deeply in our cultural, spiritual, and genetic heritage, and is truly a diet and lifestyle that significantly meet the needs of our times individually and collectively.

With one out of three children born today in the U.S. projected to develop diabetes, and the spiraling worldwide pandemic threatening the economies of nations, we need to have simple and serious solutions that are not simply palliative, but do the job effectively. As has been made abundantly clear, diet and lifestyle are the underling cause. We offer a serious and practical food and lifestyle solution to this reality. It might appear extreme, because conditions that have created diabetes are themselves ridiculously extreme. At the turn of the 1900s people ate about 15 pounds of sugar per year; now we eat up to 150 pounds per year. This is both ridiculous and extreme. It is so extreme that eating just 15 pounds per year, which is relatively normal, may itself seem radical. We must see clearly to prudence over the conventional denial thinking with such ineffective approaches as "moderation"—a term itself that gives an illusion of wisdom—in our decision to reverse diabetes. Consumption of 150 pounds of sugar per year (52 teaspoons per day) is an active Crime Against Wisdom.

Moderation Kills!

If your friend had been a smoker all of his or her life and looked to you for advice, would you tell them to cut down to only two cigarettes a day, or would you tell them to quit smoking all together? It's in this way that I'm telling you that moderation, even with the best intentions, sometimes makes it more difficult to succeed.

T. COLIN CAMPBELL, *THE CHINA STUDY*

Moderation? It's mediocrity, fear, and confusion in disguise. It's the devil's reasonable deception. It's the wobbling compromise that makes no one happy. Moderation is for the bland, the apologetic, for the fence sitters of the world afraid to take a stand to live or die. Moderation is lukewarm tea, the devil's own brew!

DAN MILLMAN, *THE WAY OF THE PEACEFUL WARRIOR*

Earlier in the book we learned about Caldwell B. Esselstyn, MD, at the Cleveland Clinic, as highlighted by T. Colin Campbell, PhD, in *The China Study*. Dr. Esselstyn's work proved that cardiovascular disease is a benign disease, and that reversing it completely is only possible when "everything in moderation" is left behind and a *prudent* diet of plant-source-only foods is applied. Diabetes, too, is a benign disease, and is therefore reversible when applying a Culture of Life cuisine and lifestyle. For many of us who are new to eating plant-source foods, this diet can *seem unusual until we get used to it.* As we move toward an organic, live-food diet, we also move from: low-nutrient to high-nutrient-dense foods; from the suffering of disease symptoms to their dissolution; dead food to vibrant, living food; maximum to minimum health care costs; below-average to above-average life span; millions dying of starvation to almost none; a translative diet of eating for comfort alone to a *transformative* diet of eating as a means and support for personal growth. Research and cultural data worldwide show that moving to a plant-source diet means the prevention and elimination of overweight, heart disease, diabetes, arthritis, hypertension, depression, and constipation, to name a few. It is a shift from an egocentric way of eating for oneself to a world-centric way of being as an Act of Love for all as well as oneself.

When it comes to prevention of disease, and particularly reversal of diabetes, the conventional understanding of moderation with its attractive appearance of intelligent balance, is anything but prudence and wisdom. I want to work with people who are determined to reverse *completely* their diabetic physiology and lifestyle back to a nondiabetic, Culture of Life existence of abundance. It has been said that a strong enough "why" can achieve any "how."

Once you recognize that as a benign disease, diabetes with all of its complications need not exist, a sense of determination will permeate your being, driving you toward a realization of a healthy physiology and lifestyle that is beyond what you may have ever imagined. This journey is an inner revolution, a mindset shift, from deprivation to abundance. You will pass through three main internal realizations as you shift into a Culture of Life anti-diabetogenic world cuisine:

1. I am not eating my standard, ego-centered diet anymore (Deprivation).
2. I am not eating my standard, ego-centered diet and I eat a Culture of Life World Cuisine (Transition).
3. I eat a Culture of Life World Cuisine and enjoy the pleasure of being healthy and free from diabetes (Abundance and Joy).

At first, you may perceive the changes in your life as deprivation, because the diabetogenic foods and lifestyle choices available are ubiquitous. Modern living will be a constant reminder to you that you have left the conventional paradigm of the Culture of Death. Your friends and family may also be an outward sign that you are in another mode of existence, and either applaud you, counsel you, or condemn you for it. The historical Buddha once said, "While a million people believe a lie, it is still a lie." The Roman stoic Lucius Seneca wrote in his essay, *On the Happy Life:*

> For it is dangerous to attach oneself to the crowd in front, and so long as each one of us is more willing to trust another than to judge

for himself, we never show any judgment in the matter of living, but always a blind trust, and a mistake that has been passed on from hand to hand finally involves us and works our destruction. It is the example of other people that is our undoing; let us merely separate ourselves from the crowd, and we shall be made whole.

Seneca was describing the importance of recognizing the power of the shadow of the Culture of Death, how we get entrapped in it and how to disentangle from it. Your life depends on understanding this. When you succeed, you naturally will be able to inspire others to also succeed in their healing. Although some friends may become distant, many new friends will come who see your light and want to be around it.

Inner Revolution

Revolution doesn't have to do with smashing something; it has to do with bringing something forth. If you spend all your time thinking about that which you are attacking, then you are negatively bound to it. You have to find the zeal in yourself and bring that out. That is what is given to you—one life to live. Marx teaches us to blame society for our frail-ties; Freud teaches us to blame our parents; astrology teaches us to blame the universe. The only place to look for blame is within: you didn't have the guts to bring up your full moon and live the life that was your potential.

JOSEPH CAMPBELL, *PATHWAYS TO BLISS*

Living in the Culture of Life requires a revolution involving an internal and external geographical reorientation. We have existed in a poor food environment for so many years and our choices in it have been making us sick and squashing our potential. We must claim excellent health for ourselves, regardless of the environment, the actions of others, or our past history.

Externally, we are looking at shifting out of conventional restaurants, and out of the center of the grocery store with its processed, adulterated foods, and into the farmer's markets, the co-ops, and the produce section of the grocery store. As pointed out in Chapter 2, buying cheap, calorie-rich, nutrient-poor processed foods in the center of the grocery store can add to the diabetogenic process. As you recall, Drewnowski found that a dollar could buy 1,200 calories of cookies or potato chips, but only 250 calories of carrots; that his dollar bought 875 calories of soda but only 170 calories of orange juice.[2] According to the USDA Economic Research Service, between 1982 and 1997, the cost increases for these (diabetogenic) foods were as follows: dairy products 47 percent; fats and oils 47 percent; meat, poultry, and fish 49 percent; sugar and sweets 52 percent. The cost increase for your Culture of Life anti-diabetogenic foods went up a staggering 93 percent, making eating a healthy diet the most costly thing at the register—but not in terms of your health. This economic reality of high-priced fresh foods is going to encourage you to frequent farmer's markets, co-ops, and locally grown foods where the costs are much lower for higher-quality foods because the prices are not controlled by agribusiness, which tends to push the high-calorie junk foods.

WHAT A DOLLAR SPENT ON FOOD PAID FOR IN 2000

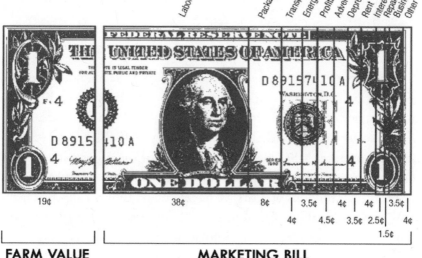

FARM VALUE   MARKETING BILL

Buying local food straight from the farmer puts you in closer touch with the origin of the food, cuts a significant portion of the time and money spent transporting and "selling" the food, saves you money, and places more dollars in the pocket of those who produce your food. Eating in the Culture of Life is about more than feeling good because of the food itself, but involves the impact of your dietary choices on the economic, agricultural, ecological, political, social, and cultural realities of your community, your nation, even the world.

This external shift creates a change *internally,* as we are reorienting ourselves to who we really are, and not what we have been told we are. The following quotes come from an agenda of economics, not conscious health concerns. Junk food, empty calories, low nutrient density, high-sugar content, and low-fiber foods can never be considered healthy by the wildest stretch of the imagination. It is time we stop listening to the economic propaganda of the Culture of Death:

> It is the position of the American Dietetic Association that all foods can fit into a healthful eating style.
>
> **ADA POSITION STATEMENT**

> All foods and beverages can fit into a healthy diet.
>
> **NATIONAL SOFT DRINK ASSOCIATION**

> Policies that declare foods "good" or "bad" are counterproductive.
>
> **GROCERY MANUFACTURERS OF AMERICA**

Despite the myths we have been told and sold, we are not by genetic constitution Mars-Bar eaters, Super-Big-Gulp drinkers, or Big-Mac snackers, nor do we suffer from a deficiency of these junk foods. None of us is suffering from a deficiency of Red Dye #40, Blue Lake #5, disodium inosinate, MSG, aspartame, or any of the other excitotoxins that have been deliberately placed in our foods to seduce and addict us for profit. For millions of years we have been physiologically, biochemically, and genetically designed to eat a diet of organic living plant foods. The overwhelming medical, sociological, and historical data corroborate this. Food is a fundamental way that we interface with our home the living planet, with our cultural ancestry (which existed *without diabetes*), and is a most important and subtle way we acknowledge an association or dissociation with who we truly are.

Living in the Culture of Life is an invitation to go on a journey to find ourselves and our God-given right to vibrant health. Commiting to a plant-source-only diet because we are determined to remove the causes of diabetes and ill health is an Act of Love and Consciousness. In this liberating and transformative process, we naturally move beyond the false identity that has been given us by advertising, including the so-called health education we have received in our schools that has been primarily financed by the dairy and meat industries so we will buy their products. Please know that this "education" we take as the truth is directly contrary to our 3.2 million years of history of the human diet (until 10,000 years ago), the message of the Bible of Genesis 1:29, and the biggest nutritional study ever done called the China Study involving 6,500 people and more than 8,000 statistically significant associations between various dietary factors and disease. All these sources, which are not motivated by profit, say the same thing: A plant-source-only diet is the healthiest and most natural diet for human beings. A plant-source diet helps us reconnect with our fundamental nature and helps heal the ecology of the planet. Because it does not create a hoarding of resources, it frees up the resources to feed everyone on the planet seven times over. In order to do this, we need the means, motivation, and support necessary to reclaim our most basic right of health and well-being.

Juice Feasting

To heal we need to move back through the Seven Stages of Disease and push the reset button on our physiology. This process may take longer than three weeks, as the precious (and not-so-precious) burdens may have taken many years to develop, especially obesity. For many of us, diabetes means a hand-in-hand compromise of our health at multiple levels over many years. We are well aware of the complications and associated conditions: cardiovascular disease (the cause of 80 percent of deaths in people with diabetes),[2] Syndrome X, hypertension, obesity, impotence, nephropathy (kidney disease), retinopathy (eye disease), neuropathy (nerve disease), infections, liver damage, gallstones, stroke, chronic pain, depression, and candida. For the majority of these health challenges, the underlying cause, and reversing mechanism, is found in diet and lifestyle. Fortunately, healing with prudent action takes a small fraction of the time it took to develop our health challenges. Depending on the condition, we course back through time about 80–120 days for each day that we Juice Feast.

Juice Feasting is a special application of nutritional healing, especially for those who are obese, that is based on the science behind many millennia of water fasting and more than 100 years of juice fasting. As the name implies, you are drinking a *lot of juice*—1 to 1.5 gallons of fresh, green, low-glycemic, organic, living juice each day. This amount of juice maintains a high metabolism, feeds the body the calories required for the day, and thus enables one to Juice Feast for 30–92 days, depending on the extent of one's health challenges. We also include superfoods and supplements during Juice Feasting as well as exercise (including weight training). These additions give a significant advantage in terms of remineralizing, rebuilding, and generally renourishing the body after so many years of diabetogenicity. The superfood concentrates help shift the body to a rebuilding, alkalizing physiology.

Pushing the Reset Button

The diabetogenic diet and lifestyle you knew in the past has created a mental and cellular memory that has covered up who you really are. With the 21-Day+ Program you have pushed the reset button and Juice Feasting keeps pushing it until you stabilize at an optimal weight and healthy physiology. It is an excellent way to reset your cellular memory, because during the Feast you are drinking the foods that you will be eating afterwards to maintain health and remain diabetes-free for the rest of your life. By drinking 12–15 pounds of juiced organic produce each day, you significantly rebuild the body with the best food possible. As you move into eating a low-glycemic diet of living foods, your whole being will ask for more of this healing and nourishing food *because you recognize it at every level as good.* Juice Feasting is exciting in that it provides excellent training at the cellular and mental levels in what to eat—and how good you can feel *when* you eat and for hours afterwards The best part is, this training occurs *while you are in the cleansing process.*

Four Aims of Juice Feasting–Cleanse, Rebuild, Rehydrate, Alkalize

As we learned from the Seven Stages of Disease, our two main underlying causes of diabetes are toxemia and inflammation. In the four aims of Juice Feasting, toxemia and inflammation are addressed by cleansing, rebuilding, rehydrating, and alkalizing. Juice Feasting also reverses another significant and common problem from our calorie-rich, nutrient-poor Western diet: nutrient deficiencies.

CLEANSE

Cleansing means weight reduction, but there are many components of weight, not just the fat around our mid-section. We have heavy-metal toxicity; uneliminated waste matter in our blood, lymph, cells, intestinal tract, and colon; toxic buildup in our organs, such as arterial plaque in our heart, calcifications in our kidneys, and stones in our liver and gallbladder; and many of us have edema, or excess water weight from the body trying to hold toxins in solution to protect the tissues. While this is not explicitly a weight loss program, Juice Feasting will accelerate your coming back in a natural way to a normal weight and eliminate one of the major co-factors in diabetes, obesity.

In order to remove all of these components of weight, we are employing several keys: physiological rest and compensation through the drinking of fresh juices; and support of the organs of elimination with personal hygiene, supplements, and exercise.

Physiological rest: Juice Feasting is a nutrient-dense, living, low-glycemic diet of liquids and superfood concentrates; it is not an extended juice fast. This is nutrition that is bioavailable with a very low amount of energy expenditure to assimilate. Russian research suggests that we use about one-third of our available energy to digest our foods; that is why people tend to fall asleep when they overeat. We require a lot of energy to digest cooked, processed, dehydrated foods, and even more so when these foods are overly constipating, as is the case with most processed, low-fiber foods. Before your body can access the nutrition from your food through the wall of the small intestine, it must be in a liquid state. In a general sense, the more food one eats, the more work must be performed by the organs making up these systems. Juice Feasting provides physiological rest for the digestive, glandular, circulatory, respiratory, and nervous systems by providing ample nutrition on all accounts, but in a form that is easy to digest. The metaphor here is your job at work. The boss tells you to go home for 30–92 days, and your paycheck is about to be doubled. After sitting around the house for a little while, you decide that it is time to do some cleaning, remodeling, and repainting after some neglect of your domicile. You are going to go through old photos, journals, and childhood memorabilia as well, and reorganize or discard some. This is Juice Feasting: time and space to clean and rebuild, with more money (nutrient-dense, bioavailable nutrition from 12–15 pounds of juiced produce each day, plus superfood concentrates) and energy. In other words, Juice Feasting is a superfood liquid diet that energizes and builds while you are continuing your normal home and work responsibilities.

Physiological compensation: "Energy saved in one department may be expended in another." As Juice Feasting coach John Rose has said in many public talks over the years:

> When we give our bodies a "solid food vacation" by only drinking freshly made juices, the energy that would have been used to convert the solid food into liquid is then redirected or re-channeled to the elimination cycle. Even though no solid food is going in, there

will be massive amounts of uneliminated waste matter coming out through the bowel. Once our colon, which is our major channel of elimination, begins to free itself from its toxic load, then every cell in our bodies will start dumping out its accumulated waste matter into our system to be eliminated.

Supporting the organs of elimination: This waste matter coming forth from all over your body must be shown the exit door in a timely manner. Otherwise you get a buildup of toxins leading to cleansing reactions and healing crises, which appear as headaches, muscle or joint pain, skin eruptions, emotional imbalance, fever, and so on. Practices are designed into Juice Feasting to move toxins out quickly through support of the organs of elimination (lymph, blood, skin, liver, kidney, and bowel), thus reducing or eliminating the discomfort that can be associated with cleansing and healing.

Personal hygiene: Enemas and colonics are often helpful. Most of the toxins you release are going to come through your bowel. You are well advised to use an enema each morning for the first 14–21 days of a Juice Feast, as this is the time that the majority of the significant cleansing occurs. Enema kits are available at most drug stores; we suggest you purchase one that is multi-use, not the single-use variety that does not hold enough liquid, is inefficient, and wasteful in its throw-away design. Colonics may be of benefit as well, as a colonic employs a deeper cleansing action with more water. Please consult your health professional or Tree of Life counselor about the appropriateness of this excellent method for moving out old matter, particularly if you are overweight and have been constipated for many years. Generally we do not recommend more than three colonics in a week over a long period of time, as they weaken the downward energy (*apana*).

Skin brushing: The skin is one of the five main elimination channels of the body, throwing off up to one pound of toxic material each day in the form of perspiration and dead skin. The skin has been called the third kidney because of its ability to rid the body of toxic waste material. Skin brushing moves lymphatic fluid under the skin, and involves using a natural-bristle brush with a long handle. The whole body (except the face) should be brushed before your morning shower. It takes two to three minutes to do this. At first, you will see something powdery coming off your skin as you brush. According to Dr. Bernard Jensen, "these are crystals of uric acid and other dried waste products that came *out* with the perspiration." Jensen continues:

> Always brush the skin when it is dry, and never expose the brush to water. Although the bristles may seem a bit stiff at first, this is because the brush is new and your skin is not yet used to the brushing. If you find the brush is too stiff, you may, just once, hold the bristles in hot water for no longer than one minute and no deeper than one-half inch. This will soften the bristles a little. However, it will not be long before you desire a stiffer brush! Your skin will love you for brushing it regularly, and you will love the way your skin feels and looks, too.[3]

The brushing motion is circular and from the feet and hands toward the heart. The skin needs to be brushed with enough pressure to create a comfortable pink color to the skin.

Hot/cool treatment: This is easy, and goes back for thousands of years. If you have ever been to a Japanese spa or to a sauna, you will experience the use of hot and cold to invigorate and help the body to cleanse. What you are achieving with the transition from hot to cold is a movement of lymphatic fluid and blood to the surface of the skin with heat, then toward the center of the body with cold, back again to the surface with heat, and so on. The way to do this at home is in the shower. Stand in the hot water for 5–8 minutes until you are nice and warm, and have rinsed off. Then begin to crank the water back toward cool for about one minute, then to hot for one minute, and so forth about seven times, ending on cool water. This will invigorate you first thing in the morning, and do wonders for helping the lymphatic fluid in your body to move, thus improving the elimination of old wastes from your system.

Supplements/cleanses: Juice Feasting employs zeolite, or Natural Cellular Defense (discussed in Chapter 4) for the removal of environmental toxins. A moderate kidney-liver-gallbladder cleanse is accomplished with 2–4 cups daily of Royal Break-Stone Tea, or for a more time-intensive and comprehensive addition, the Tree of Life has available a liver-gallbladder-parasite-fluke cleanse. See the Juice Feasting timeline below.

Exercise: We know the benefits of exercise for diabetics. During your Juice Feast, if movement is difficult, begin with just practicing a light yoga routine. This means simple stretches just to loosen up and move your body. Then shift into strolling outside, and begin walking longer distances, up to 30 minutes. This will do nicely for the first 30–45 days of a Juice Feast. When the body is in a state of cleansing, it is best to conserve most of your energy to build the vital force in order to stimulate cellular detox, but moderate exercise that moves the lymph and blood, and that leaves the body stimulated but not exhausted, is excellent. Don't overtax your body with activity. After 45–60 days, if you are continuing to Juice Feast, your coach may advise you to begin weight training, as your body is now in a state of rebuilding as much or more than a state of cleansing. The possibility of weight training is new to the world of cleansing technologies, and is made possible by Juice Feasting—drinking sufficient quantities of green vegetable juice to provide the body with the nutrient-dense building blocks necessary to build lean body mass. Everyone is unique, so you may have a need to increase the amount of juices or nutrient-dense superfoods to provide the calories and macronutrients required for this kind of building program. At this stage you will be sensitive enough to know how to make the adjustments.

REBUILD

Our body replaces its tissues and cells every one to seven years. This wide range of time depends on physiology, and varies with the sources we read.

Muscles get replaced every 6 months to 3 years. The pancreas replaces every 5–12 months. The liver replaces every 3 months. Our bones replace every 8 months to 4 years. Red blood cells replace every 90–120 days. The intestinal lining replaces every 5–30 days.

This is excellent news, and underlies the quote by Wolfe at the opening of this chapter, that you are not what you are, rather, what you are is what you can be. You have the opportunity to completely re-form your physical structure to its highest genetic potential. A healthy body helps support your optimal emotional balance, highest intelligence, and increased spiritual awareness. A Juice Feast of 92 days allows ample time for rebuilding to occur, using green vegetable juices made in a Vitamix with a nut mylk bag or in a press-style juicer such as a Green Star.

Green vegetable juices: On a Juice Feast we drink the juice from 2 pounds of *leafy* greens each day, which means that we hold greens in high regard, and as a necessity in any healing program. It took me (David Rainoshek) three years of eating a plant-based diet before I could look at a bowl of greens, or look at a glass of green vegetable juice and find my immediate response, "that's a muscle-building food," instead of seeing it as Oscar the Grouch in a can. Leafy greens are approximately 30 percent protein (amino acids, the building blocks of protein). I have had MDs argue this point with me, disagreeing that greens are so high in protein, until they see the data. We have all been socialized and taught to see greens—and vegetables in general—as sides to the "main course." If your main course is not plant foods, then you are on the main course to all manner of Western dis-eases.

What makes greens such an amazing food that we juice 2 pounds a day on a Juice Feast? According to David Wolfe in *Eating for Beauty:*

> Green leaves are the best source of alkaline minerals, contain the best fiber, have many calming, anti-stress properties, and are the best source of chlorophyll. Chlorophyll is a blood-builder and one of nature's greatest healers. Green, leafy foods are the most abundant foods on earth. In July 1940, a comprehensive study, reported

by Dr. Benjamin Gurskin, director of experimental pathology at Temple University, in the *American Journal of Surgery,* focused on 1,200 patients treated with chlorophyll. On the power of chlorophyll, Gurskin wrote: 'It is interesting to note there is not a single case recorded in which improvement or cure has not taken place.' In 1950, Dr. Howard Westcott found that just 100 milligrams of chlorophyll in the diet neutralized bad breath, body odor, menstrual odors, and foul-smelling urine and stools.

Nutrient density: Greens and superfood algaes are our most nutrient-dense foods. Nutrient density has several meanings. First, nutrient density is defined as a ratio of nutrient content (in grams) to the total energy content (in kilocalories or joules). Nutrient-dense food is opposite to energy-dense food (also called "empty calorie" food). According to the *Dietary Guidelines for Americans 2005,* nutrient-dense foods are those foods that provide the highest amounts of vitamins, minerals, enzymes, and phytonutrients per calorie.[4] For example, superfood algaes and vegetables are considered most nutrient-dense. Products containing added sugars, saturated fats, and alcohol are considered nutrient-poor. Therefore, when you eat nutrient-poor foods, you eat more food to get an equivalent amount of nutrition. Second, nutrient density is defined as a ratio of food energy from carbohydrate, protein, or fat to the total food energy. To calculate nutrient density (in percent), divide the number of calories or joules from one particular nutrient by the total number of calories or joules in the given food, and then multiply this by 100. Third, nutrient density is understood as the ratio of the nutrient composition of a given food to the nutrient requirements of the human body. Therefore, the most nutrient-dense food is the food that delivers the most nearly complete nutritional package.

Dr. Joel Fuhrman, bestselling author of *Eat to Live,* has created an excellent chart on the nutrient density calculations of various foods. It is reproduced here.

NUTRIENT DENSITY CHART

Kale	1000	Cantaloupe	120	Banana	36
Collards	916	Apple	91	Walnuts	35
Spinach	886	Peach	88	Almonds	33
Bok choy	839	Kidney beans	84	Chicken breast	32
Romaine lettuce	462	Green peas	84	Low-fat yogurt	31
Boston lettuce	412	Sweet potato	81	Apple juice	30
Broccoli	395	Soybeans	74	Egg	29
Artichoke	352	Tofu	69	Feta cheese	25
Cabbage	344	Mango	61	Whole wheat bread	25
Green peppers	310	Cucumber	59	Whole milk	23
Carrots	288	Oatmeal	55	White pasta	22
Asparagus	280	White potato	53	White bread	21
Strawberry	254	Brown rice	49	Peanut butter	21
Cauliflower	269	Salmon	48	Swiss cheese	18
Tomato	197	Shrimp	46	Ground beef	17
Cherries	197	Skim milk	43	Potato chips	13
Blueberries	155	Grapes	40	Vanilla ice cream	6
Iceburg lettuce	132	Corn	37	Olive oil	2
Orange	130	Avocado	36	Cola	0.6

Figure 1: Nutrient Density Chart (Source: Dr. Joel Fuhrman)

The first six nutrient-dense foods listed are all juiceables that one can use during Juice Feasting to rebuild every tissue in the body. How does this healing and rebuilding occur in terms of our health challenges? Consider Hering's Law of Cure. Constantine Hering was considered the "father of American homeopathy," and his Law of Cure states:

> We heal from the top down;
> We heal from the inside out;

We heal in the reverse order in which we took on our health challenges.

Therefore, we first see the accelerated healing effects of a Juice Feast in a person's face. Also, we can find in any cleansing program that things come to the surface of the skin, or our breath stinks, or our bowel movements are temporarily putrid. All of this is healing from the inside out. Finally, we heal in the reverse order that we took on our health challenges, meaning that a cut will heal in a few days, but the diabetic complications a person has developed and suffered with for decades will take a few weeks or months—still not bad considering how long many health challenges have taken to manifest.

REHYDRATE

The human adult body is approximately two-thirds water—50 percent of our body weight. In utero, the fetus body is 90 percent water, and an infant's body is 75–80 percent water. If we don't hydrate appropriately with H_2O, our water content may drop as low as 50 percent with age. Water is one of the main components of other compounds: Fat is 20 percent water, blood is 80 percent water, bone 25 percent, kidneys 80 percent, liver 70 percent, muscles 75 percent, skin 70 percent, and the brain 85 percent. This is very important when you realize that 85 percent of the brain is water, and when the brain starts to dehydrate, the neurons dehydrate and shrink. This is a significant contributor to senility.

Water acts as a universal solvent and anti-oxidant, and that is partly how it produces life on the planet. Water's ability to act as a solvent is what makes nutrition work for all living substances. Plants absorb nutrients when they are watered, just like water dissolves nutrients so they can enter our bloodstream. This is basic information, but it becomes clearer, as research has shown, that water acts as a medium that transfers and relays the tiny frequencies of information of DNA from one cell to another. If our water is polluted, meaning that what is entering our body is polluted with a set of negative frequencies, such as pesticides and herbicides, the water can't effectively relay accurate intracellular and extracellular information. If we are consuming water that is contaminated, it not only brings in poisons but it blocks adequate frequency information extracellularly and intracellularly to and from the DNA.

Water, acting as the solvent, has an electrical and mineral content that helps to regulate all the functions in the body. This is disrupted by dehydration and toxic wastes, which block the information transfer. This disturbance causes a distinct loss of electrical flow and breakdown of the cellular reactions. Dehydration also creates a buildup of extracellular acidity and toxemia, which greatly impairs the electrical energy differentiation between the cells. Because of this, it disorders the intra- and extracellular gradient. Toxemia and extracellular acidity leads to oxygen starvation, damages the DNA, and accelerates aging. It increases free-radical damage and the extracellular acidity blocks the flow of hydrogen into the cells.

It is important to understand what we call the symptoms of dehydration. One is dyspepsia, or stomach pain. This results because the cells in the lining of the stomach need to be hydrated and flushed between meals to get rid of acids and to develop a certain level of alkalinity When we are dehydrated, or we don't drink before meals, we actually cause a thinning of the stomach cell membrane buffer zone and it does not adequately protect our stomachs from the acidity that is naturally secreted. Another symptom of dehydration is rheumatoid pain, or arthritic pain, which has to do with any sort of joint pain because the joints are lubricated by water. The water creates a small film of water that helps lubricate the interface of the joint. With dehydration this lubricating film of water evaporates and the joints rub right on each other. Back pain, particularly lower back pain, and sciatica are often the result of the intervertebral discs becoming dehydrated. These discs normally create a space cushion between the vertebrae by virtue of how much water they can hold. When the discs are dehydrated, 75 percent of the upper body weight that they cushion against begins to bear down on the intervertebral spaces and put pressure on the intervertebral nerves. This often causes muscle spasms. Usually a few days after we rehydrate, the pressure on the nerves begins to alleviate. Relief from sciatic pain, in fact, may happen within an hour of rehydrating. Heart pain, or angina, is another symptom. When the body is dehydrated, the blood flow to the heart is reduced. Headaches, from toxic buildup and contracted blood vessels, are another symptom, along with dry tongue and constipation. One of the main causes of death in airplanes is dehydration, which causes clots in the legs, which then can migrate to the lungs as pulmonary embolisms.

It is estimated by some scientific sources that 75 percent of Americans are chronically dehydrated. In 37 percent of Americans, the thirst mechanism is so weak from the dehydration that it is mistaken for hunger. In fact, one of the best ways to lose weight is to drink water when you are hungry. One glass of water at bedtime can shut down midnight hunger pangs for close to 100 percent of dieters. This both treats the dehydration and gets to the cause of excess appetite, or mistaking the thirst mechanism for hunger. The disruption of the metabolic system in the body is so significant when we become dehydrated that even with mild dehydration, the metabolism will slow down as much as 3 percent. Dehydration is probably the number one trigger of fatigue in the daytime. A 2-percent drop in body water can so significantly dehydrate the neurons and the passage of neurotransmitters in brain function that we can become fuzzy-headed, develop short-term memory difficulties, have trouble with basic math, and lose focus on the computer screen. This is with only a 2-percent drop. A glass of water can significantly reverse some of the process of dehydration. A study at the University of Washington showed that drinking five glasses of water a day decreases the risk of colon cancer by 35 percent, the risk of breast cancer by 79 percent, and the risk of bladder cancer by 50 percent. This is a significant statement about the importance of water. Dehydration is something that may happen with age, so one of the main anti-aging treatments is drinking adequate water—about a half gallon (64 ounces) per day for a 150-pound person. On a Juice Feast, we drink 1-plus gallons of juice filtered through plants, which is one of our most precious and hydrating water sources.

ALKALIZE

We are constantly generating acidic waste products of metabolism that must be neutralized or excreted in some way if life is to be possible. Humans, therefore, need a constant supply of alkaline food to neutralize this ongoing acid generation. Our very life and health depend on the body's physiological power to maintain the stability of blood pH at approximately 7.46, through a process called *homeostasis*. At this slightly alkaline pH the chemical processes of the body function most efficiently and all waste products are rapidly eliminated.

The normal pH for all the tissues and fluids in the body, except the stomach, is alkaline. For example, the digestive secretions from the liver and liver bile range between 7.1 and 8.5. Bile from the gallbladder ranges from 5.0 to 7.7. If any of these pH systems are not at the optimal pH range, the digestive and metabolic enzymes in those areas and organs will function sub-optimally and we will suffer from decreased health. With the exception of the blood, all of these systems have a wide range of pH, in part so they can shift pH to maintain a balance of the blood pH. In the author's thirty-five years of experience, the healthiest blood pH is between the narrow range of 7.42 and 7.50. It is in this range that the cells operate most efficiently, especially for the brain cells. Being too alkaline can throw off body and brain function as much as being too acidic can. We focus on acidity because most people are too acidic in their blood, but we need to be mindful of both directions. The optimal urine pH for the first urine of the morning (which is the most accurate) is 6.4 to 6.8. However, if too much acidic food is eaten and the body, blood, and urine become acidic instead of alkaline, then the spleen, liver, heart, and kidneys, which are the blood-purifying organs, become overworked and ultimately weakened and susceptible to disease. Then the waste poisons can no longer be properly eliminated, and instead collect in the joints, causing arthritis and/or gout. Or they seek elimination through the skin, causing eczema, acne, sores, and boils. The condition of acidity thus may be a contributing factor to many different diseases, including piles, cancer, kidney and liver trouble, gallstones and gall bladder infections, impotency, high blood pressure and heart disease, strokes, asthma, and allergies. If the morning urine is consistently above 7.2, it is highly suggestive that the blood is too alkaline. Typical symptoms of excess alkalinity are muscle spasms, cramps, hyperreactivity, spaciness, a sense of ungroundedness, and mental imbalance.

The Culture of Death diet and lifestyle are themselves acid forming—they rob the body of alkalinizing foods and their minerals. The biggest offenders are animal foods, soft drinks, alcohol, medical drugs, and stress. To remedy the inability of the body to maintain proper acid-alkaline balance, and thus support the resolution of many diseases, it is important to increase in the diet the amount of plant-source foods that provide alkaline minerals such as organic sodium, magnesium, calcium, and potassium. This is accomplished in a very efficient manner while Juice Feasting, given the 12–15 pounds of produce we consume through alkalinizing fresh green vegetable juices each day, including one head of celery (organic sodium) and approximately 2 pounds of leafy greens.

Juice Feasting Timeline and Daily Schedule

Our timeline gives an "on-balance" view of what we are doing at each point during a Juice Feast for the further healing of a diabetic or post-diabetic physiology. Items that will create a need for adjustment of this chart are:

- The guidance of your health professional
- How long you are to Juice Feast
- Your glycemic index requirements
- Health challenges
- Affordability
- Allergies
- Physical stamina and abilities

DAYS OF THE FEAST	1–10	10–20	20–30	30–40	40–50	50–60	60–70	70–80	80–92
Fresh organic green vegetable juice (4-plus quarts/day)									
Herbal teas									
Hemp oil or flax seed oil (1–2 tablespoons/day)									
Kelp granules (¼ teaspoon/day)									
Bee pollen granules (1 tablespoon/day)									
Green superfood powder blend (1–2 tablespoons/day)									
MSM (1–3 tablespoons/day)									
Vitalzym (3–5 caps, 3 times/day)									
Natural Cellular Defense (NCD) (15 drops, 4 times/day)									
Chlorella/spirulina (1 tablespoon/day)									
E-3 Live (1–3 tablespoons/day)									
Nano B complex (½ teaspoon twice/day)									
Herbal and mineral supplements	As suggested by your health professional								

DAYS OF THE FEAST	1–10	10–20	20–30	30–40	40–50	50–60	60–70	70–80	80–92
Royal Break-Stone Tea (2-4 cups/day)									
Liver-gallbladder-fluke-parasite cleanse (for parasite cleanse only)									
Enema (in the morning)	Each day		As needed for supporting the organs of elimination						
Psyllium-bentonite shake	As needed to support organs of elimination; reduce cleansing reactions								
Dry skin brushing									
Hot/cool showers									
Yoga (15–30 minutes/day)									
Walking (30 minutes/day)									
Weight training (15–30 minutes three times/week)									

Figure 2: Juice Feasting timeline (Source: David Rainoshek, www.JuiceFeasting.com)

This timeline for Juice Feasting is used by coaches of this program; it is tailored for each client's condition and needs. Juice Feasting coaches can be contacted through NutrientDenseNutrition.com and the Tree of Life Rejuvenation Center. A few brief comments, however, should be made here. There are two specific cleanses within the Juice Feast. One is a kidney-liver-gallbladder cleanse using Royal Break-Stone Tea (also known as *Chanca Piedra*), which breaks up kidney and gallbladder stones. This is conducted during days 30–60 to give your body some time to clear out other waste matter before getting to the more sensitive liver cleansing. A parasite cleanse is done during days 60–80, as this is the point in a Feast in which there is nowhere left for the parasites to hide (because the Juice Feast is an intestinal-bowel cleanse, removing uneliminated waste matter where parasites can take up residence). Alternatively, there is the more intensive Tree of Life liver-gallbladder-fluke-parasite cleanse that can be accomplished in conjunction with Juice Feasting from days 7–49. It is important to understand that your entire physiology, diet, and lifestyle are not conducive to the maintenance of parasites by virtue of cleansing and consuming only plant-source foods. You just have to give parasites the final eviction notice with an herbal formula, and any that remain will most likely exit painlessly. This is a very important part of the cleansing and healing process.

We discussed earlier the use of enemas daily during the first three weeks of the Juice Feast, to support the elimination of waste and toxins from the body. We also discussed the introduction of weight training later in the Juice Feast, when the body is ready for muscle-building activity.

Let us briefly review a typical day of Juice Feasting. You wake up to a quart of water to assist in rehydration (the body loses 1–1.5 quarts of water during the night), and with that water you can add MSM, 15 drops of Natural Cellular Defense, and 3–5 caps of proteolytic enzyme Vitalzym. Next is an enema with warm water to release any waste matter made ready for evacuation while you rested during the night, then dry skin brushing and a warm shower. Once your warm shower is complete, you can add a hot/cool shower as described above. Take care of your oral hygiene, including the use of a tongue scraper, and exit the washroom ready for some light exercise such as yoga or walking, or a period of meditation. Then make yourself juice. If you are to be gone for the whole day without access to a juicer, make all of your juice for the day—approximately 4 quarts—in the morning. As a recovering diabetic, it is advisable to drink your juices ½ quart at a time, approximately 90 minutes apart, to maintain consistent blood sugar levels. This means that you want to have your first ½ quart of juice by

7:00–7:30 AM at the latest. Additions to your juices are green super-food powders, chlorella, kelp granules, and hemp oil.

The above Juice Feasting timeline contains numerous other aspects to the program that have been consciously designed in as a result of decades of research by live-food nutritionists. For a more detailed description of the elements of a Juice Feast, please see David Rainoshek's 92-Day Juice Feasting website at www.JuiceFeasting.com.

In summary, juice feasting:

- Addresses toxemia and deficiency through a 30–92-day nutrient-dense living liquid diet of green juices and nutrient-dense superfoods designed to cleanse, rebuild, rehydrate, and alkalize;
- Moves us back through the Seven Stages of Disease to a nondiabetic physiology if one is not already there by the end of the 21-Day+ Program because of excess weight or diabetic complications;
- Provides our bodies with every nutrient needed to address the issues of deficiency and to prevent the loss of lean body mass (muscle);
- Supports the organs of elimination to reduce cleansing reactions and healing crises;
- Allows us to continue to live a normal life so that we can continue to work, pay our bills, and take care of our family responsibilities;
- Provides ample time and opportunity for specific cleanses within the cleanse phase, such as kidney-liver-gallbladder work, heavy-metal detoxification, and a parasite cleanse;
- Trains our body and mind to ask for the foods and lifestyle choices of the Culture of Life, thus preventing the re-creation of diabetes;
- Helps support and sustain us in making the psycho-physiological shift into the Culture of Life.

Juice Recipes

We are drinking low-glycemic, Phase 1 juices made fresh at home with either a press-style juicer (such as a Green Star) or a high-speed blender (Vitamix). The juice is separated from the pulp by straining with a fine mesh bag. We are not demonizing fat, protein, or carbohydrates, and we are not eliminating any of these macronutrients. The 12–15 pounds of produce juiced fresh *each day* will contain all the protein, fat, carbohydrates, enzymes, phytonutrients, vitamins, and minerals you require. In fact, you will actually be consuming more bioavailable nutrition than you perhaps ever have in your lifetime, due to the nutrient density of the foods you are juicing, and the superfoods, essential fatty acids, and supplements you add. Here is your baseline for a Juice Feast of 4–5 quarts per day of nutrient-dense green juices made with the following ingredients:

- Base—celery, cucumber
- Leafy greens—spinach, parsley, kale, collards, Swiss chard, bok choy, watercress, beet green, cabbage, herbs (use sparingly, to avoid bitterness), dandelion, grasses, all other leafy greens
- Other vegetables—tomato, bell pepper (red, yellow, orange), nopal cactus, string beans, burdock root, Jerusalem artichoke, radish, any green sprouts
- Sweetener (use sparingly due to higher glycemic index when juiced)—parsnip, apple, sweet potato, carrot, beet
- Condiments—lemon and lime juice, cayenne powder, ginger root juice, juiced garlic, Himalayan salt, turmeric (powder or juice)

Take your juices with you wherever you go, and make sure you do not find yourself at work, on errands, or anywhere without a juice. This is the most sure way to make your head spin on a Juice Feast. Temptation to return to familiar Culture of Death habits is everywhere, and if hunger sets in on a Juice Feast, that sense of lack you will feel can bring you dangerously close to eating diabetogenic foods. Keep the wolf away from the door, and feed yourself consistently as an Act of Love and Consciousness all the way through.

Role Models Thriving on a Plant-Source-Only, Live-Food Diet

You may have never encountered live-food nutrition before, and want to know that your left ear isn't going to fall off from eating a plant-source-only diet. Many nutrition and diet books are written by people who do not look like the picture of health, and this could be an indication of the authenticity of their approach. The author has eaten a 100-percent plant-source-only diet of live, organic foods for more than thirty years, and David Rainoshek for the past five years. Both are living in vibrant health.

It is important that you seek out people who are doing well living in the Culture of Life, and you will find the names of such people in the acknowledgments at the beginning of this book. Just a few of the names you will want to become familiar with are: David Wolfe, Shazzie, Brian Clement, Viktoras Kulvinskas, John Rose, and the Boutenko family. Also seek out the members of the International Living Foods Summit. All of these people have published materials online and in books, many of which are listed in the Resources section in the appendixes.

In addition, seek out raw-food potlucks in your area, and go online using the resources suggested at the back of this book. At this very moment, you are drawing into your life the best things possible. You are a vortex of positive energy, and you have the opportunity to begin anew, becoming more than you ever thought possible. Become the continuation of those who are living the lifestyle that is achieving what you want so much to have as your daily life reality. The community of people living in the Culture of Life are some of the most vibrant, switched-on people you will ever have the pleasure of loving, and being loved by.

Further Support

The Tree of Life offers a once-a-month follow-up as support with someone knowledgeable in living the Culture of Life, or, if locally accessible, a Tree of Life branch member or potluck. See www.treeoflife.nu for a list of such groups globally. This support is not just nutrition focused, but addresses in a practical way one's emotional and spiritual life as well. Included for one year is *Alive with Gabriel* on the Internet, for helpful questions and answers.

Clinically, three to four months into the program I like to measure the HgbA1c levels, and every three months thereafter. I know we can activate the anti-diabetogenic genes and bring most people to a normal FBS in close to twenty-one days. The real task is how to stabilize participants in the diet and lifestyle of the Culture of Life. For on-site intellectual, emotional, and spiritual support and growth, at the Tree of Life we offer several valuable retreat programs in addition to the 21-Day+ Program; these are arranged according to people's needs.

The crucial reason for a one-year follow-up is that breaking free from the Culture of Death is difficult without support, when we live in a society that surrounds us by the shadow of the Culture of Death. My thirty-five years experience has shown that it may take people one to two years to transition emotionally, psychologically, and physiologically into the Culture of Life. Our experience and that of many others is that this most likely cannot be accomplished in one day. On a more humorous side, Neal Barnard, MD, relates in *Breaking the Food Seduction* that an April 2000 survey of 1,244 adults showed that when offered $1,000 to stop eating meat for a week, 25 percent of those asked would not "swap meat for cash." It was interesting that people from Hispanic and Asian backgrounds were more willing to accept this hypothetical offer (probably because fruits and vegetables are more a part of their indigenous diet), with less than 10 percent turning it down, but Caucasians and Afro-Americans turned down the $1,000 approximately 25 percent of the time.

What is the issue here? Why does meat seem so addictive, . . . because indeed it is.

Meat, as we pointed out earlier, has a high insulin index. One quarter pound of meat creates the same insulin response in the body as a quarter pound of sugar. This insulin appears to be involved in the release of dopamine, which is the pleasure-stimulating neurotransmitter that is also activated by the opiates, nicotine, cocaine, alcohol, amphetamines, and dairy (as pointed out earlier, dairy has a particular casomor-phin that is one-tenth the strength of pure morphine). When researchers from Edinburgh, Scotland, blocked meat's opiate effect, it cut the appetite for ham by 10 percent, salami by 25 percent, and tuna by a whopping 50 percent.

Not only do humans become addicted to animal products, but sheep, which are herbivores, and parrots, which are frugivores, can also become habituated to a diet of flesh. During their long sea voyages, the Nordics discovered that when the lambs on board the ships were induced to eat meat and fish, they became habituated to it. Upon arriving on land the lambs no longer desired their natural diet of grass. Horses are often fed fish and can be habituated to enjoy it, even though this is an unnatu-ral food for them. Frugivorous parrots can be taught to eat and relish animal foods, as well. In other words, these animals that were on a nat-ural live-plant-only diet became physiologically addicted to a diet of flesh foods.

As pointed out in *Breaking the Food Seduction,* sugar, as well as chocolate, releases natural opiates in the brain. In this case we are talk-ing about endorphins, which are relatives of opiates in their chemical structure. These endorphins activate the dopamine neurotransmitter system, which activates the pleasure centers of the brain. The opiate effect of sugar, according to the general research, may be triggered even by the mere taste of sugar, before the insulin-dopamine response occurs. Carbohydrate-rich foods boost another neurotransmitter, serotonin, which helps with mood and sleep.

Wheat, and particularly the gluten part of the wheat, is metabolized into at least eleven different opiates.

It is for these reasons that this year of support to break our addic-tion to the foods offered in the Culture of Death is so crucial.

ZERO POINT PROCESS INTENSIVE

The author, an internationally recognized spiritual teacher, psychiatrist, and family therapist who developed and teaches in the Zero Point Process Intensive, has this to say about it:

Zero Point assists clients in: clearing emotional and mental blocks, psychosomatic problems, food and other addictions; loving ourselves and overcoming the subtle resistance to healing from diabetes; dissolving co-dependent and unhealthy relationship patterns; and ultimately aligning with our sacred design so we may become the full living truth of who we are. The Zero Point Process Intensive opens the door to clarity and freedom from the mind's preoccupation with its own addictive psycho-emotional patterns. Zero Point helps participants awaken from the dream state that we are separate from the One. It helps one to understand that the personality is a case of mistaken identity and to be able to open to all of life. Although it is not taught as a spiritual path, it is a powerful spiritual process that supports the spiritual process of all paths and religious traditions."

The fundamental understanding that we gain in Zero Point is that *the personality is a case of mistaken identity.* To be free, we must transcend our personal, cultural, archetypical, and even our spiritual identities. We are not our thoughts, minds, or bodies. This awareness results in a completely new orientation in life. The process allows us to enter in the dual/non-dual synchronicity in which we *have* our personalities and archetypes without *being* them.

Once we understand that our thoughts have no power over us, we are free to dissolve them as needed. By dissolving what we are not, we come to the indescribable awareness of who we are. This internal change in one's cosmic world perspective opens the way to enter into the flow of a God-centered life. Life's struggles then cease. We are free to follow the flow of our destiny in a way that manifests our sacred design, our true expression in the world.

Freedom has no history, future, or present. Freedom is alone, empty, and without adjectives. What is important is to *be* the Truth in every moment, not to *seek* the Truth. Being present gives us the freedom not to be captured by the mind and its preoccupation with itself, the past, present, or future, or its relationship with the world. We are awakened from our trance and liberated from the entrapment of our stories.

The Zero Point process allows our mind to become open like the sky, which holds the sun, moon, stars, clouds, rain, snow, or just pure blue. Becoming the sky, we care not for which of these appear; we develop the room for all to pass through.

With these tools we are now empowered to embrace our destiny and our lives without fear, hesitation, or resistance. Freed from the slavery of the mind, we can live our lives in celebration, subtle non-causal joy, inner contentment, and the bliss of freedom.

GABRIEL COUSENS, MD

CONSCIOUS EATING TRAINING

The foundation of the Conscious Eating Training at the Tree of Life Café is to create food for the support of consciousness awakening. Conscious eating begins with conscious food preparation. Studies have shown that our intentions influence the smallest particles of creation. In living food, water crystalline structures take on the energy of our presence, as well as the energy of the environment wherein it is being prepared. At the Tree of Life Café, our live-food creations vibrate with a deeply healing energy that affects all levels of creation.

The focus of this six-day experiential course is to share with students the power of remaining present in our hearts while preparing food. This is the true essence of conscious food preparation. This exciting intensive guides you through the basics of conscious live-food preparation while immersing you in the Tree of Life experience.

The course content includes:

- Setting up a live-food kitchen—a practical interactive discussion
- The secrets of conscious food preparation
- Foods of Rainbow Green Live-Food Cuisine—learning the phase chart
- Introduction to ingredient balancing
- Fermented foods—a practical hands-on discussion
- Introduction to dressings, soups, crackers, and salads
- Breakfast skills class—mylks and granolas

- Basic breads and crusts
- Seed cheezes, pâtés, sauces, and marinated veggies
- Low-glycemic desserts—Phases 1.0 and 1.5
- Sacred Essene braided challah bread
- Sprouting with Effective Microorganisms (EM) and sea minerals
- Nature hike—connecting with the high desert
- Certificate of completion with closing dessert party
- Detailed class workbook—continually updated
- Volume 1 recipe booklet
- Daily guidance and support (ask us questions any time!)
- Access to the best resources (food, equipment, tuition, support)

Educational lectures are by Gabriel Cousens and the Tree of Life Café staff on the following topics:

- Rainbow Green Live-Food Cuisine
- Individualizing the diet
- Why live foods?
- Nutritional questions and answers
- Bringing it home

SPIRITUAL FASTING RETREAT

I have done fasting, yoga and meditation before, but never on the level of competence and integrity Dr. Cousens and his staff have designed to address medical, emotional and spiritual concerns in one fully integrated, lovingly supportive program.

G. L. D., PHD, TUCSON, ARIZONA

Hosted by Gabriel and Shanti Gold-Cousens, longtime experienced juice fasters, this retreat applies spiritual juice fasting to unblock the divine source of youth, vitality, and transformation. On the Spiritual Fasting Retreat, we release our resistance to healing, and open the body and mind to awakening to the Truth of who we are. Through the process of non-attachment to physical food, we open to spiritual nourishment and enjoy the spiritual feast of the four elements of air, earth (juices), water, and the sun (fire). Gabriel and Shanti participate in the group fast, teaching yoga on all levels of being. The Spiritual Fasting Retreat is the ultimate journey to the warrior within—inward and beyond to the One. During the retreat we offer the following:

- Seven days of fresh, organic juices
- Daily Shaktipat meditation with Gabriel Cousens
- Two days of live food to support reintroduction of food
- Native American sweat lodge (weather permitting)
- Daily Kali Ray Tri Yoga®
- Nature walks
- Chanting
- Spiritual discussions and seminars
- Outdoor hot tubs
- Optional whole person healing at the Tree of Life Spa

The Spiritual Fasting Retreat, with deep meditation sessions, allows you to connect to your Divine Truth and personal holy rhythm

.

Spiritual fasting is a mystical death and rebirth into the arms of God. Spiritual fasting brings you into the pleasure of the Divine. You do not know what feeling good is until you fast.

GABRIEL COUSENS, MD

SACRED RELATIONSHIPS COURSE

Know one's self as a sacred child of the Divine, and explore the universe as a sensuous, wild, passionate, abundant playground. Master the art of Sacred Relationship and invoking Divine Union in every moment. Embark upon an intimate journey unleashing the dynamic forces of love, as body, mind, and spirit merge as a continual expression of subtle ecstasy.

GABRIEL COUSENS, MD

The Sacred Relationships course is one of Gabriel and Shanti's favorite and most fun workshop to teach. Together, they weave a matrix of luminous love that inspires and supports all to find the flame of Divine Love within their own hearts. Couples explore the mysteries of intimacy as a spiritual path in which they are taught how to invoke the Divine in their relationship. Gabriel and Shanti help couples to awaken and strengthen the spiritual force in their relationships, which brings the healing of male and female energies on the planet in the process of returning to the One.

YEARLY EVENTS

To broaden the community of support and create a collectivized experience in living in the Culture of Life, the Tree of Life is host to Interdependence Day on the July 4th weekend each year with David Wolfe and Gabriel Cousens. The Tree of Life also hosts a Thanksgiving potluck, open and free to the public. In 2006, nearly 200 people gathered at Thanksgiving to celebrate their gratitude for a nutrient-dense diet of plant foods, healthy living, a better planet, and for the community of people living in the Culture of Life as an Act of Love.

Realizing Our True Potential

When we quit thinking only about ourselves and our own self-preservation, we undergo a truly heroic transformation of con-sciousness.

JOSEPH CAMPBELL

Through living in the Culture of Life we become *potentialists,* seeing the true capabilities of everyone, individually and collectively. Remember not to worry about your ability to eat a low-glycemic Culture of Life cuisine. Who you are now, and the you that will arise through the Tree of Life 21-Day+ Program and living the Culture of Life—those are two different people who will see with unique eyes. You will experience a physical, emotional, mental, and spiritual shift in yourself as you realize your own true potential at each of these levels, living with a mind, body, and spirit that asks for the best things possible to enter your life.

We eat and live in the Culture of Life as an Act of Love and Consciousness, aware that happiness is not an individual matter, that we are each a person of great import who can be vibrant and healthy, free of diabetes, and inspiring self-confidence, joy, and hope in others. We can do this just by the very simple act of living an authentic existence that acknowledges who we are—organic plant-eaters who want to move beyond the processed diabetogenic realities of "modern" living to a Culture of Life in which few are ill, we honor the inheritance of our ancestors, we create a world that is safe for the health of future generations, and all are fed the best food possible.

CHAPTER 6

Culture of Life Cuisine

I am a stronger follower of Veganism by principle, not just because of moral and aesthetic reasons. I truly believe in a Vegetarian lifestyle and I have my faith and hopes in a change of human destiny, thanks to the physical effects and benefits of a healthier diet and its influence on the character of the people. It will bring about some benefit and improvement to human society.

ALBERT EINSTEIN

To eat is a necessity, but to eat intelligently is an art.

DUC FRANCOIS DE LA ROCHEFOUCAULD

A delicious anti-diabetogenic cuisine that you can joyfully live on through the years is essential for the prevention and treatment of diabetes. For example, a 1999 study conducted in Great Britain showed that those who ate salad and raw vegetables frequently year-round had an 80 percent lower risk of Type-2 diabetes than those who ate vegetables less often.[1] The Culture of Life cuisine as taught in the Tree of Life 21-Day+ Program works. The cuisine is not a diet that you go on, but rather the delightful culinary aspect of living in the Culture of Life, for your whole life. With all the different ways of consuming foods mentioned in this book, let us recap what we have investigated. The Tree of Life 21-Day+ Program involves green juice fasting to most rapidly bring your blood sugar, HgbA1c, and other blood chemistry levels into a healthy physiological range. The program also includes eating the joyful world cuisine and learning how to prepare it, as described in this chapter. For those who are in need of additional weight loss, or further time to transform decades-old health challenges, we provide support for Juice Feasting at home with green juices, herbs, supplements, and superfood concentrates to continue the process of cleansing, rebuilding, rehydrating, and alkalizing. Juice Feasting is essentially a nutrient-dense, live-food, liquid diet that creates the space for healing to continue in an efficient manner, but is not a *cuisine* that one is to eat for the rest of one's life. In this chapter, we offer two complementary ways of eating a Culture of Life cuisine that can meet anyone's schedule, culinary culture, specific nutritional requirements, and kitchen abilities.

We offer a basic, long-term, live-foods approach as explained in the book *Rainbow Green Live-Food Cuisine,* which we call the Rainbow Green World Cuisine and developed specifically for this program. The World Cuisine is more kitchen- and time-intensive, yet enables you to create meals that meet or exceed the taste sensations and culinary delights of the diet to which you have been accustomed, and can be tailored to meet the tastes of your family, culture, and society.

The "Four Means to Get Your Greens" developed by David Rainoshek is both a complementary entry and an important functional addition to the Rainbow Green World Cuisine because it adds a convenience level that supports flexibility and mobility in your work and travel.

Concerning the glycemic index of your diet, I recommend stabilizing on Phase 1 for three to six months until your diet becomes steady and you are completely comfortable in your new physiology. Then you may move to Phase 1.5 or choose to stay at Phase 1. Thoughtfully moving from fasting, directly to the Rainbow Green World Cuisine, or to Juice Feasting and *then* to the World Cuisine (according to your physiological healing needs) and living in the Culture of Life is crucial for the long-term success of the program.

Food is a love note from God.

GABRIEL COUSENS, MD

Another essential aspect is the eating of food as a spiritually, culturally, and socially significant event when done in a spirit of awareness and sacredness. All of these aspects need to be mindfully included and balanced for long-term success. Consciousness in preparation and eating remain a vital part of the cuisine. This is especially important in the Four Means to Get Your Greens approach, where there is an easy tendency to slip into an unhealthy fast-food lifestyle. To get the fullest value out of eating, I urge you to maintain an intentional heart and mind of love, gratitude, and consciousness during the preparation and eating of your food.

I am starting this chapter by addressing your concerns about live-food preparation, showing how easy it can be to eat this way with the Four Means to Get Your Greens. Then I will describe the innovative Rainbow Green World Cuisine adapted to be a Culture of Life anti-diabetogenic cuisine.

Four Means to Get Your Greens

Those who think they have no time for healthy eating will sooner or later have to find time for illness.

EDWARD STANLEY, *THE CONDUCT OF LIFE*

You may not have a lot of time to be in the kitchen, but you want diabetes to be over with and you would rather take time to be healthy than to suffer the chronic uncontrolled disability and early death from diabetes. You know what your nutritional needs are and, after hearing about all the nutrient-dense superfoods available, the essential fats you want to include, the 1–2 pounds of leafy greens you will eat each day, and so on, you may be looking for a way to do all of this that takes minutes instead of hours, the flick of a switch instead of a culinary degree. You are in luck. Eating the best nutrient-dense live-plant-source-only cuisine that will feed you for your whole life is embarrassingly and brilliantly easy. It honors the best live-food nutritional research, and simultaneously allows for your own intuition about what you need in your cuisine to individualize your diet. The way to understand how to do this is in terms of the approximately 1 pound of leafy greens I suggest you eat each day, which until a few moments before reading this chapter sounded impossible.

The Four Means approach can be done with basic kitchen utensils— a knife, cutting board, spoon, spatula, nut mylk bag, and a high-speed blender like a Vita-Mix or K-Tec. Preparation and cleanup takes minutes, does not involve complicated recipes, is infinitely variable, nutrient-dense, super delicious, and completely portable for our active lives. This 1 pound of green leafy produce is the fundamental groundwork for your low-glycemic, nutrient-dense anti-diabetogenic Culture of Life world cuisine. In my experience at the Tree of Life, I have found that most people do well eating 1 pound of leafy greens each day, but some do well with as much as 2 pounds. This amount can vary based on whether you are a slow or fast oxidizer, or how new you are to eating a plant-source-only diet. Determining the appropriate amount of greens for you will be a matter of personal experimentation, with some investigation into your constitutional type. An excellent test to help you individualize your diet is in *Conscious Eating* by Gabriel Cousens, MD. See Chapter 3, "A Revolutionary Breakthrough in Personalizing Your Diet," and Chapter 4, "Personalizing Your Diet to Your Mind-Body Constitution" for this detailed guidance. It is important to understand that by eating 1 pound of nutrient-dense leafy greens each day in your diet, you ensure that you do not eat too much fat, or too much low-glycemic fruit, either of which, or the two in excess as a combination, will create poor blood sugar control. I call this balanced, fast-food approach Four Means to Get Your Greens. Here are the four basic means to get your greens:

One: Eat your greens
Two: Make blended green soups
Three: Make blended green smoothies with chia seeds or low-glycemic fruits, if your blood sugar is stable for six months
Four: Juice your greens into green vegetable juice (GVJ)

Food in any of these forms travels easily in a Tupperware or drinking container, can be taken on the go just about anywhere, and all Four Means can be prepared in advance at home, ready for you at every point in your day. Before I outline what a day of eating using the Four Means approach looks like, let's briefly look at the Four Means themselves.

ONE: EATING YOUR GREENS

This is the age-old way of eating a plant-source diet. Make yourself a large salad, with salad dressing, crackers, perhaps a soup, and you are good to go. Eating this way, you can realistically expect to eat ½ pound of leafy greens at a meal. The chewing involved activates a series of neural pathways, as well as increases serotonin production by two to five times, thus enhancing mood, mental clarity, and the quality of one's sleep.

TWO: BLENDED GREEN SOUPS

Soups are infinitely variable, and their great advantage is the possibility of adding things in that you would never consider eating on their own, such as whole ginger root and multiple cloves of garlic. Also, because the entire meal is blended, it is more bioavailable (the blender pre-chews it for you) as long as you chew your soup as you eat it. This form of blended salad travels well, and can be made in the morning before heading out for your day. We are not necessarily recommending that all of your meals be blended, as chewing has been shown to significantly increase serotonin production and eating whole foods helps to exercise the strength and fire of the digestive system. Therefore, when eating blended soups, chew! This goes for smoothies and juices, as well.

A blended green soup made in a high-speed blender has at its base a fat, such as sesame tahini, olives, avocado, or a salad dressing. Then you are adding in everything that you would have in a plant-source salad: leafy greens, cucumbers, celery, tomato, peppers, and so on. Next include sea vegetables such as dulse, arame, wakame, sea palm, and hijiki. Finally, spices such as whole garlic, whole ginger root, cayenne, Himalayan crystal salt or Celtic sea salt, mustard, and fresh or dried herbs of your choice. Add about ½ cup of water to your blender full of nutrient-dense green soup ingredients, and make your soup. As you eat it, know that the nutrient-dense nutrition you are getting out of this one bowl of soup is immense. During the winter, you can gradually heat these soups by setting your stove on the lowest possible setting, stirring constantly, and measuring the heat of your pot until it reaches 105-120°. Pour and serve immediately. Eating greens this way, you will find yourself with about ½ pound of greens in your bowl!

THREE: BLENDED GREEN SMOOTHIES

The key to anti-diabetogenic green smoothies is to achieve a sweet taste without the use of high-glycemic fruits. For the purposes of maintaining proper blood sugar as a diabetic or former diabetic, this means using super-low-glycemic chia seeds with your greens, in conjunction with sweet spices such as cardamom and stevia. On the Phase 1.5 cuisine, a low-glycemic fruit such as blueberries can be added in limited quantities. The way to make a blended green smoothie with chia is to add 1 cup of chia seeds to a blender of greens, add water to desired consistency, and blend a smoothie. For great smoothie recipes, see the Rainbow Green World Cuisine recipe section later in this chapter.

FOUR: JUICING YOUR GREENS

Green vegetable juice was covered in the Chapter 5 introduction to Juice Feasting. It is easy to juice a pound of leafy greens into a quart of juice, combined with celery, cucumber, lemon, Jerusalem artichoke, garlic, ginger, cayenne, curcumin, and many other low-glycemic delicious juiced ingredients. This travels, and makes for a great breakfast, mid-morning snack, afternoon pick-me-up, or even a hydrating, nutrient-dense dinner that won't put you to sleep, or keep you up at night with indigestion. You can afford to miss the fiber in this juice, as a cuisine of living plant foods will supply your digestive system with adequate fiber throughout the day, and provided that you are also practicing the first three of the Four Means. Equipment needed is your high-speed blender, knife and cutting board, nut mylk bag, and a glass quart-sized container to carry your green juice. Drink within eight hours for optimum freshness.

The Culture of Life Anti-Diabetogenic Rainbow Green World Cuisine

Preparing Rainbow Green World Cuisine is a true culinary adventure into a joyful world of health, vitality, and sumptuous tastes. If you are embarking upon the journey of live-food preparation for the first time, a wonderful treasury of new skills, equipment, ingredients, and helpful tips awaits you. This chapter is a map offering the "how to" and the help that you will need on your journey. The Mystery awaits you!

There are so many options for designing incredible Culture of Life cuisine. I invite you to use as the companion book to this recipe section *Rainbow Green Live-Food Cuisine* by Gabriel Cousens, MD, and the Tree of Life Café, which contains a wide variety of inspirational and delicious food ideas that are tailor-made for the diet and lifestyle that this book presents, and that we use in our Tree of Life 21-Day+ Program.

TASTE BALANCING

One of the main ways that we are able to help create balance and an epicurean taste experience is through a balance of flavors. The concept of taste balancing, shared with the Tree of Life Café by our former master chef, Chad Sarno, has been incorporated into our program for making gourmet, multi-cultural raw food. Taste balancing is a major key to preparing delicious food. It supports wholistic food preparation that celebrates the balance of flavors and the balance of feeding each body, from the emotional body to the spiritual body, with intention. When we feed people's physical, emotional, and spiritual bodies with comforting food, it creates balance in a variety of ways.

TASTE BALANCING TABLE			
Sweet	**Salt**	**Acid**	**Fat**
Low-glycemic fruits	Celtic sea salt	Lemon	Oils
Cherry tomatoes	Olives	Lime	Seeds and nuts
Bell peppers	Miso	Grapefruit	Seed and nut butters
Carrots	Sea veggies	Apple cider vinegar	Avocado
Beets	Kelp	Sauerkraut	Coconut pulp
Whole orange	Dulse		Olives
White miso			Purslane

In each of our foods, we like to have a taste base. That base, a balance in each dish of a sweet, salt, acid, and fat taste, gives us a foundation for making almost any ethnic dish. Again, the base components, which you will find in the majority of the recipes in this book, all have the four elements: sweet, acid, salt, and fat. For example, in a pâté, you may want to use pine nuts as a fat, carrot for sweet, a little lemon juice as the acid, and Celtic sea salt for salt. Together those elements make up your base for the pâté.

For the fat taste, we can use all sorts of oils: cold-pressed oils, walnut oil, flax, hemp, sunflower, sesame, soaked nuts and seeds, unsoaked nuts and seeds, nut butters, avocado, coconut, or olives. For acid taste, use citrus (including lemon, lime, grapefruit, and orange), apple cider vinegar, and sauerkraut. For salt, use Celtic salt, which contains eighty-two minerals. It is an uncooked, live salt. I consider miso a live food because when it is fermented, it is activated with enzymes. Miso creates a very nice salt taste, and barley miso can be used as a bouillon substitute. Olives are good for a fat and salt taste, and they are the most mineralized fruit. For sweets, do not use dried fruits, because they are too high on the glycemic index, and are mycogenic, meaning they support the growth of pathogens like candida. Instead, the Tree of Life Café tends to use the sweeter vegetables, and some of the lower-glycemic fruits. At Phase 1.5, one can occasionally use a few soaked raisins, apples, or pears, and occasionally a little orange juice. One can also use a little coconut water and the sweeter vegetables like cherry tomatoes, bell peppers, carrots, and beets. Sweet white miso is very good for a sweet and a salt.

Each culture has characteristic flavors that are achieved through the usage of specific herbs and spices. For example, in Italian and Sicilian cuisine, the key flavors are garlic, basil, oregano, and olive oil. For Thai and Balinese, the more fundamental flavors are basil, lemon grass, tamarind, galangal root, curry, cumin, and coriander. For Mexican and Spanish, use cilantro, cumin, garlic, olive oil, jalapeño, and other chiles. Moroccan and African cuisines emphasize cilantro, cinnamon, ginger, and cumin. Japanese and Chinese cuisines use ginger, garlic, and sesame. Middle Eastern cuisine features garlic, mint, oregano, cinnamon, parsley, sesame, and fenugreek. For Indian cuisine, one should use garlic, ginger, cardamom, curry mixtures, cumin, and the general masala taste, as well as sesame, saffron, cinnamon, fenugreek, turmeric, and fennel. For American cuisine, use garlic, oregano, dill, cinnamon, and chiles.

Each culture also emphasizes different foods. For example, in Italian and Sicilian cuisine, lemon, olives, tomato, and spinach are used. Thai and Balinese cuisines emphasize lime and coconut. Mexican and Spanish use lime, tomato, and avocado. Moroccan and African cuisines use olives, orange, lemon, tomato, and eggplant. Japanese and Chinese cuisines use lime, mung bean sprouts, bok choy, assorted veggies, snow peas, and cucumber. Middle Eastern and Greek cuisines use lemon, eggplant, tomato, and cucumber. Indian cuisine uses cauliflower, spinach, peas, and lemon. American cuisine features peas, carrots, lemon, and tomato.

When examining which foods, herbs, and spices work well together, especially when used to achieve certain cultural flavors, one notices a bioregional influence: plants that grow among one another often combine synergistically in the kitchen. It is, in a sense, a part of the divine blueprint of how humans are best suited to eating locally and best fed by locally grown food. For example, tomatoes and basil can be companion-planted and are complementary ingredients in cuisine.

So, if one wants to make an Italian salad, for example, use Italian produce like tomatoes, olives, and spinach, along with a little olive oil and lemon, which are common there, and then salt. Next, add the herbs that are particular to the Italian culture. If desiring a Thai dish, coconut pulp and sesame are certainly going to be used. One can use coconut with a little bit of lime, and then add the spices that are appropriate to Thai culture. To accompany these basic flavors, include peas, carrots, and cauliflower for Thai cuisine.

It is important to understand how the amounts of salt, acid, fat, and sweet complement each other and the ethnic herbs to make a complete taste. For instance, certain components emphasize certain herbs. So, if you have cilantro in a dish, then you want to add less lemon. This is because the acid in the lemon emphasizes the cilantro and brings its flavor out more. If you want to use basil instead of cilantro, you would add more lemon. Also, think about oil as a vehicle for flavor. If you just have lemon and salt and herbs, those flavors, that acid taste or the taste of salt, will go right to the taste buds. But the oil smoothes the flavors over the palate and brings them into balance. That is why the fat component is important.

The art of this culinary approach is balance. This is achieved by using fresh, seasonal ingredients that satisfy the four taste components, balancing the herbs, and finding our own unique style of putting the ingredients together into a sensational dish. In this endeavor, start with a recipe base, and then play with the elements. When you look at any of these recipes, you can see the base in them, the four tastes, and the vegetables, herbs, and spices that give the recipe a specific cultural flair. So, when creating your own Rainbow Green World Cuisine recipes from scratch, create a recipe base, with the four tastes, and then play with the herbs and spices for the particular cultural cuisine that you choose.

The Rainbow Green World Cuisine is not only the healthiest cleansing and maintenance evolutionary diet for individual health, the health of the planet, and the awakening of consciousness. It is also a joyful exploration of culinary artistry and delightful tastes.

Know Your Ingredients

This section focuses on the foods and ingredients used in our recipes at the Tree of Life Café. We emphasize foods that are nutrient-dense and low in sugar. Many of these items are available from the Health Store on the Tree of Life website: www.treeoflife.nu.

GREEN LEAFY VEGETABLES

Among the most nutrient-dense of all plant foods are the dark green, leafy vegetables, especially kale, dandelion, spinach, chard, collards, arugula, parsley, and green cabbage. These vegetables are high in alkaline minerals, protein, and chlorophyll. As such, they are regenerative and purifying.

BUYING AND STORING NUTS AND SEEDS

It is recommended that organic nuts and seeds be purchased direct by mail order from specialty suppliers (see the Resources section in this book). The nuts and seeds obtained from health food stores or conventional markets are susceptible to rancidity, as they may have been stored on the shelf, possibly for long periods of time. Ideally nuts and seeds should be stored in the freezer or refrigerator to prevent the oils from going rancid. If this is not possible, store them in a cool, dark, dry place. Be especially careful with high-oil-content nuts and seeds like Brazil nuts, macadamias, and pine/pignoli nuts. If they look yellow, it is likely that they are rancid.

BUYING OILS

As suggested in Chapter 2, people with serious ASCVD should follow Dr. Esselstyn's recommendation and eliminate olive oil and other saturated cooked or raw animal fats from their diet in their vegan approach to healing atherosclerosis. In the same context, those people diagnosed with diabetes for more than a year have, with almost 100-percent certainty, a degeneration of the endothelium of the arteries, and are most prudent to avoid or minimize the use of olive oil until the diabetic physiology has been reversed completely for two years. Even though the high-antioxidant, high-omega-3 oils are a good alternative, I do also recommend that one consider emphasizing dressings from whole pulverized nuts and seeds rather than the oils of these high quality nuts and seeds, which only contain the fat-soluble antioxidants. In general, even though these oils are beneficial, I still recommend that one keep a relatively low fat intake (approximately 15–20 percent of total calories) in the process of healing diabetes through a live-food diet. Taken in this context, because on a live-foods cuisine you can eat half as much with the same nutritional benefit, this is actually healthier and theoretically superior to having 10–15 percent of calories from fat in a cooked plant-source-only diet.

The best oils to use in salad dressings are those high in omega-3; these include walnut, flax, and hemp oils, as well as sesame oil, which is very high in antioxidants. I recommend in our Tree of Life recipes that one can try substituting these oils for olive oil.

Conventional cooking oils should be avoided, as they have been highly processed. Even "cold-pressed oils" could have been influenced by heat at some stage of processing. Recommended oils include:

- Cold-pressed flax seed oil, which should be used within three weeks from date of pressing, as it is highly susceptible to rancidity
- Hemp seed oil, which should be used within six weeks from date of pressing, as it is highly susceptible to rancidity
- Cold-pressed sesame, coconut, sunflower, and almond oils
- Coconut oil, but no more than 1–2 tablespoons per day as it has been shown to raise cholesterol levels when eaten in excess

See the Resources directory in the appendixes for recommended sources of these products.

HERBS AND SPICES

Where possible, fresh herbs and whole spices are used at the Tree of Life Café, as their flavors are so much richer and delightful than their dried counterparts. Spices such as fennel, dill, cumin, clove, cinnamon, and cardamom can be bought in whole form and easily ground in a spice mill or coffee grinder.

STEVIA

Stevia is a sweet herb native to North and South America. Only one species, *rebaudiana,* tastes sweet enough to be called "sweet leaf" in Brazil and Paraguay, where it grows wild. Stevia is a great sweetener alternative. Recent research indicates that it does not raise the blood sugar level, and may even lower it. Whole stevia leaf can be bought at health food stores or by mail order, or you can grow your own. Grind the whole leaf into a powder and add to food and teas for a sweet taste. You can also buy water-extracted stevia in liquid form from your local health food store in the supplements section. Avoid alcohol-extracted and refined forms of stevia. Unrefined stevia is dark green in color.

GOJI BERRIES

Clinical analysis shows that this unusual berry is a powerful antioxidant that contains eighteen kinds of amino acids (six times higher than bee pollen), more beta-carotene than carrots, and five hundred times the amount of vitamin C by weight than oranges. It is loaded with vitamins B-1, B-2, B-6, and E. It has been found effective in increasing white blood cells, protecting liver function, lowering cholesterol, relieving hypertension, and helping strengthen the immune system while building muscle tissue and burning body fat. Goji berries are known for enhancing longevity.

The Tibetan goji berries offered by the Tree of Life Rejuvenation Center have been grown in protected valleys in wild and cultivated areas of Inner Mongolia in million-year-old soil where pesticides have never been used. They have been dried and are packaged in a vacuum-sealed bag. In a Phase 1.5 cuisine, the berries may be eaten alone in their dried state as a snack (just a few), or they can be soaked and incorporated into recipes.

FLAX SEED

Golden flax seed is packed with nutrition and is an essential daily addition to a healthful diet. Golden flax seed has greater nutritional value than the more common brown flax seed. It contains fiber, lignans, and short-chain omega-3 fatty acids, as well as both soluble and insoluble fiber, helping to clean your intestinal tract and promote regularity. Lignans provide a powerful support to the immune system and cellular health. Long-chain omega-3 fatty acids are essential for balanced brain chemistry. Flax seed is one of the few sources of omega-3 for a plant-source-only cuisine. I recommend 3 tablespoons for slow oxidizers and 3–6 tablespoons for fast oxidizers each day. Other long-chain omega-3 sources that contain the long-chain components DHA and EPA are the product E3Live™ and the herb purslane. The conversion rate of short-chain omega-3 to long-chain is 1 percent. By adding one tablespoon of coconut oil, it increases the conversion rate to 3–6 percent, three to six times better. I do not recommend more than 1–2 tablespoons of coconut oil in a day, as excess coconut oil has been shown to raise cholesterol.

The seeds we are using can be ground in a spice mill or coffee grinder and used in many recipes, or they can simply be sprinkled on top of salads or granola or even fruit. When flax seed is soaked, the soaking water becomes thick and jelly-like, providing a versatile thickening and binding ingredient for many recipes.

CELTIC AND HIMALAYAN SALT

Light-gray Celtic sea salt consists primarily, but not completely, of sodium and chloride (33 percent sodium and 51 percent chloride). Due to a unique method of harvesting from ocean water (on the northwestern coast of France), along with gathering the naturally evaporated salt using wooden tools, it also contains up to eighty-two trace minerals not found in other sea salts. Another other excellent whole salt is Himalayan salt. Both salts are in their ionic form.

Common table salt, which I do not recommend, lacks minerals and trace elements because it is purified and refined, leaving only sodium and chloride. After refining, common table salt is mixed with iodine, bleaching agents, and anti-caking agents, which creates a pure white, free-flowing product. Even many salts labeled "sea salt" are washed or boiled, which removes minerals and trace elements, rendering them toxic to the human body. Any salt that has been heated in this manner is converted to a covalent form, which is difficult for the body to assimilate. Celtic sea salt and Himalayan salt are the most energetic and complete salts we have found. Research indicates that sea salt is used by the body for mineralization, hydration, and to restore a healthy sodium-potassium balance for the lymph, blood, and extracellular fluid.

ALMOND BUTTER AND SESAME TAHINI

Almond butter is made from raw, unsoaked almonds that have been ground. Likewise, tahini is the succulent butter ground from raw sesame seeds. Many commercial tahinis and almond butters involve exposure to intense heat in the grinding process. Thus, their labels, which identify them as "raw," are very misleading. High-quality, commercially prepared almond butter and sesame tahini that have *not* been exposed to extreme heat are available from the Tree of Life Health Store (see the Resources section).

Both almond butter and sesame tahini are versatile ingredients for many types of recipes, particularly soups and salad dressings. Tahini is especially enhancing with its creamy, dairy-like texture and rich flavor. These butters make a great snack straight out of the jar, as a dip for crudités or apple slices, or as a spread for raw bread or crackers. Research cited in this book shows that almonds are associated with up to 23 percent decrease in LDL.

HEMP SEED

The tiny shelled seed of the amazing hemp plant has a pleasant nutty flavor, similar to sunflower seeds. The seeds are packed with nutrients—they are an excellent source of the essential fatty acids (EFAs), delivering these EFAs in a balanced 3.75:1 ratio. Hemp seed contains the rare fatty acid gamma-linolenic acid (GLA). Hemp seed is a source of complete protein, containing all the essential amino acids. It is equal to flax seed as a source of short-chain omega-3 fatty acids.

Unfortunately, most hemp seeds are irradiated upon import; however, the Tree of Life is able to supply truly live, organic hemp seeds (see the Resources directory), which we call hemp nuts. Hemp seed is great with granola, sprinkled on salads, and is especially tasty in tomato-based sauces. Hemp seed is a delicious substitute for other nuts and seeds in most any recipe.

OLIVES

The healthiest olives are those that are water-cured or cured in Celtic sea salt. Olives are rich in monounsaturated fat, with high proportions of essential amino acids, vitamins E and A, beta-carotene, calcium, and magnesium.

COCONUT OIL

Mature coconuts are used in the creation of health-enhancing coconut oil that is mostly solid at room temperature, so it is often referred to as coconut butter. Raw, unprocessed coconut oil smells fragrant like fresh coconuts, while most commercial coconut oils, including the brands commonly found in health food stores, are often deodorized and heat-processed, and therefore are not recommended. Cold-pressed coconut oil is available from the Health Store on the Tree of Life website.

The saturated fats in coconut oil are medium-chain fats (triglycerides, or MCTs) and therefore unlike most other sources of saturated fats (long-chain triglycerides), which are stored in the body as fat reserves. The high MCTs found in coconut oil are easy to digest, even for people who typically have trouble digesting fats. In fact, MCTs actually assist the body in metabolizing fat efficiently. As such, coconut oil provides a readily available fuel source. Saturated fats are also an important building block for all the cells of the human body. Coconut oil helps convert short-chain omega-3 fats to long-chain omega-3 fats.

Coconut oil has a high (50 percent-plus) lauric fatty acid and caprylic acid content, from which it derives its anti-parasitical, anti-viral, and anti-fungal properties. Those with intestinal problems such as candida or other systemic infections can therefore benefit from the daily inclusion of coconut oil in their diet. Coconut oil can be added to nut mylks, dressings, desserts (acting as a thickener when chilled), and even soups. I do not recommend more than 1–2 tablespoons of coconut oil daily because of its tendency to raise cholesterol in higher amounts. Coconut oil also makes an excellent skin lotion and massage oil.

A NOTE ABOUT NAMA SHOYU AND BRAGG'S AMINO ACIDS

These soy-based condiments are a popular flavoring agent for many raw-food chefs. They are not used, however, in the Rainbow Green World Cuisine because soy is difficult for the body to process and the products are likely to be contaminated by GMO crops. It has also been shown that during the heat of processing (yes, all soy products are cooked) of these products there is a formation of naturally occurring MSG.

Food Preparation Equipment

High-quality food preparation equipment is essential for optimizing the health-giving properties of the recipes in this book. The purchase of quality equipment for the living-foods kitchen requires a small investment, but the durability and the results are well worth the initial cost. Most of the items listed here are available from the Health Store on the Tree of Life website: www.treeoflife.nu.

SELECTING A CHEF'S KNIFE

A good chef's knife is your most important tool in the kitchen. Purchase the best-quality knife you can afford. A high-carbon steel blade is recommended, as it is the most durable material. Try it out in the store if possible, noticing how it feels in your hand. A good knife should have balance—like an extension of your arm.

Ceramic knives are an excellent alternative to steel because they do not lead to browning in fruits and vegetables due to oxidation caused by the metal, nor is there any subtle metallic taste imparted to the food. They will also last months, or even years, without sharpening. Ceramic is a very hard material, but brittle; these knives are susceptible to breakage if care is not taken in their use and handling.

For mincing fresh herbs, a cleaver with a slightly rounded blade is essential. Use a rocking motion, moving back and forth across the herbs, finely chopping them.

BLENDER

A high-speed blender is essential in the living-foods kitchen. Household blenders are unable to adequately process or achieve the desired smoothness when blending hard nuts and seeds—the motors will quickly burn out with this type of use. I recommend the Vita-Mix Super 5000 (the most versatile blender), the K-Tec HP3 blender, and the Tribest single-serving blender (great for traveling).

JUICER

The selection of a juicer for your living-foods kitchen should be carefully considered. Most home juicers are of the centrifugal type. The quality of the juice extracted from this type of juicer is less than ideal because as the centrifugal mechanism spins at high speed, it shreds the produce, which therefore oxidizes more rapidly. Centrifugal juicers also tend to waste produce because they are unable to fully break down the cell wall and extract all the juices.

The best type of juicer is one that masticates the produce at low speeds and therefore preserves the health-giving qualities of the juice. Masticating juicers produce a very dry pulp, as the juices are completely extracted, thus providing a greater return on your investment. The Green Star juicer is perhaps the best masticating juicer currently available. It is capable of juicing all types of produce, including green leafy vegetables (even grasses), and can effectively homogenize nuts and seeds for pâtés. I recommend the Green Star as it is efficient for juicing greens and homogenizing ingredients. You can also make green vegetable juice with a high-speed blender, by blending your produce with a little water, and straining the juice out through a nut mylk bag (a fine mesh bag) over a bowl or pitcher.

FOOD PROCESSOR

A high-quality food processor enables you to process vegetables in a variety of forms; it will also allow the processing of nuts and seeds to a variety of consistencies. Look for one with 8- to 10-cup capacity. Cuisinart is a time-honored favorite brand, although there are many good food processors on the market today.

DEHYDRATOR

When looking for a dehydrator it is important to choose one that is fan-operated, which provides even drying temperatures throughout. It should also allow for temperature selection and control. Many home models lack quality temperature controllers.

The Tree of Life Café recommends the Excalibur dehydrator because of its efficient fan-operated system, accurate temperature control, and ease of use and cleaning. The Excalibur has up to nine trays that slide in and out of the dehydrator without disturbing other levels, as would be the case with the common circular stacking models. See the tips in the next section on dehydration.

COFFEE GRINDER OR SPICE MILL

A coffee grinder can be used to grind whole spices, and it works perfectly for grinding your daily flax seed. A quality spice mill may be more effective for grinding hard spices to a fine powder and will simultaneously provide air-tight storage for your whole spices. In this case, purchase a spice mill for each type of whole spice you use, such as black and white peppercorns, nutmeg, coriander, cardamom, cinnamon, cumin, caraway, and anise.

SPIRAL SLICER (SALADACCO)

A spiral slicer, also called a Saladacco, is essential, if you want to create pasta-like "noodles" from a variety of vegetables such as zucchini, carrot, squash, and root vegetables. It is easy to make both flat ribbon "noodles" and super-thin angel hair "pasta" with this clever tool. This and the mandoline are primarily for higher-end cuisine preparations.

MANDOLINE

A most versatile kitchen tool, the mandoline is simple to use and will perfectly slice veggies and fruits thick or thin. With the switch of a blade, you can instantly julienne, grate, or shred. Essential for making vegetable "pasta" for live-food lasagna and other wide "noodle" dishes.

Miscellaneous Tips

DEHYDRATION

Low-temperature food dehydration is a technique that warms and dries food yet will not destroy enzymes. It has been suggested by Edward

Howell in his book *Food Enzymes for Health and Longevity* that food enzymes are destroyed when the food temperature reaches 115–120°. However, recent research by the Excalibur Dehydrator Company suggests that it is actually better to begin the dehydration process at 145° for the initial stage of the drying process. The reasoning is that as the food is dehydrating, it literally "sweats out" the moisture it contains, and thus creates cooling.

This information changes how I think about the entire process of food dehydration. It means that the safest way to dehydrate is to begin drying at 145° for a maximum of three hours for foods with a high water content. After this the temperature is set in the "normal" range of 110–115° through the completion of the drying process. By doing this we are limiting the potential of bacterial growth by reducing the time the food spends in the dehydrator. The longer that a food is in the dehydrator, the more potential exists for the enzymes to be destroyed, even at lower temperatures. Low-temperature dehydration for sustained time, as practiced for years by the live-food community, may not be safe because sustained low-temperature dehydration encourages bacterial growth and fermentation. At the Tree of Life we feel that the new approach is both safer and more efficient.

This technique of dehydration is only recommended for the Excalibur dehydrator because of the way it dries food. First the Excalibur has the Parallexx™ Horizontal-Airflow Drying System, which evenly distributes air, eliminating "hot" spots. Also, a thermostat controls the temperature in the Excalibur, so that, when it reaches the set temperature, the heating element shuts off. The advantage to this is that when the temperature is higher, moisture is evaporates from the food (instead of being trapped inside by hardening of the outer surface). Then as the temperature goes down, moisture is able to pass from the inside to the outside of the food as the outer moisture is evaporated. In this way the food dries much more quickly and evenly so there is less chance of bacterial growth.

The Excalibur dehydrator comes equipped with Teflex sheets. These non-stick sheets are used whenever the food to be dehydrated is of a more liquid-like consistency that could spill through the plastic net sheet that is normally used on the dehydrator tray.

THROW OUT YOUR MICROWAVE!

A microwave oven decays and changes the molecular structure of the food by the process of radiation, making it a "radiation oven." The Soviet Union banned the use of microwave ovens in 1976. Yet, more than 90 percent of American homes have microwave ovens. Because microwave ovens are so convenient and energy efficient, as compared to conventional ovens, very few homes or restaurants are without them. The general perception, even among health professionals, is that whatever a microwave oven does to foods cooked in it doesn't have any negative effect on either the food or the consumer of the food. This is far from the truth. The author actually cured two people from what was diagnosed as "chronic fatigue" by having them literally throw out their microwave. The following five pieces of information, although not conclusive, are highly suggestive of the potential risks of using microwave ovens.

The first is a piece of news about a lawsuit in Oklahoma in 1991 concerning the hospital use of a microwave oven to warm blood needed in a transfusion. The case involved a hip surgery patient, Norma Levitt, who died from a simple blood transfusion. It seems the nurse had warmed the blood in a microwave oven. The implication is that the microwaving of the blood to be transfused transformed the structure of the previously compatible blood, making it incompatible for transfusion.

The second is a report on microwaved baby formula, from *The Lancet* of December 9, 1989:

Microwaving baby formulas converted certain trans-amino acids into their synthetic cis-isomers. Synthetic isomers, whether cis-amino acids or trans-fatty acids, are not biologically active. Further, one of the amino acids, L-proline, was converted to its d-isomer, which is known to be neurotoxic (poisonous to the nervous system) and nephrotoxic (poisonous to the kidneys). It's bad enough that many babies are not nursed, but now they are given fake milk (baby formula) made even more toxic via microwaving.

The third is a report on eating microwaved food, showing that eating microwaved food changes blood chemistry. Titled "Comparative Study of Food Prepared Conventionally and in the Microwave Oven," published by Raum and Zelt in 1992, at 3(2):43, it states:

> One short-term study found significant and disturbing changes in the blood of individuals consuming microwaved milk and vegetables. Eight volunteers ate various combinations of the same foods cooked different ways. All foods that were processed through the microwave ovens caused changes in the blood of the volunteers. Hemoglobin levels decreased and overall white cell levels and cholesterol levels increased. Lymphocytes decreased.

The fourth piece of information concerns the carcinogens created when the food is microwaved. In Dr. Lita Lee's book, *Health Effects of Microwave Radiation—Microwave Ovens,* and in the March and September 1991 issues of *Earthletter,* she stated that every microwave oven leaks electromagnetic radiation, harms food, and converts substances cooked in it to dangerous organ-toxic and carcinogenic products. Further research summarized in this article reveal that microwave ovens are far more harmful than previously imagined.

The fifth interesting piece of information is the Russian investigations published by the Atlantis Raising Educational Center in Portland, Oregon. Carcinogens were formed in virtually all foods tested. No test food was subjected to more microwaving than necessary to accomplish the purpose, that is, cooking, thawing, or heating to ensure sanitary ingestion. Here's a summary of some of the results:

- Microwaving prepared meats sufficiently to ensure sanitary ingestion caused formation of d-Nitrosodienthanolamines, a well-known carcinogen.
- Microwaving milk and cereal grains converted some of their amino acids into carcinogens. Thawing frozen fruits converted

their glucoside and galactoside containing fractions into carcinogenic substances.

- Extremely short exposure of raw, cooked, or frozen vegetables converted their plant alkaloids into carcinogens.
- Carcinogenic free radicals were formed in microwaved plants, especially root vegetables.

Russian researchers also reported a marked acceleration of structural degradation leading to a decreased food value of 60 to 90 percent in all foods tested. Among the changes observed were:

- Deceased bio-availability of vitamin B complex, vitamin C, vitamin E, essential minerals, and lipotropics factors in all food tested.
- Various kinds of damage to many plant substances, such as alkaloids, glucosides, galactosides and nitrilosides.
- The degradation of nucleo-proteins in meats.

SALTING AND MASSAGE

The technique of salting, as indicated in many recipes, helps to soften hard vegetables such as cabbage, kale, or broccoli. Salt causes the vegetables to release moisture as it breaks down the cell walls. Digestion is made easier when these fibers are broken down. Foods that are high in cellulose will wilt slightly, creating a texture similar to cooked food.

Green leafy vegetables can be "massaged" by using the hands directly to rub the salt into the greens. This effect is further enhanced by adding a small amount of an acid, such as lemon juice or apple cider vinegar. It is recommended that only Celtic sea salt or Himalayan salt be used for all food preparation.

SOAKING AND SPROUTING

Many nuts, seeds, and grains must be soaked or sprouted before they can be used in live-food cuisine. Soaking the seeds and nuts removes the enzyme inhibitors they contain, thereby activating a food's full nutritional potential. Below is a chart to guide you in this process.

SOAKING AND SPROUTING GUIDELINES

Seed Type	Dry Measure	Soaking Time	Sprouting Time	Yield	Length@ Harvest	Tips
NUTS						
Almonds	1 cup	12 hours			None	Store in water in refrigerator.
Pecans	1 cup	1–2 hours				
Walnut	1 cup	1–2 hours				
Macadamia		Do not soak				Yellow seeds indicate rancidity.
Pine nuts		Do not soak				Yellow seeds indicate rancidity.
In-shell Pistachio		Do not soak				
SEEDS						
Hulled Pumpkin	1 cup	4 hours	24 hours	2 cups	1/8 inch	
Hulled Sunflower	1 cup	4 hours	24 hours	2.5 cups	1/4–1/2 inch	Can spoil if not used promptly.
Hulled Buckwheat (careful, soaking/ sprouting too long will cause fermentation)	1 cup	15 minutes	24 hours	2 cups	1/8inch	Use only raw groats.
White Hulled Sesame	1 cup	4 hours				
Black Sesame	1 cup	4 hours				
Hemp Seeds	1 cup	Do not soak				
Golden/ Brown Flax Seeds	1 cup seed, 1 cup water	8 hours				

SOAKING AND SPROUTING GUIDELINES

Seed Type	Dry Measure	Soaking Time	Sprouting Time	Yield	Length@ Harvest	Tip
SEEDS						
Golden/ Brown Flax Seeds (for grinding)	1 cup	Do not soak, just grind and eat dry				
GRAINS						
Rye	1cup	6 hours	5–7 days	3 cups	4 inches	
Spelt	1 cup	6 hours	5–7 days	3 cups	4 inches	Spelt is a primitive wheat.
Wheat	1 cup	6 hours	5–7 days	3 cups	4 inches	
Kamut	1 cup	6 hours	5–7 days	3 cups	4 inches	
Barley	1 cup	6 hours	5–7 days	3 cups	4 inches	
Amaranth	1 cup	3 hours	24 hours	3 cups	1/8 inch	
Millet	1 cup	3 hours	12 hours	3 cups	0–1/8 inch	
Quinoa	1 cup	3 hours	24 hours	3 cups	1/4 inch	
GREEN SPROUTS						
Buckwheat	1 cup	6 hours	5–7 days	3 inches		
Sunflower	1 cup	7 hours	5–7 days	3 inches		
SMALL VEGETABLE						
Alfalfa	3 tablespoons	5 hours	5 days	4 cups	2 inches	
Clover	3 tablespoons	5 hours	5 days	4 cups	2 inches	
Fenugreek	1/4 cup	6 hours	5 days	4 cups	2 inches	Good to dissolve mucus
Kale	1/4 cup	5 hours	5 days	4 cups	1 inch	
Mustard	3 tablespoons	5 hours	5 days	4 cups	1.5 inches	Spicy
Radish	3 tablespoons	6 hours	5 days	4 cups	2 inches	Spicy

SOAKING AND SPROUTING GUIDELINES

Seed Type	Dry Measure	Soaking Time	Sprouting Time	Yield	Length@ Harvest	Tips
MISCELLANEOUS						
Sun-dried Tomato	1 cup	3–4 hours				Warm water speeds up the soaking process.
Raisins	1 cup	3 hours				Warm water speeds up the soaking process.
Dulse Sea Vegetable	1 cup	2 minutes				Massage in water and drain immediately to retain minerals.
Wakame	1 cup	2 hours				**Quite chewy, chop well.**
Sea Palm	1 cup	15 minutes				

Data resourced from: http://www.supersprouts.com

Basic Daily Menu Flow on the Rainbow Green World Cuisine

Using the Rainbow Green World Cuisine approach, Tim and Michela Casey (the Tree of Life Café managers) and I have designed a menu that is flexible, simple, and based on a typical day. This menu is a basic layout you can apply, using the recipes here and other Phase 1 recipes from *Rainbow Green Live-Food Cuisine* to create a cuisine that works with your time and culinary expertise.

BREAKFAST

One of the following: salad, soup, green smoothie, or green vegetable juice

Green superfood powders and blends, depending on your

constitutional needs (A variety of these powders and blends are available in the marketplace.)
Tea

SNACK

1 pint green vegetable juice (if you need higher protein, add nuts and seeds, or 1–2 tablespoons of high-protein concentrates such as chlorella or spirulina, or a green superfood powder blend. (A variety are available in the marketplace.)

LUNCH

Either salad or soup
Entree
Pâté, crackers, or nut mylk
Tea

SNACK

1 pint green vegetable juice (if you need higher protein, add nuts and seeds, or 1–2 tablespoons of high-protein concentrates such as chlorella or spirulina, or a green superfood powder blend), or
Veggie sticks and pâté, or
Sushi rolls

DINNER

Either salad or soup. If you like, include any items below, but dinner should be light.
Entree
Pâté, crackers, or nut mylk
Tea
Dessert once a week
If you need higher protein, add nuts and seeds, or 1–2 tablespoons of high-protein concentrates such as chlorella or spirulina, or a green superfood powder blend

Entrees

Broccoli with Bell Pepper and Cheeze

Veggies:

2 cups broccoli, sliced or chopped

1 cup red bell pepper, julienne-cut

Seed cheeze in blender:

1 cup sunflower seeds

¼ cup olive oil (or other recommended oil to taste)

2 tablespoons lemon juice

½ teaspoon black pepper

¼ teaspoon Celtic or Himalayan salt

one-half bunch fresh cilantro

¼ teaspoon cayenne

¼ teaspoon hing (Hing is an Ayurvedic spice that tastes like onion. It
  has anti-flatulence properties.)

2 teaspoons cumin

kalamata olive water, to desired consistency (Note: This is the soak
  water that the olives are marinating in.)

Toss the bell pepper and broccoli, and set aside. In food processor,
process the seeds to a butter or as much as possible. Add olive oil,
lemon juice, water, hing, black pepper, cayenne, and salt. Process to a
creamy consistency. Massage into broccoli and bell pepper, and mix.
Eat as is or serve in a flax wrap burrito-style. Serves 1–2.

Flax Wraps

1 cup flax seed, ground, unsifted

1 cup seed flour, ground and sifted

2 tablespoons poppy seed, whole

½ teaspoon Celtic or Himalayan salt

½ cup blessed water, a little at a time to a dough-like texture that can be
  patted and rolled out with a rolling pin

Grind flax in blender, and toss into bowl. Grind and sift dried seed pulp
from mylks into bowl (see the section on seed and nut mylks, below) to

create a "seed flour." Combine all dry ingredients together. Add water a little at a time. Roll out dough and cookie-cut six-inch circles. Roll out each circle again to achieve a very thin tortilla-style wrap. This is a basic flax wrap. Other dried herbs can be added for a "savory wrap." Serves 1–2.

Sushi Nori or Cucumber Rolls

Sushi filling:

2 cups walnuts

Red and yellow bell pepper

2 tablespoons sesame oil

2 tablespoons lemon or lime juice

2 tablespoons ginger juice

½ teaspoon Celtic or Himalayan salt

¼ teaspoon freshly ground black pepper

dash cayenne

4–6 tablespoons fresh cilantro and/or basil, minced

Optional:

1 teaspoon lemongrass, ground in the spice mill

1 kaffir lime leaf, ground in the spice mill

For filling:

Process nuts in food processor. Add oil, lemon or lime juice, salt, and pepper. Add lemongrass, lime leaf, and fresh herbs.

Julienne red bell pepper and yellow bell peppers. Use sunflower sprouts, red clover, alfalfa, and/or julienned greens.

For rolling:

Place filling on the bottom half of the nori sheet. Place bell peppers and sprouts over the top of filling. Begin rolling the filling in sheet to form a tube. Use a little water to seal the edges. Cut and serve.

For cucumber rolls:

Take both ends off of the cucumber. Use a vegetable peeler to peel all the skin off, discard. Use the vegetable peeler to peel the whole length of the vegetable. Keep peeling to get long thin strips of cucumber the same width of the vegetable peeler blade. Lay these strips overlapping each other approximately ¼ to ½ inch, achieving a 6- or 7-inch width sheet. You can place nori over this and roll, or roll without nori the same as the directions above for rolling.

Nori is a wonderful food. We often cut the sheets into quarters and fill them with a bit of salad, then fold over like a taco shape and enjoy. Serves 4.

Taco Shells

Use one of the basic cracker recipes. After 4 hours of drying, flip the crackers off of the telex and onto a cutting board, cookie-cut the cracker with a six-inch cookie cutter (or use a Rubbermaid 1-gallon circular jug top, for example). You may need to use a knife to cut through the dry parts. Shape the circle into a half-moon taco shell shape, using a washcloth folded into quarters as a spacer. With this method you should be able to fold two shells over one cloth. Lay the shells on their side and dehydrate the remaining time. Fill shells with greens, guacamole, and salsa. Serves 4.

Guacamole

2 avocados, diced and mashed
2 tablespoons lime juice
¼ cup minced cilantro
1 teaspoon cumin
¼–½ teaspoon Celtic or Himalayan salt
Dice avocado and add remaining ingredients. Mash a bit to achieve a
  creamy texture. Serves 2–4.

Tomato Salsa

1½ cup ripe tomatoes, diced
1½ cup cucumbers, deseeded and diced
1 cup cilantro, finely chopped
1 tablespoon olive oil
1 tablespoon lime juice
dash cayenne
dash Celtic or Himalayan salt

Chop all ingredients and add lime juice, oil, spices, and salt. Serves
   1–2.

Strawberry Salsa

1 cup strawberries, sliced
1 cup cucumbers, deseeded and diced
1 cup tomatoes, diced
1 cup cilantro, finely chopped
dash cayenne
1 tablespoon lime juice
¼ teaspoon Celtic or Himalayan salt
1 tablespoon olive oil

Chop and dice all ingredients and toss into bowl. Add remaining
   ingredients and mix. Serves 2.

Pizza

Pizza crust:

Use either bread recipe: Form dough into a ball and place in the center
of a teflex sheet. Press the center of the ball into the sheet and form into
a pizza crust shape. To avoid any cracks in the dough, use the palm of
one hand to press and the other hand to guide the shape. If a crack
begins to form, quickly attend to it by pressing it back together. Serves 4.

Pizza cheeze:

Use the Seed Cheeze recipe (see Nuts and Seed Cheezes) with the
optional Italian seasoning and thyme. Or, as an alternative to the
cheeze, use the Basil Pesto recipe, below.

Marinara:

1 red bell pepper
2 cups sun-dried tomato
½ cup sun-dried tomato water
¼ cup olive oil (or other recommended oil to taste)
1 clove garlic
2–4 tablespoons Italian seasoning
½ teaspoon black pepper
¼ teaspoon Celtic or Himalayan salt

Place all ingredients in blender and process on high speed. Serves 4.

Topping:

  2 bell peppers, diced

  1 zucchini, diced

  1 clove garlic, minced

  one bunch of basil

  ¼ cup kalamata olives, pitted and minced

  3 tablespoons Italian seasoning

  2 tablespoons cold-pressed stone-ground olive oil

  1 tablespoon kalamata olive water

  ½ –1 teaspoon black pepper

  ¼ teaspoon Celtic or Himalayan salt

Dice all ingredients and place into bowl. Toss in all herbs and spices and let marinate for a few minutes. Serves 4 when used as pizza topping.

Basil Pesto

  2 cups walnuts

  ½ cup olive oil (or other recommended oil to taste)

  ½ teaspoon Celtic or Himalayan salt

  ½ teaspoon black pepper

  2 cups basil

In food processor, process nuts with the S-blade until fine. Add remaining ingredients and process until very smooth. Serves 4 when used as pizza topping.

Indian-Flavored Shish Kabobs

Marinated vegetables:

  1 zucchini, sliced on a diagonal

  1 yellow bell pepper, cut into large panels

  1 broccoli, in large florets

  1 red bell pepper, cut into large panels

  1 tomato, sliced

Cut all veggies to proper size and marinate 4 hours with Indian-Style Sauce (below). Place marinated veggies on a shish kabob, alternating with walnut savory balls. Dehydrate on 145° for 2 hours. Serve over coconut rice. Serves 4.

Indian-Style Sauce

1 cup olive oil (or other recommended oil to taste)

2 cups Brazil nuts

6 tablespoons lemon juice

2 tablespoons coriander seeds, ground

2 tablespoons ginger, minced

2 tablespoons cumin, ground

½ teaspoon turmeric powder

½–¾ teaspoon Celtic or Himalayan salt

½ teaspoon hing

1 teaspoon freshly ground black pepper

½ teaspoon cayenne

½ cup ginger juice

one-half bunch cilantro

one-half bunch basil

Optional Thai version:

Add 1 tablespoon lemongrass and 1 lime leaf

Place all ingredients in blender and blend on high speed. Serves 4 when used as marinade for vegetables.

Coconut Rice

1 mature coconut removed from shell and peeled, processed with S-blade in food processor to a fine consistency

½–1 teaspoon Celtic or Himalayan salt

1 teaspoon black pepper

dash cayenne

Toss the food-processed coconut and spices together. Serves 4 when served with Indian-Flavored Shish Kabobs.

Indian-Style Savory Balls

½ cup almonds, soaked
½ cup sunflower seeds, soaked
½ cup hemp seeds
½ cup celery, minced
¼ cup fresh lemon juice
1 tablespoon fresh ginger, grated
½ teaspoon Himalayan or Celtic salt
2 teaspoons cumin
1 teaspoon coriander
dash turmeric
dash cayenne
dash hing
dash mustard seed
dash fenugreek

Process all nuts and seeds in food processor and place into bowl. Add remaining ingredients and mix to a texture that can be formed into balls. Hint: Use an ice cream scoop that is 1½ inch in diameter to portion size. Dehydrate on 145° for 2 hours. Serves 4 when served in combination with Indian-Flavored Shish Kabobs.

Walnut Savory Balls

1 cup walnuts, soaked
1 cup sunflower seeds, soaked
¼ cup fresh basil or cilantro
1 tablespoon fresh ginger, grated
½ teaspoon Celtic or Himalayan salt
dash hing
dash cayenne
dash turmeric

Place nuts and seeds in food processor and process to a fine texture. Add remaining ingredients and process to a formable texture. Form into balls and dehydrate on 145° for 2 hours. Serves 4.

Stringbean Dhal

1 cup stringbeans

1 cup avocado

¼ cup water

1 tomato

2 tablespoons olive oil (or other recommended oil to taste)

2 teaspoons salt

1 teaspoon cumin

¼ teaspoon turmeric

⅛ teaspoon cayenne

⅛ teaspoon coriander

⅛ teaspoon mustard seeds

In the blender, combine two stringbeans with the remaining ingredients until smooth. Add additional water for consistency.

Cut remaining stringbeans in 2-inch lengths. In a mixing bowl, combine sauce and beans, and mix well. Serves 2.

Herbed Stringbeans

¾ pound stringbeans

2 tablespoons olive oil (or other recommended oil to taste)

1½ tablespoon fresh parsley

1 tablespoon fresh mint

ground pepper to taste

1 tablespoon lemon juice

2 teaspoons lemon zest

½ teaspoon salt

Place beans in large bowl, add salt, and massage until beans are softened, around 5 minutes.

Whisk together remaining ingredients and toss with beans. Serve at room temperature. Serves 2.

Rice and Cabbage

¾ cup long-grain brown rice
1⅓ cup water
2 tomatoes
One-third head coarsely chopped cabbage
ground pepper, salt, cilantro, and dill, for seasoning to taste

Simmer rice and water around 15 minutes, then add remaining ingredients and continue simmering until cabbage it soft, 5–10 minutes. Serves 2.

Mexican Rice

½ cup uncooked brown or wild rice
1 cup cold water
1 garlic clove, crushed (optional)
2 tablespoons olive or coconut oil
1 tablespoon miso
¼ onion, coarsely chopped (optional)
1 small Roma tomato, chopped
⅛ small jalapeño pepper
2 soaked sun-dried tomatoes, blended
½ teaspoon cumin seeds, ground
salt to taste

Add oil to a pot on medium, then add uncooked rice and brown in the oil. Stir to keep from burning, for 5 minutes. Add garlic (optional). Add water and remaining ingredients, and stir well. Cover and simmer on medium-low heat for 20–30 minutes. Ready when rice is fluffy and water is absorbed. Serves 2.

Brown Rice in Palm Oil

4 cups water
2 cups brown rice
1 tablespoon red palm oil
1 garlic clove, minced (optional)

1 tablespoon cumin, ground

½ teaspoon cayenne (to taste)

1 teaspoon salt

In a pot, sauté garlic in palm oil for 2 minutes on medium heat.
Add spices and water, and bring to boil. Add rice. Cook with no lid
on medium heat until water bubbles through top of rice. Then cover
and steam rice on low until water is absorbed, around 25 minutes.
Serves 4.

Millet, Peas, and Indian Spice

2 cups green split peas

4 cups water

2 stalks celery, chopped

½ onion, chopped (optional)

1 teaspoon coconut oil

2 tablespoons curry powder

2 teaspoons cumin, ground

1 garlic clove, pressed (optional)

1½ teaspoon salt

dash of cayenne (optional)

1¼ cup millet, hulled

Bring the water, with the peas, ¼ cup onion (optional), spices, and oil to
a boil and simmer 35 minutes. Stir in the millet. Cover and steam for 20
minutes. Remove from heat. Stir in ¼ cup onion (optional) and the
celery. Let sit 10 minutes, covered. Toss with 2 tablespoon coconut oil,
and serve. Serves 4.

Lentils and Rice

1½ cup uncooked long-grain brown rice

3 cups water

1 medium onion, diced

⅓ cup dried brown lentils

¼ teaspoon dried red chili flakes

½ teaspoon salt

1 large bay leaf

Heat oil in pot on medium heat. Add onion and chili, and stir until onion is clear. Add the rice and lentils, and stir for 5 minutes. Add water and spices, bring to a boil, then steam on medium-low heat, covered, for 50 minutes. Remove from heat, keeping the lid on for 10 minutes to absorb the steam. Serves 2.

Rice and Black-Eyed Peas

1½ cup uncooked long-grain rice

2 cups freshly cooked black-eyed peas

3½ cups water

1 onion, diced

2 tablespoons coconut oil

1 bay leaf

½ teaspoon salt

black pepper and cayenne to taste

Boil 3 cups of the water. Add rice, bay leaf, and ¼ teaspoon salt. Boil again, cover, and let steam on simmering heat for 45 minutes. Remove, let sit with cover on 10 minutes, then remove bay leaf.
In a pan, heat coconut oil on medium heat, and add in onions, ¼ teaspoon salt, and the peppers. Stir until onion browns. Then toss in the peas, ½ cup water, and rice. Serves 4.

Amaranth

1 cup amaranth

3 cups water

1 small garlic clove, minced (optional)

1 medium onion, diced (optional)

1 tablespoon coconut or olive oil

salt and pepper to taste

dried chili flakes or cayenne powder to taste

In a pot, combine first four ingredients. Bring to a boil, and reduce to a simmer. Cover and steam amaranth for 25 minutes. Remove lid and stir in remaining ingredients. Serves 2.

Amazingly Versatile Rice Dish

4 cups water

1 cup brown rice

1 cup lentils or beans

1 medium onion, chopped (optional)

2 cloves garlic, minced (optional)

3 tablespoons olive oil (or other recommended oil to taste)

2 tablespoons spices according to taste (see below)

In a pot, warm the oil, then add the onion, garlic, and spices. Sauté until golden brown, then add remaining ingredients. Bring to a boil, then reduce heat to medium-low. Cover and simmer 30–35 minutes or until water has evaporated. Remove and ladle into a blender and blend. Only fill halfway each time you blend. The blending is what makes this velvety and smooth.

Spice options:

Indian: Use curry powder, chili powder, cinnamon, or cumin

Mediterranean: After cooking, add in chopped tomatoes, basil, parsley, oregano, and a squeeze of lemon juice

Or just toss with some Moroccan olive soak water (the juice that the olives come bottled in)

Dhal

2 cups water

1 cup red lentils

1 cup chopped cabbage

2 tomatoes, chopped

1 hot green chili pepper, chopped or whole (optional)

1 tablespoon olive or coconut oil

1 teaspoon cumin seeds, ground

¼ teaspoon turmeric powder

salt and lime to taste

one-quarter bunch cilantro, chopped

Wash lentils, and cook in the water on medium-low heat for 20 minutes. In separate pot, heat the oil on medium heat, then add cumin, stirring 30 seconds. Add chili and cabbage, and sauté until softened. Set aside.

When lentils are soft, mash them or blend with water and add into the cabbage pot. Add turmeric and salt. Remove from heat. Toss in cilantro, tomatoes, and lime juice. Serves 2.

Spiced Kidney Beans

4 cups cooked kidney beans

2 tablespoons olive or coconut oil (or other recommended oil to taste)

1½ onion, chopped (optional)

2 inches ginger root, peeled and minced

4 cloves fresh garlic, peeled and minced

6 large tomatoes, chopped

1–2 teaspoons salt

½ tablespoon curry powder

½ teaspoon turmeric powder

¼ teaspoon paprika

¼ teaspoon cumin seeds, ground

½ cup sun-dried tomatoes, dry, ground in a coffee grinder or blender (to thicken)

one-half bunch fresh cilantro or parsley, chopped

½ lemon or 1 lime, juiced (optional)

Toss all ingredients in a large mixing bowl. To enhance flavor, let sit before serving (as long as you can, up to overnight in the fridge). Serves 2.

Ginger Juice

2–4 inches of ginger, peeled and chopped

1 cup water

Blend in a high-speed blender and strain through a nylon mesh seed or nut mylk bag, cheesecloth, or a natural-fiber seed or nut mylk bag.

Salads

Option 1

one bunch kale, chard, or collards, destemmed and chopped, or bok choy, napa or other cabbages, massaged with ½ teaspoon salt

Option 2

one bunch spinach or other favorite greens (arugula, lettuces, mustard greens, lamb's quarters, dandelion, or other wild greens), tossed with ingredients listed below and

¼–½ teaspoon Himalayan or sun-dried sea salt

Add:

1 bell pepper (red, orange, or yellow)

1 avocado and/or ¼ cup hemp seed

3–4 tablespoons lemon juice or 2 tablespoons apple cider vinegar

3 tablespoons hemp, olive, or sesame oil

Optional for Any Salad

Sea vegetables, dulse (whole or flakes), nori (whole or torn sheets)

Superfoods, spirulina, or other green powders

Fresh herbs

Roots (burdock and/or radish)

Olives, whole or pitted

Spices (cumin, caraway, curry, coriander, turmeric) or other favorite spices

Dash of hing, cayenne, black pepper, and/or chipotle

Massage and serve. Serves 1.

Kale Salad with Chipotle

Base:

two bunches of kale, destemmed

one-half bunch parsley, minced and massaged with

½ teaspoon Celtic or Himalayan salt

Add:

1 avocado

1 bell pepper, julienned

small handful of whole dulse cut with scissors

2–3 tablespoon of hemp or high-quality cold-pressed olive oil

3 tablespoons lemon or lime juice

½ –1 tablespoon cumin

¼ teaspoon chipotle

dash hing

dash chlorella or other green powders

Serves 1 or 2.

Spinach Salad with Spirulina

Base:

one bunch spinach, chopped and washed

two handfuls of baby lettuce

Add:

1 avocado, diced

1 bell pepper, julienned

2–3 tablespoons hemp oil

2–3 tablespoons lemon

1 tablespoon spirulina or other green powders

3–4 olives

¼ teaspoon turmeric

¼ teaspoon cayenne

dash hing

¼ teaspoon Celtic or Himalayan salt

A little ground sesame or flax on top is also nice. Creates a small
medium bowl of salad for 1 or 2.

Cabbage Salad with Caraway Sesame Tahini

Base:

half head cabbage, shredded or chopped, massaged with

½ teaspoon Celtic or Himalayan salt

Add:

one bunch cilantro

1 avocado, diced

1 bell pepper, julienned

Dressing:

In blender, combine the following ingredients:

¼–½ cup ground sesame seed

1 clove garlic, minced

2–3 tablespoons sesame oil

2–3 tablespoons lemon

2–3 tablespoons blessed water or olive brine, to desired consistency

1 tablespoon caraway

¼ teaspoon cayenne and/or black pepper

¼ teaspoon Celtic or Himalayan salt

Building the salad:

Massage dressing into salad ingredients, and top with:

handful of red clover, alfalfa, or sunflower greens, or

1 tablespoon green powder superfood, or

dulse flakes or kelp powder

Creates a small medium bowl of salad for 1 or 2.

Sea Vegetable Salad with Sesame Tahini

Base:

one bunch dinosaur kale, massaged with

¼ teaspoon Celtic or Himalayan salt

Add:

1 cup whole dulse, cut into strips with scissors

1 tablespoon kelp powder

one bunch cilantro or parsley

½ cup chopped spinach

1 avocado, diced, or hemp seed

1 bell pepper, julienned

1 tablespoon spirulina

Dressing:

In blender, combine the following ingredients:

¼–½ cup sesame seed, ground

1 clove garlic, minced

2–3 tablespoons sesame oil

2–3 tablespoons lemon juice

2–3 tablespoons blessed water or olive brine, to desired consistency

¼ teaspoon turmeric

¼ teaspoon cayenne and/or black pepper

¼ teaspoon Himalayan or Celtic salt

Option: ¼ cup unchopped fresh herb basil or cilantro

Building the salad:

Massage dressing into salad ingredients, and top with a handful of red clover, alfalfa, or sunflower greens. Serves 1 or 2.

Wild Greens Salad with Cactus Pad Dressing

Base:

one bowl full of baby greens

one or two handfuls of wild greens (lamb's quarter, dandelion, or wild mustard)

Add:

1 avocado, diced

1 bell pepper, julienned

¼ cup young raw nopal cactus pad, diced or julienned (Note: Remove thorns by scraping surface of pad and rinsing.)

Dressing:

Combine the following ingredients:

1 young raw nopal cactus pad (Note: Very young cactus pads without thorns may be blended without the scraping technique.)

¼ cup hemp seed

¼ cup cilantro, fresh, unchopped

2–3 tablespoons hemp, sesame, or cold-pressed olive oil

2 tablespoons lemon

3 tablespoons blessed water

¼ teaspoon Celtic or Himalayan salt

Toss all ingredients in blender and blend on high speed.

Building the salad:

Massage dressing into salad ingredients. Serves 1 or 2.

Quinoa and Black Bean Salad

1 cup cooked quinoa (see chart)

2 scallions, sliced thin

½ cup chopped tomatoes

½ cup chopped celery

½ cup chopped red bell pepper

1 cup cooked black beans (see chart)

Toss in a large mixing bowl.

Dressing:

Whisk together:

4 tablespoon olive oil

2 tablespoon lemon juice

1 small clove garlic, minced (optional)

salt and pepper to taste

one-half bunch cilantro, minced

Toss with quinoa and bean mixture. Serves 4.

Diabetes Healing Bean Salad

4 cups green beans (cooked or raw)

2 cups black beans (cooked)

2 cups kidney beans (cooked)

2 cups chickpeas (cooked)

2 cups celery, diced

2 cups red bell pepper, diced

1 red onion, thinly sliced (optional)

⅔ cup lemon juice (option: apple cider vinegar)

⅓ cup olive oil (or other recommended oil to taste)

25 drops stevia (optional)

salt and pepper to taste

Warm together in a large pot for 5 minutes while stirring. Remove from heat, let sit 30 minutes to 1 hour. Serve warm or chilled. This dish will last a few days in the fridge. Serves 6 generously.

Sumptuous Salad

3 cups cooked grains of choice (cooled)

1 cup cooked beans of choice (cooled)

2 cups diced vegetables of choice (colored bell peppers, celery, spinach, cucumber, tomato)

1 cup nuts or seeds, chopped

¼ red onion (optional)

one-half bunch minced herb of choice (cilantro, basil, oregano, thyme, parsley)

2 tablespoons olive oil (or other recommended oil to taste)

1 teaspoon salt

1 clove garlic, minced

1 teaspoon lemon or lime juice

This is a great quick and easy salad and the beans are a great source of protein! This fast and healthy complete meal serves 4.

Quinoa Salad

3 cups water

1½ cup quinoa

1 tablespoon coconut oil (or other recommended oil to taste)

¼ teaspoon salt

Combine in saucepan, bring to a boil, cover, and steam for 15 minutes. The quinoa will be translucent. Remove from heat and stir in 2 tablespoons coconut oil. Leave the lid off and set aside.

In a medium bowl, combine:

2 celery stalks, diced

¼ red onion, diced (optional)

2 tomatoes, diced

one bunch cilantro, chopped

one-half bunch parsley, chopped

1 tablespoon coconut oil

1 clove of garlic (optional)

1½ tablespoons lemon juice

Season with salt and pepper to taste. Toss in the cooked quinoa and serve warm or chilled. Serves 2.

Brown Rice and Bean Salad

1 cup cooked brown rice

½ cup cooked beans of choice

1 tomato, chopped

1 green onion, chopped (optional)

½ avocado, chopped

dash cayenne

½ cup cilantro, chopped

½ lime, juiced

salt and pepper to taste

6 large butter lettuce leaves, whole, to serve as a wrap for the salad

Mix all ingredients in a large mixing bowl. Serve in lettuce leaves and eat as a wrap.

Dressings

Tomato Dressing

½ cup sun-dried tomato, rehydrated

½ cup sunflower seeds

½ cup blessed water

¼ cup sun-dried tomato water

2 tablespoons olive oil or sesame oil

1 tablespoon lemon

½ tablespoon ginger

dash Celtic or Himalayan salt

dash cayenne

dash hing

Toss all ingredients into blender and blend to a creamy texture.

Tahini Dressing

1 cup sesame seeds

½ cup kalamata olive brine or ½ cup blessed water with a dash of salt

3 tablespoons lemon juice

2–3 tablespoons tomato soak water

2 tablespoons ginger juice

3 tablespoons olive oil (or other recommended oil to taste)

1 tablespoon sesame oil

1 tablespoon cumin

¼ teaspoon black pepper

dash Celtic or Himalayan salt

dash cayenne

dash hing

Blend all ingredients together in high-speed blender. Makes 2–3 servings.

Avocado Caraway Dressing

1 avocado

3 tablespoons lemon juice

3 tablespoons ginger juice

2 tablespoons caraway

¼ teaspoon black pepper

dash to ¼ teaspoon Himalayan or Celtic salt

dash cayenne

dash hing

1 cup kalamata olive water or blessed water with a dash of Celtic or Himalayan salt

Blend all ingredients together in high-powered blender. Serves 1–2.

Dulse Dressing

1 avocado
3 tablespoons lemon juice
3 tablespoons dulse flakes
2 tablespoons ginger juice
¼ teaspoon black pepper
dash to ¼ teaspoon Celtic or Himalayan salt
pinch cayenne
1 cup blessed water

Blend all ingredients together in high-powered blender. Serves 1–2.

Cumin Caesar Dressing

1 avocado
3 tablespoons lemon juice
3 tablespoons ginger juice
2 tablespoons olive oil (or other recommended oil to taste)
1 tablespoon cumin
¼ teaspoon black pepper
dash to ¼ teaspoon Himalayan or Celtic salt
dash cayenne
dash hing
1 cup kalamata olive water or blessed water with a dash of celtic or Himalayan salt

Blend all ingredients together in high-speed blender. Serves 1–2.

Creamy Italian Dressing

1 cup tomato
1 avocado
¼ cup olive oil

1 tablespoon Italian seasoning

2 tablespoons lemon juice

¼ teaspoon black pepper

dash hing

dash Himalayan or sun-dried sea salt

one-half bunch fresh oregano

Blend tomato with olive oil, lemon juice, avocado, hing, spice, salt, and pepper. Chop oregano. Mix into dressing and blend lightly. Serves 1–2.

Thai-Style Caesar Dressing

1 avocado

3 tablespoons lime juice

½ kaffir lime leaf and/or few sprigs of cilantro for variation

1 teaspoon minced lemon grass or a sprig of basil, for variation

2 tablespoons stone-crushed cold-pressed olive oil (or other recommended oil to taste)

2 tablespoons ginger juice

¼ teaspoon black pepper

dash to ¼ teaspoon Celtic or Himalayan salt

pinch cayenne

1 cup blessed water

Blend all ingredients together in high-speed blender. Serves 1–2.

Sea Vegetable Caesar Dressing

1 avocado

3 tablespoons lemon juice

2 tablespoons kelp

2 tablespoons hemp oil or stone-crushed cold-pressed olive oil

2 tablespoons ginger juice

¼ teaspoon black pepper

dash to ¼ teaspoon Celtic or Himalayan salt

pinch cayenne

1 cup blessed water

Blend all ingredients together in high-speed blender. Serves 1–2.

Hemp Seed Dressing

½ cucumber

¼ cup hemp oil

2 tablespoons ginger juice

2 tablespoons lemon juice

dash Himalayan or Celtic salt

½ cup hemp seed

¼ cup basil

2 tablespoons oregano, fresh

Blend cucumber with lemon juice, ginger juice, and hemp oil. Add hemp seed and blend. Chop basil and oregano. Mix into dressing. Serves 1–2.

Creamy Italian Dressing with Brazil Nuts

½ cucumber

¼ cup olive oil

¼ cup fresh basil, chopped

2 tablespoons fresh oregano, chopped

2 tablespoons ginger juice

2 tablespoons lemon juice

½ cup Brazil nuts

dash Celtic or Himalayan salt

Blend cucumber with lemon juice, ginger juice, and olive oil. Add Brazil nuts and blend. Mix chopped basil and oregano into dressing. Serves 1–2.

Sweet Pepper Dressing

1 bell pepper, seeded

1 tomato

½ cup hemp or olive oil

one-quarter bunch cilantro

2 tablespoon lemon juice

dash Himalayan or Celtic salt

dash hing

Blend bell pepper with lemon juice, salt, hing, and oil. Chop cilantro and pulse-blend into dressing. Serves 1–2.

Hummus

3 cups cooked garbanzo beans (see chart)

1–3 cloves of garlic (optional)

6 tablespoons lemon juice

2 tablespoons tahini or sesame oil

2 tablespoons dill weed, minced

1 tablespoon cumin seeds, ground

1 teaspoon salt

1/8 teaspoon cayenne

5 drops stevia (optional)

In a food processor combine all ingredients and process until desired texture. Serve with vegetable sticks, flax crackers, or on salads. Serves 2.

Soups

Spinach Vegetable Medley Soup

In bowl:

1 bell pepper (red or yellow), diced

2 ribs of celery, diced

one-half bunch or 2 cups spinach, minced with S-blade in food processor

1 avocado, diced

one-half bunch of cilantro or basil, S-bladed to mince

¼ cup sun-dried tomato, blended to a creamy texture in blender

2 tablespoons pumpkin seed, whole

1 tablespoon Italian seasoning

1 tablespoon cumin

1 tablespoon hemp, coconut, sesame, or cold-pressed olive oil

1 tablespoon lemon or ½ tablespoon apple cider vinegar

1 tablespoon sun-dried tomato water

½ tablespoon kalamata olive brine or apple cider vinegar

¼–½ teaspoon Himalayan or Celtic salt

dash cayenne

dash hing

1 cup rooibos, nettle, or dandelion tea

2–4 tablespoons non-soy adzuki or chick pea miso (optional)

For superfood option, add 1 tablespoon spirulina, green powder, and/or 1 tablespoon of maca root powder

To make tea:

½ cup dry tea

3 cups hot water

Steep for 20 minutes.

Toss all prepared ingredients into a pot. Warm to 100°, and serve. Serves 1–2.

Note: This soup can be made in many different varieties by substituting various greens, herbs, and spices.

Hemp Spinach Basil Soup

1 small zucchini

1 rib of celery

1 bell pepper

one-half bunch spinach

one-quarter bunch of basil

¼ cup hemp seeds

½ cup olive brine, or 1 tablespoon of apple cider vinegar and ½ cup water

2 tablespoons hemp, sesame or stone-ground cold-pressed olive oil

2 tablespoons lemon juice

2 tablespoons ginger juice

dash cayenne

pinch of chipotle

¼ teaspoon Himalayan or sun-dried sea salt

Place all ingredients in blender and blend on high speed. Chop basil and blend in lightly. Serves 1–2.

Classic Tomato Soup

1–2 cups sun-dried tomato

2 medium tomatoes

¼ cup sun-dried tomato water

¼–½ cup hemp seeds or sunflower seeds

2 tablespoons hemp oil or stone-ground cold-pressed olive oil

2 tablespoons lemon juice

2 tablespoons ginger juice

dash Himalayan or sun-dried sea salt

dash hing

dash black pepper

blessed water to desired consistency

Toss all ingredients into blender and blend on high speed. Serves 1–2.

Gazpacho

2 medium tomatoes

1 bell pepper

1 young raw nopal cactus pad, spines removed, or

½ cucumber

¼ cup hemp oil or stone-ground cold-pressed olive oil

dash Himalayan or Celtic salt

dash black pepper

dash hing

dash cayenne

Toss all ingredients into blender and blend on high speed. Serve 1-2.

Super Green Cactus Chia Soup

1 young raw nopal cactus pad, spines removed

4 cups greens (kale, spinach, lamb's quarters, baby lettuces, or other favorite greens)

¼ cup hemp oil or stone-ground cold-pressed olive oil

¼ cup chia seeds or hemp seeds

2–4 tablespoons lemon juice

2–4 tablespoons ginger juice

1–3 teaspoons kelp powder

1–3 teaspoons maca root powder

dash black pepper, cayenne, turmeric, and hing

dash Himalayan or sun-dried sea salt

1 cup blessed water to desired consistency

Toss all ingredients into blender and blend on high speed. Serves 1–2.

Aloe Vera Stringbean Soup

1 cup aloe vera, outside skin removed

1 cup stringbeans

2 cups greens (collards, kale, baby lettuces, spinach, or chard)

1 cup cilantro, chopped, loosely packed

¼ cup hemp oil or stone-ground cold-pressed olive oil

2–4 tablespoons lemon juice

2–4 tablespoons ginger juice

1–3 teaspoon kelp powder or other green superfood powders

dash black pepper, cayenne, and hing

dash to ¼ teaspoon Celtic or Himalayan salt

1 cup blessed water to desired consistency

Toss all ingredients into blender and blend on high speed. Serves 1–2.

Aloe Vera Cactus Pad Burdock Cilantro Soup

1 cup aloe vera, diced

1 cup cactus pad, diced

1 cup celery

1 cup cilantro, chopped, loosely packed

¼ cup burdock

2 teaspoons lemon juice

3 tablespoons stone-ground cold-pressed olive oil

1 tablespoon pumpkin seed oil
dash to 1¼ teaspoon Celtic or Himalayan salt
dash cayenne
dash black pepper
dash hing

Place all ingredients in blender and blend on high speed. Serves 1.

Velvety Red Lentil Soup

2 yellow onions, diced (optional)
2 cups red lentil (or any lentil desired)
6 cups water
2 cups chopped vegetables of choice (celery, red bell pepper,
   spinach, kale)
1 tablespoon olive oil
1 teaspoon ground pepper
salt to taste

In a pot, warm oil. Add the onions, and sauté until golden brown. Add the remaining ingredients. Bring to a boil, reduce heat to medium-low. Cover and simmer 25 minutes.

Remove from heat and ladle into a blender, and blend (only halfway full for each blending cycle). The blending is what makes this soup velvety smooth. Serves 4.

Simple Lentil Soup

4 cups lentils, washed and picked through for any pebbles
In a pot, cover lentils plus a couple inches above, with water. Add:
4 tomatoes, chopped
1 big onion, chopped (optional)
3 stalks celery, chopped
1 cup olive oil (or other recommended oil to taste)
1 or more cloves garlic, minced (optional)
salt and pepper to taste
1–2 bay leaves

Bring to a boil until lentils are tender, 30–60 minutes. Toss in chopped
parsley and shallots if desired before serving.

To make this thicker or have a more intense flavor, add at the start your
own tomato paste:

½ cup dry sun-dried tomatoes, blended to a paste in a blender or clean
coffee grinder

Crackers and Breads

Tools needed: Blender for grinding, large mixing bowl, food processor,
S-blade, knife, cutting board, spice grinder or coffee grinder, dehydrator, dehydrator trays, teflex dehydrator sheets, and off-set spatula for
spreading crackers.

Herby Chile Pepper Flax Crackers

4 cups golden flax, ground, soaked in sun-dried tomato water or
blessed water

4 cups nuts or seeds, soaked, ground with S-blade or added whole if
seed is small

4 cups sun-dried tomato, ground to a puree

½ cup poppy seed, whole

½ cup Italian seasoning

two bunches cilantro or basil or other fresh herbs, minced with S-blade

3 tablespoons cumin seed, ground in spice or coffee grinder

1 tablespoon kelp, powder

1 teaspoon chipotle

¼ teaspoon cayenne

1 teaspoon black pepper

3½ teaspoons Himalayan or Celtic salt

Grind and soak flax in blessed water or sun-dried tomato water for 10
minutes in a large bowl. Mince herbs with the S-blade. Toss into the
bowl. Grind soaked nuts or seeds with S-blade to a fine consistency,
toss into the bowl, or if using whole seed toss into the bowl whole.
Grind sun-dried tomato to a puree, and toss into the bowl. Add salt,

kelp, and spices. Stir. Spread on teflex dehydrator trays. Dehydrate for 4 hours. Flip the crackers and dehydrate for 12 more hours. Crackers will keep up to 3 weeks if stored in a cool dry environment. Creates 9 trays of crackers.

Seedy Tomato Herb Crackers

Seeds and spice:

2 cups flax seed, whole, soaked

2 cups nuts or seeds, soaked, ground with S-blade or added whole if seed is small

½ cup ground flax seed

¼ cup poppy seed

¼ cup thyme

¼ cup Italian seasoning

one bunch fresh herbs (marjoram, oregano, or basil)

1½ teaspoon Celtic or Himalayan salt

¼ teaspoon hing

pinch cayenne and/or chipotle

1 cup sun-dried tomato, soaked, ground

Mix all ingredients in a bowl, spread on Teflex dehydrator sheets, and dehydrate for 4 hours. Flip and dehydrate for 12 more hours. Creates 2½ trays of crackers.

Sun-Dried Tomato Bread

Base:

2 cups fresh nut/seed pulp or flour

2 cups sun-dried tomato, S-bladed to a puree

one bunch basil

one bunch of oregano or marjoram

½ cup poppy seed

½ cup Italian seasoning

¼ cup thyme

1 tablespoon olive oil

½ teaspoon Celtic or Himalayan salt

dash to ¼ teaspoon hing

Add:

2 cups flax, ground, massaged into base to a dough-like texture

If using dried nut or seed flour, possibly add more liquid elements: ½–1 cup kalamata olive brine and/or sun-dried tomato water, added a little at a time to reach a cookie-dough consistency.

Mold the dough into a loaf. Slice ⅜ to ½ inch thick. Lay on mesh trays and dehydrate for 2 hours. Creates 1 dehydrator tray of bread. Serves 4.

Savory Bell Pepper Bread

Base:

2 cups fresh nut/seed pulp or flour

2 bell peppers, minced (red or yellow, or mixed)

one to two bunches cilantro or basil, S-bladed

one bunch fresh oregano or marjoram

½ cup poppy seeds

1 cup dried Italian seasoning

½ teaspoon salt

½ teaspoon hing

dash to ¼ teaspoon cayenne or chipotle

1 tablespoon olive oil

Add:

2 cups golden flax, ground

If using dried nut or seed flour, possibly add more liquid elements: ½–1 cup kalamata olive brine and/or sun-dried tomato water, added a little at a time to reach a cookie-dough consistency.

Mold dough into a loaf. Slice ⅜ to ½ inch thick. Lay on mesh trays and dehydrate for 2 hours. Creates 1 dehydrator tray of bread. Serves 4.

Green Smoothies

Basic Green Blender Full

3 bell peppers (red, orange, or yellow, or mixed)

½–1 avocado

3 cups greens (spinach, kale, collards, cilantro)

2 tablespoons lemon juice

2 tablespoons ginger juice

2 cups blessed water

Toss all ingredients into the blender and blend to a creamy consistency. Creates one full Vita-Mix blender. Serves 1–2.

Aloe Vera and Lemon Smoothie

2 cups aloe vera

1 tablespoon lemon juice

1 teaspoon blessed water

Toss in blender and blend on high speed. Serves 1.

Chia Smoothie

1 cup chia seeds

7–8 cups blessed water

Optional: 1 cup ice

Optional ingredients: Add superfood nutrition with cinnamon, nutmeg, star anise, licorice root powder, mesquite, carob, stevia, superfood green powders, spirulina, chlorella, blue green algae, and/or maca. Also, 2–4 cups of any fresh green can be added to make a super chia green smoothie. (Note: If adding greens, use less water.)

Place seeds in blender, with any or all of the optional ingredients listed. Fill halfway with water, add ice, and blend to a creamy consistency. As machine is running, use the remaining water to top off container. Creates one full Vita-Mix of smoothie. Serves 1–2.

Cinnamon Chia Smoothie

1 cup chia seeds

2–3 tablespoons cinnamon

1 tablespoon carob

½ nutmeg, micro-planed

1 teaspoon cardamom

½ teaspoon Celtic or Himalayan salt

¼ teaspoon stevia, whole leaf, powder, or ½–1 dropper of liquid

8 cups blessed water, or 7 cups blessed water plus 1 cup ice

Toss all dry ingredients in, fill halfway with water (and ice, if using), and blend. Fill remaining space with water and blend completely. Serves 1–2.

Breakfast Grains

Millet Breakfast Mix

This is an alkaline grain.

½ cup cooked millet (see chart)

2 tablespoons chopped, walnuts, almonds, or pecans

Nut mylk to cover

Flavor with your favorite spices, such as: cinnamon, cardamom, vanilla, coconut flakes, and coconut oil. Add a pinch of salt, and sweeten with licorice root powder or stevia. Serves 1.

Oatmeal

1 cup rolled oats

1 cup water

1 tablespoon coconut oil

dash salt

Boil water in saucepan, add salt. Add oatmeal and oil. Stir on medium heat for 5 minutes or according to directions on box. Serves 1.

Seed and Nut Mylks

General directions for making seed and nut mylks:

2 cups soaked or unsoaked seeds or nuts

8 cups blessed water

Place seeds or nuts in the blender. Fill blender halfway with water. Blend to a creamy consistency. While the machine is on, add more water all the way to the top. Place mesh bag over the container and pour all mylk through the bag, straining the mylk, into a bowl. Transfer and store in a glass container. Serves 4, in 16-ounce glasses, as is or chilled.

Mylk is delicious plain. As an option, pour the mylk back into blender and add spices (cinnamon, nutmeg, star anise, cardamom, licorice root powder, mesquite, or carob). You can also add superfood green powders, spirulina, chlorella, blue green algae, and/or maca to boost the nutritional content.

Mylk will keep 2–3 days if stored in a glass jar or pitcher.

Sesame Mylk

8 cups sesame seeds

2–3 tablespoons cinnamon powder

1 tablespoon maca root powder

1 tablespoon mesquite

pinch of Celtic or Himalayan salt

Pumpkin Seed Mylk

8 cups pumpkin seeds

1 tablespoon green superfood powder

1 tablespoon blue green algae

pinch of Himalayan or sun-dried sea salt

Almond Mylk

8 cups almonds
2–3 tablespoons cinnamon
½ teaspoon nutmeg
pinch of Himalayan or Celtic salt

Walnut Mylk

8 cups walnuts
2–3 tablespoons star anise, ground and sifted
dash of licorice root powder
pinch of Himalayan or Celtic salt

Seed and Nut Cheezes

Seed Cheeze

Basic:

one bunch fresh herb, cilantro or basil, S-bladed in food processor
2 cups sunflower seeds or soaked walnuts, ground with an S-blade

Add:

4–6 tablespoons stone-ground cold-pressed olive oil or hemp oil
2 tablespoons lemon juice
2 tablespoons kalamata olive brine
2 tablespoons sun-dried tomato water
¼–½ teaspoon Celtic or Himalayan salt
dash cayenne or chipotle
dash hing or 1 clove of garlic

Optional:

¼ cup Italian seasoning
2 tablespoons thyme

Process herbs in food processor with S-blade, and set aside. Grind sunflower seeds in food processor to a fine texture. Add remaining ingredients and herbs to the food processor container, and process to a creamy texture. Serves 4.

Brazil Nut, Olive, and Herb Cheeze

1 cup sunflower seeds

1 cup Brazil nuts

¼ cup olive oil (or other recommended oil to taste)

2–4 tablespoons lemon juice

½ tablespoon black pepper

¼ cup oregano or dill, fresh, chopped

2 tablespoons thyme or Italian seasoning, dried

¼–½ teaspoon Celtic or Himalayan salt

dash hing

1 cup kalamata olives, minced

kalamata olive brine water or blessed water, to desired texture

Process nuts and seeds to a butter, or as much as possible. Add olive oil, lemon, kalamata olive brine, hing, black pepper, salt, and dried herbs. Process to a creamy consistency. Pour or scoop into a bowl, then mix in olives and fresh herbs by hand. Serves 4.

Under the Sea Pâté

1 cup hemp seeds

1 cup almonds

¼ cup celery and/or bell pepper, diced

2–4 tablespoons lemon juice

2 tablespoons olive oil (or other recommended oil to taste)

¼–½ teaspoon Himalayan or Celtic salt

1 teaspoon freshly ground black pepper

½ cup dulse

1 tablespoon kelp

Process almonds and hemp seeds in food processor. Add lemon juice, oil, and spices. Mix in by hand the celery and bell pepper. Serves 4.

Almond Cilantro Cheeze

1 cup sunflower seeds

1 cup almonds

¼ cup olive oil (or other recommended oil to taste)

¼ cup lemon juice

¼–½ teaspoon Himalayan salt

½ tablespoon black pepper

dash hing

one-half bunch cilantro

Add liquid elements to desired consistency. Mince the cilantro with S-blade and set aside. Process the nuts and seeds to a fine consistency. Add olive oil, lemon juice, spices, and salt. Process to a creamy consistency. Then mix in the cilantro. Serves 4.

Dill Brazil Cheeze

1 cup sunflower seeds

1 cup Brazil nuts

¼ cup olive oil (or other recommended oil to taste)

¼ cup lemon juice

¼–½ teaspoon Himalayan or Celtic salt

½ tablespoon black pepper

one bunch dill

dash of hing

Mince the dill with S-blade and set aside. Process the nuts and seeds to a fine consistency. Add oil, lemon juice, salt, and spices. Process to a creamy texture. Then mix in the dill. Serves 4.

Desserts

Muesli and Granola

4 cups nuts and/or seeds (walnuts, pumpkin seed, sesame seed, sunflower seed, hemp seed)

2–8 tablespoons sweet spice (cinnamon, pumpkin pie spice, fennel, anise, or star anise)

2–4 tablespoons coconut or sesame oil

½–1 teaspoon Himalayan or Celtic salt

Optional: orange or lemon zest and/or essential oils

Serve as is, with nut mylk if desired, for muesli. For granola: spread on teflex and dehydrate on 108 degrees overnight to a crunchy texture. Serves 4.

Cardamom Bars with Two Icings

Base:

1 cup hemp seeds, unsoaked, whole

1 cup brown sesame seeds, soaked, whole

1 cup sunflower seeds, soaked, whole

Keep the seeds whole. Toss into a bowl.

Cream:

1 cup coconut cream (dried mature coconut meat that has been blended into a cream)

¼ cup coconut cream oil blended with

½ cup warm water

¼ cup cardamom

½ tablespoon mesquite

1 teaspoon stevia, powdered

½ teaspoon Himalayan or Celtic salt

Combine and blend.

Cardamom icing:

1 cup coconut cream butter

¼ cup hot water

2 tablespoons cardamom

½ teaspoon licorice root powder

pinch Himalayan or Celtic salt

pinch stevia

Place all ingredients in blender and blend on high speed, to a smooth and spreadable consistency.

White licorice icing:

¾ cup coconut cream butter

3 tablespoons hot water

¾ teaspoon licorice root powder

pinch Himalayan or Celtic salt

pinch stevia

Place all ingredients in blender and blend on high speed, to a smooth and pourable consistency.

Building the bars:

To the blended cream, add the whole seeds. Press mix into a flat rectangular glass container. Create cardamom icing and spread over the surface of the mix. Create white licorice icing and drizzle over the top of the cardamom icing. Chill, cut rectangles, and serve. Serves 4–8, depending on size of bars. Bars will keep up to 4 days, refrigerated.

Star Anise Bars with Lemon Icing

Base:

1 cup brown sesame seeds, soaked, whole

1 cup sunflower seeds, soaked, whole

1 cup chia seeds, unsoaked, mixed into the base

½–1 cup of water to rehydrate chia seeds

Toss all seeds into a bowl.

Cream:

1 cup coconut cream and

¼ cup coconut oil, blended with

½ cup warm water

5 tablespoons star anise, ground and sifted

½ tablespoon mesquite

1 teaspoon stevia, powdered

½ teaspoon Himalayan or Celtic salt

Combine and blend.

Lemon icing:

½ cup coconut cream butter

2 tablespoons hot water

2 tablespoons lemon juice

pinch stevia

Optional: ¼ teaspoon lemon zest or a drop of lemon essential oil

Place all ingredients in blender and blend on high speed, to a smooth, spreadable consistency.

Building the bars:

Toss all seeds into a bowl and mix. Massage in the blended cream. Press into a flat glass rectangular container. Create lemon icing and spread over the mix. Chill, cut rectangles, and serve. Serves 4–8, depending on size of bars. Bars will keep up to 4 days, refrigerated.

Cinnamon Bars

Base:

1 cup walnuts, soaked, S-bladed

1 cup hemp seeds, unsoaked

1 cup chia seeds, unsoaked, mixed into the base

½–1 cup of water to rehydrate chia seeds

Toss all seeds into a bowl.

Cream:

1 cup coconut cream

¼ cup coconut oil, blended with

½ cup hot water

¼ cup cinnamon

½ tablespoon mesquite

1 teaspoon stevia, powdered

½ teaspoon Himalayan or Celtic salt

Combine and blend.

Building the bars:

Food process walnuts with S-blade to a finer consistency, then toss into bowl. Add hemp seeds and chia seeds, whole, with the water. Massage in the cream. Pack into a flat rectangular glass container. Serves 4–8, depending on size of bars. Bars will keep up to 4 days, refrigerated.

Lemon Coriander Bars with Coriander Icing

Base:

1 cup hemp seeds, unsoaked, whole

1 cup brown sesame seeds, soaked, whole

1 cup sunflower seeds, soaked, whole

Toss all seeds into a bowl.

Cream:

1 cup coconut cream

¼ cup coconut oil, blended with

½ cup hot water

½ cup poppy seed

¼ cup coriander

½ tablespoon mesquite

1 teaspoon stevia, powdered

½ teaspoon Himalayan or Celtic salt

Combine and blend.

Coriander icing:

1 cup coconut cream butter

2 tablespoons hot water

2 tablespoons lemon juice

5 tablespoons corianders

1 teaspoon licorice root powder

pinch Himalayan or Celtic salt

pinch stevia

Place all ingredients in blender and blend on high speed, to a smooth
and spreadable consistency.

Decoration:

coriander, ground, sifted

Building the bars:

Toss base seeds, whole, into the bowl. Massage in the blended cream.
Pack into a flat glass rectangular container. Create icing in blender and
spread over the mix. Decorate with ground and sifted coriander. Serves
4–8, depending on size of bars. Bars will keep up to 4 days,
refrigerated.

Grain Cooking

GRAIN (1 CUP DRY)	CUPS WATER	COOK TIME	CUPS YIELD
Amaranth	2½	20–25 min.	2½
Buckwheat groats *	2	15 min.	2½
Millet 3–4	20–25 min.	3½	
Quinoa**	2	15–20 min.	2¾
Rice, brown, basmati	2½	35–40 min.	3
Rice, brown, long-grain	2½	45–55 min.	3
Rice, brown, short-grain	2–2½	45–55 min.	3
Rice, brown, quick	1¼	10 min.	2
Rice, wild	3	50–60 min.	4
Spelt	3–4	40–50 min.	2½

BASIC COOKING DIRECTIONS

For all grains start by measuring the grains and water into a pot. If you are cooking 1 cup of grains, use a 2-liter (or 2-quart) pot.

Add ½–1 teaspoon Celtic or Himalayan salt if desired.

Cover, and bring to a boil on high heat.

Turn heat to medium-low for the specified cooking time.

Check the grains after this period of time. If they are still hard, cover again and continue steaming for 5–10 minutes. If the water has evaporated, add ¼ cup water before steaming.

If soft, turn off heat and let sit covered for 10 minutes. Fluff and serve.

Notes:

* Buckwheat groats are an exception to the above directions, because they are porous and absorb the water quickly. They do best if water is boiling before they are added. Cover and return to a boil once groats are in pot. Turn heat to low and steam for the specified time.

** Quinoa is always best prepared by first rinsing in a fine strainer for 2 minutes to remove what is called the *saponens,* a natural protective coating that will give a bitter flavor if not rinsed off before cooking.

Bean and Legume Cooking

BEAN (1 CUP DRY)	CUPS WATER	COOK TIME	CUPS YIELD
Adzuki (Aduki)	4	45–55 min.	3
Anasazi2½–3	45–55 min.	2¼	
Black beans	4	1 hr.–1½ hrs.	2¼
Black-eyed peas	4	1 hr.	2
Cannellini (white kidney beans)	3	45 min.	2½
Cranberry bean	3	40–45 min.	3
Fava beans, skins removed	4	40–50 min.	1⅔
Garbanzo beans (chickpeas)	3½	1–3 hrs.	2
Great northern beans	4	1½ hrs.	2⅔
Green split peas	4	45 min.	2
Yellow split peas	6	1–1½ hrs.	2
Green peas, whole	3	1–2 hrs.	2
Kidney beans	2¼	1 hr.	2¼
Lentils, brown	2	45 min.–1 hr.	2¼
Lentils, green	3	30–45 min.	2
Lentils, red	4	20–30 min.	2–2½
Lima beans, large	4	45 min.–1 hr.	2
Lima beans, small	4	50–60 mins.	3
Lima beans, Christmas	2½	1 hr.	2
Mung beans	3	1 hr.	2
Navy beans	3	45–60 min.	2⅔
Pink beans	3	50–60 min.	2¾
Pinto beans	4	1½ hrs.	2⅔

BASIC COOKING DIRECTIONS

Begin by washing beans and discarding any discolored or deformed ones. Check for small rocks and twigs to be removed.

Beans cook quicker if soaked overnight for 8 hours, covered a couple inches over with water. Strain the soak water off before cooking.

Sometimes beans will take longer to cook. This may be due to the use of hard water, or the beans may have been dried for a longer period of time. If this is the case, soaking them for 24 hours and changing the water two or three times during the soaking period speeds up the cooking.

Soaking also aids in breaking down the complex sugars (oligosaccharides), which challenge the digestive system and cause gas.

Some herbs that help in the digestion of beans can be added during cooking. For example: bay leaves, cumin, winter or summer savory, fresh epazote (available in Hispanic markets). Many people from India maintain the tradition of chewing on dried fennel seeds or drinking a cup of fennel tea at the end of a legume meal to aid the digestion.

As a general rule of thumb, 1 cup of dried beans will yield about 2½ to 3 cups of cooked beans.

Quick-Soak Method for Dried Beans: When time is limited, you can wash and pick over beans and put them in a stock pot with water to cover by 3 inches. Bring to a boil and boil for 10 minutes to remove toxins. Then cover and allow to soak for 1 hour. Discard the soak water, add fresh water, and cook until tender.

Cooking Dried Beans in a Pressure Cooker: For pressure-cooked beans you can soak overnight or use the quick-soak method, or skip this step altogether. Once ready, put the beans in the pressure cooker with three times as much water as beans. Cook at 15 pounds of pressure for 30 minutes for small beans, and 40 minutes for large beans (lima, fava, etc.).

Cooking Fresh Beans: Two methods are used: boiling and steaming.

To boil the beans, drop the shelled beans into boiling water to cover, and boil gently for 5–10 minutes. Flavor while cooking with onion, garlic, herbs of your choice, and a dash of salt added to the water.

To steam the beans, put around an inch of water in the bottom of a pot, and put beans into a steamer basket that fits in the pot. Cover the pot, and steam the beans over boiling water for 5–10 minutes.

Fava Beans: These beans require a bit of different handling before cooking. They are usually peeled after cooking, as leaving the skins on will give a the beans a bitter flavor. To peel, use a paring knife and peel one end, then squeeze the opposite end and the bean will slip out easily.

These are general guidelines. Some varieties of grains and beans will require different cooking times than those specified in the chart. This will depend on the variety of the bean. The variation will only be a matter of a few minutes. If you are cooking packaged beans with directions, always follow the recommendations on the package for the variety you have.

Those new to natural foods can choose to discover how easy it is to prepare good, wholesome meals that rely on whole grains and legumes as the center of their meals. Here is a useful website to begin your discovery: http://www.vegparadise.com/charts.html

Summarizing Thoughts

People suffer from preventable evils, and the people perish for lack of knowledge.

THE GOLDEN VERSES IN FRAGMENTA PHILOSOPHORUM GROECORUM

It is important to reiterate that this program is a logical extension of past research that extends back to the 1920s, when Dr. Max Gerson healed Albert Schweitzer from Type-2 diabetes with a live-food diet. Over a period of thirty-five years, I have seen a variety of people heal diabetes naturally with live foods and fasting. Other live-food clinics have achieved similar results. Research reported in the literature by Dr. James Anderson, and by Dr. Neal Barnard, have validated the importance of a plant-source-only diet in the amelioration of diabetes. All we have done differently with our 21-Day+ Program is to take the next logical and common-sense step. As Ralph Waldo Emerson said, "Society is always taken by surprise by any new example of common sense." The common sense in this case, is that we understand the power of live foods and green juice fasting to create a rapid genetic upgrade. We have found that by taking the next evolutionary step, supported by clinical experience and employing a diet that is based on those principles, clients move away from a phenotypic expression of diabetes to a phenotypic expression of health and well-being. I have done the obvious and common-sense move by making the green juice fast and live-food plant-source diet the prudent approach to healing diabetes naturally. Consistently with this approach, within 1 to 4 days clients are off all medications. In one week the FBS number for many people comes into normal range, and in three weeks, the FBS is normal for the majority of people. Depending on the degree of complications, FBS may take longer to come into a nondiabetic range, but the end result is a normal fasting blood glucose level. As with all human issues of healing, one is not able to issue a 100 percent guarantee, but our clinical experience at this point has been that this is the case for 90 percent of our clients within three weeks, if they are fully attentive to the program.

Most people also see their blood chemistry, cholesterol, and C-reactive protein return to normal on the 21-Day+ Program.

As a scientist, I share in this book a theory that with the live foods and green juice fasting one is rapidly turning on the anti-aging and anti-diabetic genes. This has yet to be proven conclusively. But then again, it took thirty years to prove that smoking causes lung cancer. The second part of that belief is that, as a scientist, I realize we do not have enough controlled data to make a definitive statement about this program and its theory. I am looking for the funding for this next step. I am planning to conduct a study of 200 people in the diabetic program including both the U.S. and Israel to further explore this question. I feel there is enough data, and the issue is important enough, given the pandemic nature of diabetes, to release our preliminary results at this time. I do so with an awareness that much more research is needed to validate this theory and the results.

It is clear that the 21-Day+ Program gives a desirable result. The big question is the human question—can people sustain themselves in the Culture of Life with a high degree of success? With highly motivated people there is a high success rate, but as this is applied to a pandemic level in many cultures and economic realities, I am looking very closely at support programs that will be desirable and thus successful for all circumstances. This will require a lot of creativity to apply this logical, common-sense breakthrough to cultures worldwide. It is one thing to develop a successful health program, but something else to create a program that is feasible for all.

The causal levels come out of the Culture of Death, which is naturally promoting a Culture of Death diet, which leads people to a place where they feel at a point of no return once the diabetes genes are activated. The sensible and important awareness is that there is always the potential of a return. Paracelsus said: "No physician can ever say that any disease is incurable. To say so blasphemes God, blasphemes Nature, and depreciates the great architect of Creation. The disease does not exist, regardless of how terrible it may be, for which God has not provided the corresponding cure."

In this context, the current so-called "normal" standard American diet is immoderate and detrimental, as it directly contributes to the manifestation of diabetes. Previous "moderate" diets have been shown to ameliorate and control diabetes to a limited degree. None of these diets have been particularly successful beyond marginally ameliorating diabetes. For example, Dr. Barnard's research team compared the Physician's Committee for Responsible Medicine vegan approach to the control diet using ADA guidelines. With the ADA approach, they found a 0.4 percent drop in A1c levels. This is very mild. The vegan program did three times better with an average drop of 1.2 points in five-and-a-half months. What we are finding with the Tree of Life 21-Day+ Program is a major change—for the one Type-1 diabetic highlighted in our results, a 196 percent drop in his HgbA1c level from 11.8 percent to 6.0 percent in three months, a drop of 5.8 points (or 14.5 times more than the ADA controls). This dramatic change does not come as a result of practicing the conventional moderation approach of the Culture of Death, which in essence is a way of making denial seem reasonable. To make this kind of significant change requires a lifestyle and diet that is dramatically and excitingly different, resulting in powerful results in a short period of time. This requires leading a life of love, purpose, meaning, and self-value, and choosing a diet and lifestyle that reflect these values. Of course, this is the diet and lifestyle of the Culture of Life.

The essential question that is asked of participants is *"Do you love yourself enough to want to heal and save your life?"* The results revealed in this book, for those who have answered this question in the affirmative, show that the conventional paradigm for diabetes—as stated by the ADA and most medical schools, as incurable—is a self-defeating myth. In all fairness, the conventional paradigm also teaches that proper diet and exercise help slow the progression of this "incurable" disease, but those adhering to the conventional paradigm do not offer the proper diet to do the job. We have activated a new paradigm that previous research has pointed toward, by taking the next logical step, going deeper into the underlying causes by seeing diabetes as a symptom of the Culture of Death.

By the Culture of Death, we are talking about a culture founded on predatory competition in which people are economic commodities. *Wealth* is for the few versus *health* for the many. It is a culture of separateness, domination, and resulting exploitation. In this culture people have lost their soul connection. This is connected to the 80–90 percent obesity in diabetics, for as previously said, there is never enough food for a hungry soul. There is a food environment characterized by heavy marketing of excitotoxin-rich processed junk foods, refined carbohydrates such as white sugar and white flour with alloxan, heavy use of animal fats and trans fats, agrochemical-laden foods, and heavy-metal toxicity. These characteristics combine to result in a negative synergy that has precipitated diabetes at pandemic levels, when it was relatively rare before 1940. This is not an accident—the Culture of Death is an active and thoughtless Crime Against Wisdom.

The Culture of Life manifests as cooperation, health, harmony, and compassion, combined with production of healthy, natural, organic foods that preserve soil and minimizes the pollution of both people and planet. The Culture of Life helps us reconnect to our heart and soul in a way that brings the presence of light, love, and the Divine back into the core of our human experience. Instead of a "moderate" diet, the Culture of Life cuisine is a *prudent,* common-sense diet of extremely low-glycemic, low-insulin-index foods, organic, high mineral, hydrating, live, with no animal or trans fat, 15–20 percent high EFA plant-based fats, high fiber, and thoughtful, prudent food intake.

The healing of diabetes at the pandemic level requires the healing of the ecology of the planet and the consciousness of the people. To heal oneself requires the ability to love oneself enough to have the intention to reconnect with the Culture of Life which is our birthright. In that way we perform an Act of Love for oneself as an individual person, and as part of the living planet. This results in the healing of the planet and all species. The healing of diabetes in this context is an Act of Love, Compassion, and Consciousness.

APPENDIX 1

About the Tree of Life

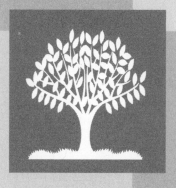

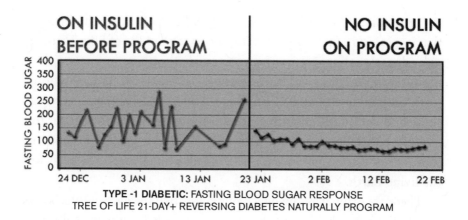

TYPE -1 DIABETIC: FASTING BLOOD SUGAR RESPONSE
TREE OF LIFE 21-DAY+ REVERSING DIABETES NATURALLY PROGRAM

The Tree of Life Rejuvenation Center is an ecologically based health and spiritual center and community dedicated to the awakening of consciousness through worldwide educational, humanitarian activities and specialized retreat programs. The Center, located on 174 pristine acres in the exquisite high-desert mountains of Patagonia, Arizona, is indeed an Oasis for Life: We are the only center in the world offering 100-percent organic, live-food, plant-source cuisine, much of which is cultivated on our own land, which borders the Coronado National Forest and flows from the majestic 6,300-foot Red Mountain. The Patagonia Mountains are majestic, yet calming and very peaceful, and offer spectacular views of the water valley as well as breathtaking walking and hiking trails.

The Tree of Life Rejuvenation Center is a sanctuary for holistic healing that inspires openness and awakening. People from ninety countries have taken shade under our Tree; they have touched its earth, breathed its pure air, and reconnected to life in new and unimaginable ways—always with soul-enriching experiences. They return to their homes around the globe rejuvenated, inspired, and empowered.

A Beacon of Light for the Culture of Life

Welcome to the Culture of Life, and to the "family" that is at the core of the Tree of Life experience. At the Tree of Life Rejuvenation Center, we are dedicated to helping you enjoy choices in cuisine and lifestyle that inspire and empower your transition to the Culture of Life. Through our educational programs and your experience here in our majestic mountain valley, you will learn about the choices that naturally bring forth optimal health and spiritual joy. You will also experience what thousands of our guests attest to: a unique, healthy foundation for living, a renewed connection with yourself, and a strong, unshakable sense of self-esteem and love for Self and all living beings, as well as for the living Earth.

There are many ways by which our guests find the Tree of Life. Some people come to enhance and support their already healthy lifestyles and to ensure their healthy futures. Some are seeking more joy, peace, and a deeper soul connection to the Divine, while others simply wish to experience the joy of a vegan vegetarian spiritual retreat that is in alignment with their personal lifestyle. There are also those who are suffering the results of years of damaging lifestyle and dietary choices, and visit out of their need to address a serious, life-threatening degenerative illness. They may also feel a lack of joy and peace, a separation from love and Self, and a disconnection from the experience of the soul. Still others are experiencing environmental stress and degradation firsthand in the form of chemical imbalances and toxicity, and while they may not be diagnosed, they have very little energy and enthusiasm for life.

Taking shade under our tree means having a place to rejuvenate, to rest the body, mind, and soul, and to escape the chaos of the world. This new way of living, with a foundation of compassionate action and conscious eating, consistently nourishes one's being with the pleasure, happiness, inner peace, and love that is our divine birthright.

We invite you with love to embrace and enjoy the Tree of Life experience, and to join us in reconnecting with the Culture of Life. However you choose to experience our Center, whether through a personal or family vacation, an apprentice program, a workshop or specific training, you are making the choice to improve, maintain, or enhance your health, and creating a foundation for lifelong joy, health, and happiness. We celebrate you and your journey to wellness and spiritual pleasure!

Our Programs

The Tree of Life Experience is a dynamic, ongoing program for cultivating personal harmony and revitalization. Our guests find inspiration and wonder in the high desert setting, enhanced by our simple, gentle yet effective approach to whole-person awakening.

During your Tree of Life Experience you will cultivate valuable skills and new perspectives that inspire your new beginning. Our programs embody the essence of the Culture of Life: they encourage connection with all aspects of Self and environment while fostering spiritual development and connection with the Divine. Our programs also promote sustainability and address your health and that of our planet on a foundational level.

At the Tree of Life Rejuvenation Center, we are sensitive to people who are transitioning into the Culture of Life and provide guidance to support a positive and uplifting experience. We also offer post-program assistance to help you maintain the Culture of Life and continue to experience the joy and inner peace of this beneficial lifestyle upon returning home for your self and your communities.

PILGRIMAGE... TO YOURSELF

Expansive, clear skies and majestic, star-filled nights are a stunning backdrop for a healing and educational community that features:

- Meditation temple
- Live-food café
- The Tree of Life Spa
- Non-chlorinated swimming pool and hot tubs
- Ecologically sound strawbale lodging
- Awakened Living Shoppe
- Two-acre organic garden for our healthy cuisine
- Kali Ray TriYoga® classes
- The largest outdoor Chartres labyrinth on the globe
- Inipi (Native American sweat lodge)
- A Children's Peace Garden

- Nature trails and mountain views
- World-famous bird watching region

The Tree of Life Rejuvenation Center is natural and purposefully simple. We celebrate living close to the earth and remain intentionally "back-to-nature" with dirt roads, pathways, and minimal artificial lighting. Our guests enjoy comfortable weather year-round in our tranquil and natural setting. During the summer months of July–September, Patagonia, Arizona, is regularly 8–15 degrees cooler than Tucson or Phoenix.

RETREATS, WORKSHOPS, AND TRAININGS

Our offerings include:

Reversing Diabetes Naturally:
21 Day+ Program
One-year follow-up
Four-six times per year

Spiritual Juice Fasting:
10 days
Three to four times a year

Detoxification Fasting Program:
10, 17, or 24 days
Begins weekly

Zero Point Process:
4 days
Four to six times a year

Conscious Eating Intensive:
6 days
Four to six times a year

Sacred Relationships:
4 days
One to two times a year

Inter-Dependence Celebration:
4 days
Once a year

Whole Person Healing:
3 days, per doctor's availability

EDUCATION AND APPRENTICESHIP PROGRAMS

Our offerings include the following (see our Tree of Life Educational Programs brochure for more details):

Spiritual Live Food Apprentice Program:
10 weeks
Five cycles each year

Spiritual Veganic Farming Apprentice Program:
12 weeks
Four cycles each year

Spiritual Sprouting Apprentice Program:
One-month cycle, year-round

Spiritual Nutrition Accreation for a Master's Degree Awarded by the University of Integrative Science Program:
Two to three years
Offered each year; open enrollment

Essene Priesthood and Priestesshood:
Two to three years
Offered each year; open enrollment
All Culture of Life Programs include:

- Ecological straw-bale structures
- Use of the facilities, swimming pool, hot tubs, all meals and/or juicing, hiking trails, meditation temple, labyrinth, day and evening seminars (excluding specific workshops and programs), far-infrared sauna
- Daily Kali Ray TriYoga® group classes with pranayama and meditation

- 100-percent organic, plant-source live-food cuisine and juice with group and community blessings of meals
- Conscious living food preparation and sprouting classes
- Nature and wild food hikes
- Mishpacha (guest support groups): Two times each week guests share their ongoing experiences with our friendly staff.
- Bi-weekly nutritional Q&A sessions: In these sessions you can ask questions about nutrition, diet, live foods and making the live foods lifestyle work for you.
- Evening spiritual programs (Check website for frequency)
- Agni Hotra: Sunset Ceremony for Healing the Planet
- Satsang: This is a special time to gain support by asking questions that pertain to your spiritual life.
- Shaktipat Meditation (weekly): Brings a sense of inner peace, builds spiritual power, and activates the next evolutionary phase in spiritual life
- Homa (weekly): Ancient Indian ceremony designed to burn up that which no longer serves you
- Chanting: Opens the heart, allowing love to permeate your very being
- Shamanic Kabbalat Shabbat: Ancient Essene ceremony to invoke joy, peace and harmony
- Native American sweat lodges, or Inipi (monthly)
- Women's Circles near the time of new moons

Plus! The Children's Peace Garden, which offers children ages 3–7 who accompany their parents to the Tree of Life their own experience of the Culture of Life. Held in an uplifting greenhouse! We support a whole-family approach to the Culture of Life.

As a part of whole-person awakening, many guests elect:

- Bodywork and healing energy practices at the Tree of Life Spa that stimulate and soothe the senses, balancing the internal with the external
- Whole-person healing consultations

- Lymph and deep-tissue massages
- Far-infrared sauna
- Ozone steambox
- Oxy-Rebounding
- Body wraps
- Facials
- Private Kali Ray TriYoga® sessions for enhancing the flowing motion of Kundalini

For more information on our programs or for reservations, fill in the "Call-Me-Now" form at www.treeoflife.nu, or call toll-free 1-866-394-2520.

Culture of Life Retreats and Workshops

TREE OF LIFE REVERSING DIABETES NATURALLY

This 21-Day+ Program is described throughout this book.

SPIRITUAL AND YOGA FASTING RETREATS

The *New York Times* calls Gabriel Cousens "a green juice fasting and detoxification Guru." This ten-day revitalizing spiritual juice fast renews body and soul, and reconnects you to your inner truth and sacred design! Continual support is provided by Gabriel Cousens and Shanti Golds-Cousens, who have experience guiding thousands of fasters worldwide. Includes Shaktipat meditation, Kali Ray TriYoga®, spiritual Q&A, chanting, sweat lodge (weather permitting), organic green juice, and support for breaking the fast with live-food meals.

DETOXIFICATION AND CLEANSING FASTS

Harper's Magazine says we offer "one of the world's ten best detoxification retreats!" Our ten-, seventeen-, and twenty-four-day packages enliven every cell in your system! Fresh organic green juice, innovative, non-invasive cleansing technologies, and the natural way of yoga and meditation turn on the genes for youth and euphoria. The plan allows the body's innate wisdom to restore beauty and balance through a variety of massage therapies, oxygen-enhanced rebounding, air-and-sun bathing, ozone therapies, hydrotherapy, infrared sauna, colon therapies, nature walks, and more. Toxins are removed from reproductive cells, and we experience weight reduction and rejuvenation. Includes some individually designed support. The fasts start every Tuesday!

ZERO POINT PROCESS INTENSIVE

Awaken from the dream of a separate "self" so that you may live without fear in the chaos of the world and embrace your true destiny! In this extraordinary training program you will learn how to turn off the mind and become free from unhealthy habits and negative emotions, self-images, and phobias, allowing you to reconnect with the authentic Self. This course is part of the Six Foundations for Spiritual Life, which prepare you to hold the grace of liberation and open you to living in the pleasure of the Divine Presence. This four-day, all-day, intensive course taught by world-recognized spiritual teacher Gabriel Cousens, who trained as a psychiatrist and family therapist, is Gabriel's approach to Jnana Yoga—Yoga of the Mind. It can bring us to direct knowing and clarity that "the personality is a case of mistaken identity." Learn how to let go of the mind's addictive emotional patterns, obsessions, and thought forms! Live in celebration and experience the non-causal joy, inner contentment, and bliss of who we are!

WHOLE-PERSON HEALING

This expertly designed health evaluation and personal treatment program, created by Gabriel Cousens, MD, is a foundation for optimal strength, vitality, and long-term wellness. Whole-Person Healing targets your individual health needs. We offer individualized guidance on nutrition and lifestyle change, and create a superior supplement plan designed to help you realize harmony in body-mind-spirit quickly and effectively. This program offers a level of self-awareness that makes it possible to heal more rapidly from diseases such as depression, diabetes, arthritis, chronic fatigue, hypoglycemia, candida, fibromyalgia, and chronic degeneration, and to create your own health.

CONSCIOUS EATING INTENSIVE

This exciting six-day course in the basics of live-food preparation is an immersion into the conscious eating lifestyle. We will show you how to create the deeply healing and delightful cuisine that is the foundation of the Culture of Life. Join us for an incredible journey into the food that supports the blossoming of wellness and spiritual life! Includes three lectures and Q&A sessions.

SPA AT THE TREE OF LIFE

An ideal day-long retreat for vegans and vegetarians who wish to enjoy spa treatments in a spiritually conscious community and our 100-percent organic, plant-source live food. The Spa at the Tree of Life is a treat for mind, body, and spirit, and a delightful reprieve from the busy life! Infuse your spirit with love and joy at the place where thousands around the globe have initiated their awakening to the Culture of Life. This is a wonderful gift for you and your loved ones.

SACRED RELATIONSHIPS

Unleash the dynamic force of couples' love and embark on a journey into the unknown frontier of intimacy as a spiritual path. In this four-day, three-night workshop for couples, lead by Gabriel and Shanti, you become skilled and empowered in the art of Sacred Relationship and learn how to invoke Divine Union in every moment. Cultivate deep listening skills, practice connecting through shared body movement with a special Couples Yoga created by Shanti and Gabriel, and experience the ecstasy of subtle spiritual energies merging into one powerful, devotional, and synergistic energy. Join us and begin to realize the universe as the sensuous, wild, passionate, and abundant playground of intimacy that it truly is!

Support Connections for Wellness

We are available at any distance, via the Tree of Life website www.tree-oflife.nu and the other websites shown below.

Alive with Gabriel: Remain supported and connected with our network of internet/telecommunication media, symposia, audio, video, and articles at www.AlivewithGabriel.com. Each *Alive with Gabriel* monthly program (called *Wake Up with Gabriel* when it is in the morning), presented by Gabriel Cousens, features a variety of practical and invaluable information about spirituality, nutrition, and healthy lifestyles to help you sustain the Culture of Life.

The Tree of Life Awakened Living Shoppe: Located at the Tree of Life Rejuvenation Center, the Awakened Living Shoppe offers vegan, organic foods and supplements, books, and other products to support a healthy awakened life. We cheerfully help with questions and phone orders; call toll-free 1-866-394-2520 (local 1-520-394-2520) x212. Internet orders can be placed by visiting www.AwakenedShoppe.com

Branches of the Tree of Life Association: Become a beacon of light in your own community, and a branch of our ever-expanding global Tree of Life network by hosting monthly potlucks and seminars following the regularly scheduled *Alive with Gabriel* or *Wake Up with Gabriel* live Internet telecasts. Becoming a branch, which requires certain criteria be met, also comes with several benefits.

Superfood Juice Feasting: For those who have long-term weight loss, detoxification, and healing needs. Visit www.treeoflife.nu and www.JuiceFeasting.com for more information.

TO REACH US:

For more information on our programs or for reservations, fill in the "Call-Me-Now" form at www.treeoflife.nu, or call toll-free 1-866-394-2520 (local 1-520-394-2520).

Tree of Life Rejuvenation Center
P.O. Box 778 (mail)
686 Harshaw Road (shipping)
Patagonia, AZ 85624 USA
Toll-free 1-866-394-2520; local 1-520-394-2520
E-mail: info@treeoflife.nu
Website: www.treeoflife.nu

APPENDIX 2

The Tree of Life at the Dead Sea

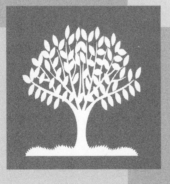

Serving the Middle Eastern and European communities, the Center is located thirty minutes from the holy city of Jerusalem and forty-five minutes from Tel Aviv International Airport. The Center is active for intensive programs of 21 Day+ cycle for two or three times a year as well as a base for ongoing Conscious Eating courses, Sacred Relationships workshops, and a base for Gabriel and Shanti to teach in Europe and the Middle East.

Program Highlights

The Tree of Life at the Dead Sea offers on-site Reversing Diabetes Naturally 21-Day+ Program with One-Year Follow-Up, as described in this book.

This whole-Person Rejuvenation is the ultimate healing vacation by the Dead Sea.

The powerful Tree of Life transformational workshops are offered, featuring:

- Spiritual Juice-Fasting Retreat (9 days)
- Individualize Your Spiritual Nutrition Cuisine
- Zero Point Process (4 days)
- Conscious Eating (5 days)

Participants are welcome to join each of the above segments separately or take the whole twenty-one-day cycle as a profound, multi-layer transformation that we call the Whole-Person Rejuvenation. From our experience, the magnitude of each step of the program is enhanced greatly when done in one sequence.

The Spiritual Resident Program is for those who wish to simply be in a retreat setting within a spiritual community. This program offers full accommodation with three organic live-food meals a day, and daily attendance to TriYoga classes, meditation, and Shaktipat meditation.

A key part of this program is *seva,* or service, where you are invited to volunteer and serve in the kitchen, help our production crew, or serve in other ways.

This program is best suited for those who have already taken the Tree of Life's workshops in the past, for those who travel on a modest budget, or for those who want an extended time to heal and meditate in an optimal setting. Spaces are limited and subject to vacancy.

We offer an Overview of Nearby Sites, tours for people coming to the ancient Holy Land that can be arranged. Visited sites include:

- Dead Sea, 10 minutes away
- Jerusalem, 30 minutes
- Qumran, ancient Essene site, 15 minutes
- Metsada (Masada) Mountain, 45 minutes
- Tel Aviv, 80 minutes away, rated as one of the world's top cities of interest due to its diversity of culture and art

For further information, international air and road travel, and registration, please call Ya'ara at +972-50-226-7596. Or e-mail treeoflife.israel@gmail.com. Or see our website at http://www.treeoflife.org.il.

Continuing Education
Opportunities and Resources

RAINBOW GREEN LIVE-FOOD CUISINE DVD

This dynamic, hands-on DVD has been created to support you in the journey of healing and awakening with Rainbow Green Live-Food Cuisine. The full-length video includes:

- An in-depth interview with author and wholistic physician Gabriel Cousens, MD, which highlights the key principles of Rainbow Green Live-Food Cuisine
- A series of Rainbow Green Live-Food Cuisine recipe demonstrations with the personable and talented Tree of Life Café chefs
- Introduction to the Tree of Life Rejuvenation Center and the Secrets of Rejuvenation

ORDERING INFORMATION

To order books and videos/DVDs, please contact the Tree of Life:

Website: www.treeoflife.nu
e-mail: orders@treeoflife.nu
Phone: (520) 394-2520 x 203

TREE OF LIFE'S FREE E-WELLNESS NEWSLETTER

Subscribe online at www.treeoflife.nu and receive wholistic healing, sociopolitical, spiritually uplifting articles by Gabriel Cousens, MD, and news from the Tree of Life every month.

SPIRITUAL AND NUTRITIONAL WORKSHOPS

We invite you to join us at the Tree of Life Rejuvenation Center to be supported in living the Rainbow Green Live-Food Cuisine lifestyle. We offer a variety of workshops, detoxification programs, and lifestyle learning opportunities. Please visit us on line at www.treeoflife.nu or call us at (520) 394-2520 x 206.

VEGAN LIVE-FOOD CULINARY ARTS APPRENTICESHIP PROGRAM

This unique ten-week apprenticeship program offers those interested in the art and science of live-food preparation an opportunity to receive personal and career training with the talented Tree of Life Café chefs. Participants become certified chefs in the sophisticated Rainbow Green Live-Food Cuisine.

MASTER'S DEGREE PROGRAM IN SPIRITUAL NUTRITION

This two-year correspondence program with one four-week residency intensive and one four-day intensive is offered through the University of Integrative Learning under the Provostship of Gabriel Cousens, MD, at the Tree of Life Rejuvenation Center. Faculty and staff include Gabriel Cousens, MD, MD (H), Diplomate in Ayurveda, David Wolfe, JD, John Phillips, MS, Shanti Golds-Cousens, MA, Philip Madeley, and Tim and Michela Casey.

JUICE FEASTING PROGRAM ONLINE

The website www.JuiceFeasting.com is an online 92-Day Juice Feasting resource designed by David Rainoshek, MA, to serve as a dynamic instructional course on plant-source live-food nutrition. More than 6,000 hours of thorough research support the 350-plus scientifically referenced documents on nutrition, with hundreds of videos and graphics, all organized to provide the best information and inspiration possible for engaging in a Culture of Life diet and lifestyle with intellectual and emotional confidence.

GLOSSARY

ACE inhibitor —Type of drug used to lower blood pressure. It may also help prevent or slow the progression of kidney disease in people with diabetes.

acute—Happening for a limited period of time and/or coming on abruptly.

adrenal glands—Two organs sitting on top of the kidneys that make and release hormones such as adrenaline (epinephrine).

albuminuria—Having an excess amount of protein called albumin in the urine. Albuminuria may indicate kidney disease.

aldose reductase inhibitor—A class of drugs under investigation as a way to prevent eye and nerve damage in people with diabetes.

alpha cell—A type of cell in the pancreas that makes and releases the hormone glucagon.

angiopathy—A disease of the blood vessels (arteries, veins, and capillaries) that occurs when someone has diabetes for a long time.

antigens—Substances that cause an immune response in the body. The body perceives the antigens to be harmful and thus produces antibodies to attack and destroy the antigens.

arteriosclerosis—A group of diseases in which the artery walls get thick and hard, slowing blood flow.

artery—A large blood vessel that carries blood from the heart to other parts of the body.

atherosclerosis—One of many arteriosclerosis diseases in which fat builds up in the large and medium-size arteries.

autoimmune process—A process by which the body's immune system attacks and destroys body tissue that it mistakes for foreign matter.

beta cells—Cells that make the hormone insulin, which controls blood glucose levels. Beta cells are found in areas of the pancreas called the Islets of Langerhans.

bladder—A hollow organ that urine drains into from the kidneys. From the bladder, urine leaves the body.

blood glucose—The main sugar that the body makes from the food we eat. Glucose is carried through the bloodstream to provide energy to all of the body's living cells.

blood glucose monitor—A machine that helps measure the amount of glucose in the blood.

blood pressure—The force of the blood against the artery walls. Two levels of blood pressure are measured: the highest, or systolic, occurs when the heart pumps blood into the blood vessels, and the lowest, or diastolic, occurs when the heart rests.

blood sugar—See blood glucose.

blood urea nitrogen (BUN)—Waste product produced by the kidneys. Raised BUN levels in the blood may indicate early kidney damage.

callus—Thick, hardened area of the skin, generally on the foot, caused by friction or pressure. Calluses can lead to other problems, including serious infection and even gangrene.

capillary—The smallest blood vessel in the body.

capsaicin—A colorless irritant that gives hot peppers their hotness. Used for an ointment made from chili peppers to relieve the pain of peripheral neuropathy.

carbohydrate—One of three main groups of foods in the diet that provide calories and energy. (Protein and fat are the others.) Carbohydrates are mainly sugars (simple carbohydrates) and starches (complex carbohydrates, found in whole grains and beans) that the body breaks down into glucose.

cataract—Clouding of the lens of the eye.

cholesterol—A substance similar to fat that is found in the blood, muscles, liver, brain, and other body tissues. The body produces and needs some cholesterol for hormone synthesis. However, too much cholesterol can make fats stick to the walls of the arteries and cause a disease that decreases or stops circulation.

chronic—Lasting a long time. Diabetes is an example of a chronic disease.

creatinine—A chemical in the blood that is eliminated through urine. A test of the amount of creatinine in the blood and/or urine indicates whether the kidneys are working properly.

corn—A thickening of the skin of the feet or hands, usually caused by pressure against the skin.

diabetes mellitus—A disease that occurs when the body cannot use glucose adequately or has none of its own to use. This is caused by a deficiency of the pancreatic hormone insulin, which results in a failure to metabolize sugars and starch. Sugars accumulate in the blood and urine, and the byproducts of alternative fat metabolism disturb the acid–base balance of the blood, causing a risk of convulsions and coma. It is also a disturbance of protein and fat metabolism.

diabetes pills—Pills or capsules that are taken by mouth to help lower the blood glucose level. These pills may work for people whose bodies are still making insulin.

diabetic eye disease—A disease of the small blood vessels of the retina of the eye in people with diabetes. In this disease, the vessels swell and leak liquid into the retina, blurring the vision and sometimes leading to blindness.

diabetic ketoacidosis—High blood glucose with the presence of ketones in the urine and bloodstream, often caused by taking too little insulin or during illness. It can be life threatening.

diabetic kidney disease—Damage to the cells or blood vessels of the kidney. Often fatal five years after beginning dialysis.

diabetic nerve damage—Damage and pain to the nerves of a person with diabetes. Nerve damage may affect the feet and hands, as well as major organs.

dialysis—A method for removing waste such as urea from the blood when the kidneys can no longer do the job. There are two types of dialysis: hemodialysis and peritoneal.

diphtheria—An acute, contagious disease that causes fever and problems for the heart and nervous system.

diuretic—A drug that increases the flow of urine to help eliminate extra fluid from the body.

endocrine glands—Glands that release hormones into the bloodstream and affect metabolism.

end-stage renal disease (ESRD)—The final phase of kidney disease.

epinephrine—A hormone, also called adrenaline, secreted by the adrenal glands and helping the liver release glucose. The principal blood-pressure-raising hormone. Used medicinally as a heart stimulant and muscle relaxant in bronchial asthma.

EKG—A test that measures the heart's action. Also called an electrocardiogram.

fasting blood sugar (FBS)—the blood sugar level taken first thing in the morning before eating.

fats—One of the three main classes of foods and a source of energy in the body. (Protein and carbohydrates are the other two.)

fiber—Substance in food plants that helps the digestive process, lowers cholesterol, and helps control blood glucose levels.

flu—An infection caused by the influenza virus. A contagious viral illness that strikes quickly and severely. Signs include high fever, chills, body aches, runny nose, sore throat, and headache.

gangrene—Death or pervasive decay of body tissue, usually caused by loss of blood flow.

gastroparesis—A form of nerve damage that affects the stomach.

gestational diabetes—A type of diabetes that can occur in pregnant women who have not been known to have diabetes before. Although gestational diabetes usually subsides after pregnancy, many women who've had gestational diabetes develop Type-2 diabetes later in life.

gingivitis—A swelling and soreness of the gums that, without treatment, can cause serious gum problems and disease.

glaucoma—An eye disease characterized by increased pressure in the eye.

glomeruli—Tiny blood vessels in the kidneys where the blood is filtered and waste products are eliminated.

glucagon—A hormone that raises the blood glucose level. When someone with diabetes has a very low blood glucose level, a glucagon injection can help raise the blood glucose quickly.

glucose—A sugar in our blood and a source of energy for our bodies.

glucose tolerance test—A test that shows how well the body deals with glucose in the blood over time; used to see if a person has diabetes. A first blood sample is taken in the morning before the person has eaten; then the person drinks a liquid that has glucose in it. After one hour, a second blood sample is taken and then, one hour later, a third.

glycogen—A substance composed of sugars that is stored in the liver and muscles and releases glucose into the blood when needed by cells.

glycosylated hemoglobin test—A blood test that measures a person's average glycosylated hemoglobin in the red blood cell in the three-month period before the test.

glycosylation—The process in which glucose binds to, chemically alters, and damages proteins. These altered proteins are called advanced glycation end products (AGEs). Over time, AGE proteins may accumulate in the cells and interfere with normal cell functioning. Glycosylation is accelerated in people with diabetes, and complications with eyes, kidneys, and the circulatory system are associated with AGE proteins.

HDL (high-density lipoprotein)—A combined protein and fatlike substance that lowers cholesterol and usually passes freely through the arteries. Sometimes called "good cholesterol."

heart attack—Damage to the heart muscle caused when the blood vessels supplying the muscle are blocked, such as when the blood vessels are clogged with fats (a condition sometimes called hardening of the arteries).

hemodialysis—A mechanical way to remove waste products from the blood. See also dialysis.

hemoglobin (Hgb)—The substance in red blood cells that carries oxygen to the body's cells.

HgbA1C—A test that sums up how much glucose is non-enzymatically bound to the hemoglobin during the past three months.

high blood glucose—A condition that occurs in people with insulin resistance, pre-diabetes, and diabetes when their blood glucose levels are too high. Symptoms include having to urinate often, being very thirsty, losing weight, and a general accelerated aging process.

high blood pressure—A condition where the blood circulates through the arteries with too much force on the artery walls. High blood pressure tires the heart, harms the arteries, and increases the risk of heart attack, stroke, and kidney problems.

hormone—A chemical that special cells in the body release to help other cells work. For example, insulin is a hormone made in the pancreas to help the body use glucose as energy.

human insulin—Laboratory-made insulins that are similar to insulin produced by the human body.

hyperesthesia—One of different changes in nerve function in extremities, expressed with numbness and tingling.

hyperglycemia—See high blood glucose.

hypertension—See high blood pressure.

hypoglycemia—Also called low blood glucose. A condition independent of diabetes in which there is an imbalance in the endocrine system in which the blood sugar drops rapidly or too low. The problem is usually with pancreatic, adrenal, or thyroid imbalances.

immunization—Sometimes called vaccination; a shot or injection that theoretically protects a person from getting an illness by making the person "immune" to it. Evidence does not necessarily support the theory.

impaired glucose tolerance (IGT)—Blood glucose levels that are higher than normal but not so high as to be considered diabetes.

implantable insulin pump—A small pump placed inside the body to deliver insulin on demand from a handheld programmer.

impotence—A condition where the penis does not become or stay hard enough for sex. Some men who have had diabetes a long time become impotent if their nerves or blood vessels have become damaged.

influenza—See flu.

inject—To force a liquid into the body with a needle and syringe.

insulin—A hormone that helps the body use blood glucose for energy. The beta cells of the pancreas make insulin. When people with diabetes can't make enough insulin, they may have to inject it from another source.

insulin-dependent diabetes mellitus (IDDM)—See Type-1 diabetes.

insulin pump—A beeper-sized device that delivers a continuous supply of insulin into the body.

insulin reaction—A response to a too-low level of glucose in the blood; also called hypoglycemia.

insulin receptors—Sites on the outer part of a cell that allow the cell to join with insulin.

insulin resistance—Occurs when the different functions of the insulin hormone are blocked. It may force the pancreas to overproduce up to four times the amount of insulin to compensate. May result in inflammation, scarring, and destruction of the beta cells of the pancreas from exhaustion and burn-out.

intensive therapy—A method of treatment for Type-1 diabetes in which the goal is to keep the blood glucose levels as close to normal as possible. Also recommended for Type-2 diabetes.

ketoacidosis—See diabetic ketoacidosis.

ketones—Chemical substances that the body makes when it doesn't have enough insulin in the blood. When ketones build up in the body for a long time, serious illness, acidosis, or coma can result.

ketosis—A condition when ketone bodies build up in body tissues and fluids. Ketosis can lead to ketoacidosis.

kidney—One of the twin organs found in the lower part of the back. The kidneys purify the blood of all waste and harmful material. They also control the level of some helpful chemical substances in the blood.

kidney disease—Also called nephropathy, kidney disease can be any one of several chronic conditions that are caused by damage to the cells of the kidney.

lente insulin—An intermediate-acting insulin.

low blood glucose—A condition that occurs in people with diabetes when their blood glucose levels are too low from excess insulin or oral hypoglycemics. Symptoms include feeling anxious or confused, feeling numb in the arms and hands, and shaking or feeling dizzy.

LDL (low-density lipoprotein)—A combined protein and fatlike substance. Rich in cholesterol, it tends to stick to the walls in the arteries. Sometimes called "bad cholesterol."

meal plan—A guide to help people get the proper amount of calories, carbohydrates, proteins, and fats in their diet.

microalbumin—A protein found in blood plasma and urine. The presence of microalbumin in the urine can be a sign of kidney disease.

nephropathy—See diabetic kidney disease.

neuropathy—See diabetic nerve damage.

non-insulin-dependent diabetes mellitus (NIDDM)—See Type-2 diabetes.

Neutral Protamine Hagedorn (NPH) insulin—An intermediate-acting insulin

obesity—Excessive accumulation and storage of fat in the body. The degree of overweight when people have 20 percent or more extra body fat for their age, height, sex, and bone structure.

oral glucose tolerance test (OGTT)—A test to see if a person has diabetes. See also glucose tolerance test.

pancreas—Organ in the body that makes insulin so that the body can use glucose for energy. The pancreas also makes enzymes that help the body digest food.

parasthesia—One of different changes in nerve function in extremities, expressed with numbness and tingling.

periodontitis—Gum disease in which the gums shrink away from the teeth. Without treatment, it can lead to tooth loss.

peripheral neuropathy—Nerve damage associated with diabetes that usually affects the feet and legs.

peritoneal dialysis—A mechanical way to clean the blood of people with kidney disease.

plaque—A film of mucus that traps bacteria on the surface of the teeth. Plaque can be removed with daily brushing and flossing of teeth.

polydipsia—Great thirst that lasts for long periods of time.

polyphagia—Great hunger.

polyunsaturated fats—Fat that comes from vegetables.

polyuria—Excessive, frequent urination.

protein—One of the three main classes of food. (Fats and carbohydrates are the other two.) Proteins are found in many foods, including greens, legumes, and algae. Leafy greens are 30 percent protein.

proteinuria—Presence of too much protein in the urine; may signal kidney disease.

pumice stone—A special foot care tool used to gently file calluses as instructed by one's health care team.

regular insulin—A fast-acting insulin.

retina—Center part of the back lining of the eye that senses light.

retinopathy—See diabetic eye disease.

risk factors—Traits that make it more likely that a person will get an illness. For example, a risk factor for developing Type-2 diabetes is having a family history of diabetes.

saturated fat—Fat that comes from animals.

secondary diabetes—Diabetes that develops because of another disease or because of taking certain drugs of chemicals.

self-monitoring blood glucose—A way for people with diabetes to find out how much glucose is in their blood. A drop of blood from the fingertip is placed on a special coated strip of paper that "reads" (often through an electronic meter) the amount of glucose in the blood.

sorbitol—A sugar alcohol produced by the body, which, if levels get too high, may cause damage to the eyes and nerves.

stroke—Damage to a part of the brain that happens when the blood vessels supplying that part are blocked, such as when the blood vessels are clogged with fats (a condition sometimes called hardening of the arteries).

sucrose—Table sugar; a form of sugar the body must break down into a simpler form before the blood can use it.

support group—A group of people who share a similar problem or concern. The people in the group help one another by sharing experiences, knowledge, and information.

syringe—Device used to inject medications or other liquids into the body tissues. An insulin syringe has a hollow plastic or glass tube with a plunger inside. The plunger forces the insulin through the needle into the body.

transcutaneous electric nerve stimulation (TENS)—A treatment for painful neuropathy.

triglyceride—A type of blood fat.

Type-1 diabetes—Also known as IDDM. A condition in which the pancreas makes so little insulin that the body can't use blood glucose as energy. Type-1 diabetes most often occurs in people younger than age 30 and must be controlled with daily insulin injections.

Type-2 diabetes—Also known as NIDDM. A condition in which the body either makes too little insulin or can't use the insulin it makes to use blood glucose as energy. Type-2 diabetes has typically occurred in people older than age 40, but increasingly in children today, and can often be controlled through meal plans and physical activity plans. Some people with Type-2 diabetes have to take diabetes pills or insulin.

U-100—A unit of insulin, meaning 100 units of insulin per milliliter or cubic centimeter of solution.

ulcer—A break or deep sore in the skin. Germs can enter an ulcer so that it may be hard to heal.

ultralente insulin—A long-acting insulin.

urea—One of the chief waste products of the body. When the body breaks down food, it uses what it needs and throws the rest away as waste. The kidneys flush the waste from the body in the form of urea, which is in the urine.

urine testing—A test of urine to see if it contains glucose and ketones.

vaccination—A shot given to theoretically protect against a disease.

vitrectomy—An operation to remove the blood that sometimes collects at the back of the eyes when a person has eye disease.

yeast infection—A vaginal, blood, sinus, or colon infection that is usually caused by a fungus. Women who have this infection may feel itching, burning when urinating, and pain, and some women have a vaginal discharge. Yeast infections occur more frequently in women with diabetes because of the high blood glucose.

ABOUT THE AUTHOR

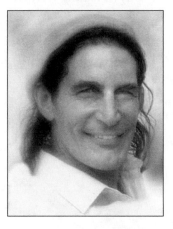

GABRIEL COUSENS, MD

Gabriel Cousens, MD, MD(Homeopathy), DD, Diplomate American Board of Holistic Medicine, Diplomate in Ayurveda, a holistic medical doctor with thirty years of success in healing diabetes naturally, is the founder and director of the Tree of Life Foundation and Tree of Life Rejuvenation Center in Patagonia, Arizona. A graduate of Amherst College, where he published his first scientific paper in the *Journal of Biochemical and Physics Acta* and was captain of an undefeated football team, Cousens received his MD from Columbia Medical School in 1969 and completed his psychiatric residency in 1973.

A bestselling author and the creator of the Tree of Life 21-Day+ comprehensive program for diabetes, Dr. Cousens uses the modalities of nutrition, naturopathy, Ayurveda, and homeopathy blended with spiritual awareness in the healing of body, mind, and spirit. He facilitates the spiritual, nutritional, and lifestyle support tele-seminars, "Alive With Gabriel," and has given seminars on nutrition through the U.S., Canada, Central and South America, all of Western Europe, Turkey, Greece, Israel, and South Africa. Through his books, media, and body-mind-spirit transformative programs at the Tree of Life Rejuvenation Center, Dr. Cousens is recognized as the leading medical authority in the world of live-food nutrition and a renowned spiritual teacher. He recently established a 21-Day+ Healing Diabetes Naturally Program in Israel.

Dr. Cousens, who has two children and two grandchildren, is married to Shanti GoldsCousens. He can be reached at www.TreeOfLife.nu, healing@treeoflife.nu, and (520) 394-2520.

ABOUT THE RESEARCH ASSISTANT

DAVID RAINOSHEK, MA

David Rainoshek, MA, a graduate of the Tree of Life master's program, was Dr. Cousens's research assistant for *There Is a Cure for Diabetes*. He advises and coaches 92-Day Juice Feasts for clients and retreats worldwide. For information on his 92-Day Juice Feasting program, visit www.JuiceFeasting.com.

NOTES

Chapter 1: Diabetes Pandemic: World, Nations and Cultures, Cities

1. International Diabetes Federation. "Diabetes epidemic out of control." December 4, 2006.
   http://www.idf.org/home/index.cfm?node=1563

2. World Health Organization. *Preventing Chronic Diseases: A Vital Investment*, 2005.
   http://www.who.int/chp/chronic_disease_report/en/index.html

3. World Health Organization, 2007.

4. International Diabetes Foundation, "Diabetes deaths to increase dramatically over next ten years" Brussels, 05 October 2005.
   http://www.idf.org/home/index.cfm?unode=7952D720-102D-4842-8487-FB94FEC5B275

5. World Health Organization, 2007.

6. World Diabetes Foundation, "Diabetes facts." http://www.worlddiabetesfoundation.org/composite-35.htm

7. Burkitt, D, and Trowell, H. *Western Diseases: Their Emergence and Prevention*. Cambridge: Harvard University Press, 1981.

8. Vahouny, G, and Kritchevsky, D. *Dietary Fiber in Health and Disease*. New York: Plenum Press, 1982.

9. Murray, M T. "Diabetes Mellitus," *Natural Medicine Journal*, April 1998, p. 5.

10. In a cross-section of U.S. adults age 40–74 years tested from 1988 to 1994, 33.8 percent had Impaired Fasting Glucose (IFG), 15.4 percent had Impaired Glucose Tolerance (IGT), and 40.1 percent had pre-diabetes (IGT or IFG or both). Applying these percentages to the 2000 U.S. population, about 35 million adults age 40–74 would have IFG, 16 million would have IGT, and 41 million would have pre-diabetes.

11. Kitagawa, T, Owada, M, Urakami, T, and Yamauchi, K. "Increased incidence of non-insulin dependent diabetes mellitus among Japanese schoolchildren correlates with an increased intake of animal protein and fat." *Clin Pediatr* (Phila.), 1998, 37:111–115.

12. Pan American Health Organization. *Health in the Americas*. Washington, D.C., 1998.

13. Stem, M P, and Mitchell, B D. "Diabetes in Hispanic Americans." *Diabetes in America*. Washington, D.C., National Institutes of Health, 1995, 2nd ed., pp. 631–659.

14. Jackson, D Z. "Diabetes and the trash food industry." *Boston Globe,* January 11, 2006.

15. CDC, National Center for Health Statistics, Division of Health Interview Statistics, data from the National Health Interview Survey, 2004–2005.

16. http://www.cdc.gov/brfss/training/interviewer/01_section/09_ diabetes.htm

17. *USDA Agriculture Fact Book,* 2001–2002.

18. *Medscape,* "There Is a Strong Relationship Between Diabetes Mortality and Family Income." http://www.medscape.com/ viewarticle/416943

19. International Diabetes Federation. Online Press Release April 2005. http://www.idf.org/home/index.cfm?node=1398

20. Motala, A A, Omar, M A, and Pirie, F J. "Diabetes in Africa. Epidemiology of type 1 and type 2 diabetes in Africa." *J Cardiovasc Risk,* April 2003, 10(2):77–83.

21. International Diabetes Federation, African Region. http://www.idf.org/home/index.cfm?node=46

22. Mokhtar, N, Elati, J, Chabir, R, Bour, A, Elkari, K, Schlossman, N P, Caballero, B, and Aguenaou, H. "Diet culture and obesity in northern Africa." *J Nutrition,* 2001, 131:887S–892S.

23. *Alternative Medicine,* February 2007, p. 64.

24. Cherewatenko, V. *The Diabetes Cure.* New York: Harper Resource, 2000, p. 13.

25. Ibid.

26. *USDA Agriculture Fact Book,* 2001–2002.

27. University of Wisconsin-Milwaukee Graduate School, "Solving A Diabetes Mystery: Leslie Schulz is providing new insight into the high rate among Pima Indians in Arizona." http://www.uwm.edu/Dept/Grad_Sch/Publications/ResearchProfile/ Archive/Vol21No1/schulz.html

28. American Diabetes Association. "Total Prevalence of Diabetes and Pre-Diabetes." http://www.diabetes.org/diabetes-statistics/ prevalence.jsp

29. Steinbrook, R. "Facing the diabetes epidemic: Mandatory reporting of glycosylated hemoglobin values in New York City." *New Eng J Med,* February 9, 2006, 354(6):545–548. http://content.nejm.org/cgi/content/full/354/6/545?ck=nck

30. International Diabetes Federation, "Did you know?" http://www.idf.org/home/index.cfm?node=37

31. International Diabetes Federation, "The human, social and economic impact of diabetes." http://www.idf.org/home/index.cfm?node=41

32. McLarty, D G, Kinabo, L, and Swai, A B M. "Diabetes in tropical Africa: a prospective study, 1981–7. II. Course and prognosis." *BMJ,* 1990, 300:1107–1110.

33. Joslin, E P. *The Treatment of Diabetes Mellitus.* 4th ed. Philadelphia: Lea and Febiger, 1928, p. 384.

34. International Diabetes Federation. "The human, social and economic impact of diabetes." Op. cit.

35. Centers for Disease Control and Prevention. *National Diabetes Fact Sheet.* Washington, D.C., U.S. Department of Health and Human Services and the Centers for Disease Control and Prevention, 1998.

36. These estimates of the economic cost are supported by the findings in a study by the Lewin Group, Inc., for the American Diabetes Association and are 2002 estimates of both the direct (cost of medical care and services) and indirect costs (costs of short-term and permanent disability and of premature death) attributable to diabetes.

37. Stein, R. "A Regular Soda a Day Boosts Weight Gain: Non-Diet Drinks Also Increase Risk of Diabetes, Study Shows." *Washington Post,* August 25, 2004. http://www.washingtonpost.com/wp-dyn/articles/A29434-2004Aug24.html

38. McVitamins, "High-fructose corn syrup."

Chapter 2: Diabetic Lifestyle Habits and Risk Factors

1. Hu, F B, Li, T Y, Colditz, G A, Willett, W C, and Manson, J E. "Television watching and other sedentary behaviors in relation to risk of obesity and type 2 diabetes mellitus in women." *JAMA,* 2003, 289:1785–1791.

2. Olshansky, S J, Passaro, D J, Hershow, R C, et al. "A potential decline in life expectancy in the United States in the 21st century." *New Eng J Med,* March 17, 2005, 352(11):1138–1145. http://content.nejm.org/cgi/content/abstract/352/11/1138?ck=nck

3. Pollan, Michael. "You Are What You Grow." *New York Times,* April 22, 2007.

4. Whitaker, JD. *Reversing Diabetes.* New York: Warner Books, 2001, p. 116.

5. Wolfe, D. *Eating for Beauty.* San Diego: Maul Brothers Publishing, 2002, pp. 33–38.

6. Snowdon, D A, and Phillips, R L. "Does a vegetarian diet reduce the occurrence of diabetes?" *American Journal of Public Health,* 1985, 75:507–512.

7. Tsunehara, C H, Leonetti, D L, and Fujimoto, W Y. "Diet of second-generation Japanese American men with and without NIDDM." *Am J Clin Nutr,* 52 (1990):731–738.

8. Ibid.

9. "Position of The American Dietetic Association: Vegetarian Diets." *J Am Diet Assoc,* June 2003, 103(6):748–765.

10. Ellis, F R, and Montegriffo, V M E. "Veganism, clinical findings and investigations." *Am J Clin Nutr,* 1970, 23:249–255.

11. Berenson, G, Srinivasan, S, Bao, W, Newman, W P Tracy, R E, and Wattigney, W A. "Association between multiple cardiovascular risk factors and atherosclerosis to children and young adults. The Bogalusa Heart Study." *New Eng J Med,* 1998, 338:1650–1656.

12. Key, T J, Fraser, G E, Thorogood, M, et al. "Mortality in vegetarians and nonvegetarians: Detailed findings from a collaborative analysis of 5 prospective studies." *Am J Clin Nutri,* 1999, 70(Suppl.):516S–524S.

13. Bergan, J G, and Brown, P T. "Nutritional status of "new" vegetarians." *J Am Diet Assoc,* 1980, 76:151-155.

14. Appleby, P N, Thorogood, M, et al. "Low body mass index in non-meat eaters: The possible roles of animal fat, dietary fibre, and alcohol." *Int J Obes,* 1998, 22:454–460.

15. Dwyer, J T. "Health aspects of vegetarian diets." *Am J Clin Nutr,* 1988, 48:712–738.

16. Key, T J, and Davey, G. "Prevalence of obesity is low in people who do not eat meat." *BMJ,* 1996, 313:816–817.

17. Stein, R. *The Washington Post,* November 14, 2006. http://www.washingtonpost.com/wp-dyn/content/article/2006/11/13/AR2006111300824_pf.html

18. Lindahl, O. "Vegan Regimen with Reduced Medication in the Treatment of Bronchial Asthma," *Journal of Asthma,* 1985, 22:44.

19. Culhane, J. "PCBs: The Poison that Won't Go Away." *Reader's Digest,* December 1980, pp. 112–116.

20. International Medical Veritas Association. "Diabetes and Mercury Poisoning," October 2006. http://imva.info/med_dia_mercury_poisoning.shtml

21. Robbins, J. *Diet for a New America*. Tiburon, Calif.: H J Kramer, 1987, p. 333. Cited in "Infant Abnormalities Linked to PCB Contaminated Fish," *Vegetarian Times,* Nov. 1984, p. 8.

22. Robbins, ibid., p. 334. Cited in Jacobsen, S. "The effect of intrauterine PCB exposure on visual recognition memory." *Child Development,* 1985, Vol. 56.

23. Vaarala, O, et al. "Cow's milk formula feeding induces primary immunization to insulin in infants at genetic risk for Type-1 diabetes." *Diabetes,* 1999, 48:1389–1394.

24. LaPorte, R E, Tajima, N, Akerblom, H K, et al. "Geographic differences in the risk of insulin-dependent diabetes mellitus: The importance of registries." *Diabetes Care,* 1985, 8(Suppl. 1):101–107.

25. Perez-Bravo, F, Carrasco, E, Gutierrez-Lopez, M D, et al. "Genetic predisposition and environmental factors leading to the development of insulin-dependent diabetes mellitus in Chilean children." *J Mol Med,* 1996, 74:105–109.

26. Kostraba, H N, Cruickshanks, K J, Lawler-Heavner, J, et al. "Early exposure to cow's milk and solid foods in infancy, genetic predisposition, and risk of IDDM." *Diabetes,* 1993, 42:288–295.

27. LaPorte, R E, Tajima, N, Akerblom, H K, et al. Op. cit.

28. Virtanen, S M, Laara, E, Hypponen, E, et al. "Cow's milk consumption, HLA-DQB1 genotype, and Type-1 diabetes." *Diabetes,* 2000, 49:912–917.

29. "American Gastroenterological Association Medical Position Statement: Guidelines for the Evaluation of Food Allergies," *Gastroenterology,* 2001, 120:1023–1025.

30. National Digestive Diseases Information Clearinghouse. "Lactose Intolerance," *National Institute of Diabetes and Digestive and Kidney Diseases,* March 2003.

31. Taylor, C. "Got Milk (Intolerance)? Digestive Malady Affects 30–50 Million," *The Clarion-Ledger,* 1 Aug. 2003.

32. "Cow's Milk Protein May Play Role in Mental Disorders," *Reuters Health,* 1 Apr. 1999.

33. Carrell, S. "Milk Causes Serious Illness for 7M Britons. Scientists Say Undetected Lactose Intolerance Is to Blame for Chronic Fatigue, Arthritis and Bowel Problems," *The Independent,* 22 June 2003.

34. Lewinnek, G E, Kelsey, J, White, A A III, et al. "The significance and a comparative analysis of the epidemiology of hip fractures." *Clin Ortho Rel Res,* 1980, 152:35–43.

35. Recker, R R, and Heaney, R P. "The effect of milk supplements on calcium metabolism, bone metabolism and calcium balance." *Am J Clin Nutr,* 1985, 41:254–263

36. *Postgraduate Medicine Journal,* 1978, 54:244.

37. Campbell, T C. *The China Study.* Dallas: Benbella Books, 2004, p. 7.

38. Ursin, G, Bjelke, E, Heuch, I, et al. "Milk consumption and cancer incidence: A Norwegian prospective study." *Br J Cancer,* 1990, 61:456–459.

39. Cramer, D W, Harlow, B L, Willett, W C, Welch, W R, Bell, D A, Scully, R E, Ng, W G, and Knapp, R C. "Galactose consumption and metabolism in relation to the risk of ovarian cancer. *The Lancet,* 1989, 2(8654):66–71.

40. Fairfield, K M, Hunter, D J, Colditz, G A, Fuchs, C S, Cramer, D W, Speizer, F E, Willett, W C, and Hankinson, S E. "A prospective study of dietary lactose and ovarian cancer." *Intl J Cancer,* 2004, 110(2):271–277.

41. Larsson, S C, Bergkvist, L, and Wolk, A. "Milk and lactose intakes and ovarian cancer risk in the Swedish Mammography Cohort." *Amer J Clin Nutr,* 2004, 80(5):1353–1357.

42. Mettlin, C. "Milk drinking, other beverage habits, and lung cancer risk" *Intl J Cancer,* April 15, 1989, 43(4):608–612.

43. Mettlin, C, Selenskas, S, Natarajan, N, et al. "Beta-carotene and animal fats and their relationship to prostate cancer risk. A case-control study." *Cancer,* 1989, 64:605–612.

44. Chan, J M, and Giovannucci, E L. "Dairy products, calcium, and vitamin D and risk of prostate cancer." *Epidemiol Revs,* 2001, 23:87–92.

45. Plant, J A. *The No-Dairy Breast Cancer Prevention Program.* New York: St. Martin's Press, 2001, p. 74.

46. Plant, J A. *The No-Dairy Breast Cancer Prevention Program.* New York: St. Martin's Press, 2001, p. 75. Cited in: Kliewer, E V, and Smith, K R, "Breast cancer mortality among immigrants in Australia and Canada," *J Natl Cancer Inst,* 1995, 87(15):1154–1161. See also Cancer Research Campaign, *Factsheet 6.2, Breast Cancer—UK,* 1996.

47. McManamy, J. "Depression and Diabetes." http://www.mcmanweb.com/article-42.htm

48. *San Antonio Express News,* "Scientists Examine Link Between Diabetes, Depression." June 16, 2000.

49. Golden, S H, Williams, J E, Ford, D E, et al. "Depressive Symptoms and the Risk of Type 2 Diabetes." *Diabetes Care*, 2004, 27:429–435.

50. Yoon, J W, et al. "Effects of environmental factors on the development of insulin-dependent diabetes mellitus." Department of Microbiology and Infectious Diseases, Julia McFarlane Diabetes Research Unit, University of Calgary, Alberta, Canada. *Clin Invest Med*. Sept. 1987, 10(5):457–469.

51. Banu Priya, C A Y, et al. "Toxicity of Fluoride to Diabetic Rats." International Society for Fluoride Research, *Fluoride*, 1997, 30(1):51–58. http://www.fluoride-journal.com/97-30-1/301-51.htm

52. Professor I M Trakhtenberg. (From Russian translation.) "Chronic Effects of Mercury on Organisms." (Poisons, especially mercury and its compounds, reacting with SH groups of proteins lead to the lowered activity of various enzymes containing sulfhydryl groups. This produces a series of disruptions in the functional activity of many organs and tissues of the organism.)

53. Timoshina, I V, Liubchenko, P N, and Khzardzhian, V G. *Ter Arkh*, 1985, 57(2):91–95. (Article in Russian. Examination of the exocrine function of the pancreas in 52 workers exposed to lead, including 36 with the symptoms of intoxication (mild in 33 and marked in 3) revealed the primarily hyposecretory response of acinar cells stimulated with pancreozymin and secretin, while the hyposecretory and dyspancreatic responses were recorded less frequently. The endocrine function of the pancreas was revealed to be also lowered, which was confirmed by the decreased fasting blood insulin content and low blood insulin content after glucose intake as well. The changes in pancreatic function are among the pathogenetic mechanisms of the abdominal syndrome observable during lead intoxication.)

54. Urinary cadmium, impaired fasting glucose, and diabetes in the NHANES III Pathophysiology/Complications. National Health and Nutrition Examination Survey. *Diabetes Care*, Feb. 2003.

55. Satarug, S, Haswell-Elkins, M R, and Moore, M R. "Safe levels of cadmium intake to prevent renal toxicity in human subjects." *Br J Nutr*, Dec. 2000, 84(6):791–802.

56. Fahim, M A, Hasan, M Y, and Alshuaib, W B. "Cadmium modulates diabetes-induced alterations in murine neuromuscular junction." *Endocr Res*, May 2000, 26(2):205–217.

57. Jin, T, Nordberg, G, Sehlin, J, Wallin, H, and Sandberg, S. "The susceptibility to nephrotoxicity of streptozotocin-induced diabetic rats subchronically exposed to cadmium chloride in drinking water." *Toxicology*, Dec. 1999, 142(1):69–75.

58. Gumuslu, S, Yargicoglu, P, Agar, A, Edremitlioglu, M, and Aliciguzel, Y. "Effect of cadmium on antioxidant status in alloxane-induced diabetic rats." *Biol Trace Elem Res,* May 1997, 57(2):105–114.

59. Ya Wen Chen, et al. *Chem Res Toxicol,* 2006, 19(8):1080–1085. (Institute of Toxicology, Department of Laboratory Medicine, and Department of Orthopaedics, College of Medicine, National Taiwan University, Taipei, Taiwan, and Departments of Traumatology, Surgery, and Emergency Medicine, National Taiwan University Hospital, Taiwan.)

60. International Medical Veritas Association. "Diabetes and Mercury Poisoning." http://imva.info/med_dia_mercury_poisoning.shtml

61. Ibid.

62. Tseng, C H, et al. "Long-term arsenic exposure and incidence of non-insulin-dependent diabetes mellitus: A cohort study in arseniasis-hyperendemic villages in Taiwan. *Environ Health Perspect,* Sept. 2000, 108(9):847–851.

63. Rahman, M, et al. "Diabetes mellitus associated with arsenic exposure in Bangladesh." *Am J Epidemiol,* 1998, 148(2):198–203.

64. Berkson, L. *Hormone Deception.* New York: Contemporary Books, 2000, p. 312.

65. Shirng-Wern Tsaih, et al. "Lead, Diabetes, Hypertension, and Renal Function: The Normative Aging Study." Harvard Medical School, Boston, Massachusetts. *Environmental Health Perspectives,* 2004, 12(11).

66. "Fluoride in Drinking Water: A Scientific Review of EPA's Standards," National Research Council, 2006.

67. The information in this section is gathered from the National Vaccine Information Center (NVIC), a national, nonprofit educational organization founded in 1982. NVIC is the oldest and largest consumer organization advocating for vaccine safety and informed consent protections in the mass vaccination system.

68. National Vaccine Information Center, "Juvenile Diabetes and Vaccination: New Evidence for a Connection," http://www.909shot.com/Diseases/juvenilediabetes.htm

69. Ibid.

70. Ibid.

71. Centers for Disease Control, *Pharmacoepidemiology and Drug Safety,* 1998, 6(2):S60.

72. So Jung Lee, et al. "Caffeine Ingestion Is Associated With Reductions in Glucose Uptake Independent of Obesity and Type 2 Diabetes

Before and After Exercise Training." *Diabetes Care,* 2005, 28:566–572.

73. "Cigarettes: What the warning label doesn't tell you." *The American Council on Science and Health,* 1996

74. Targher, G, et al. "Cigarette smoking and insulin resistance in patients with non-insulin resistance in patients with non-insulin-dependent diabetes mellitus." *J Clin Endocrinol Metab,* 1997, 82:3619–3624.

75. Targher, G, Alberiche, M, Zenere, M B, et al. "Cigarette smoking and insulin resistance in patients with non-insulin dependent diabetes mellitus." *J Clin Endocrinol Metab,* 1997, 82:3619–3624.

76. Kelley, D E, Goodpaster, B, Wing, R R, and Simoneau, J A. "Skeletal muscle fatty acid metabolism in association with insulin resistance, obesity, and weight loss." *Am J Physiol,* 1999, 277:E1130–E1141.

77. Gutierrez, D. "Exercise shown to powerfully decrease cigarette cravings." News Target.com, April 4, 2007. http://www.newstarget.com/021769.html

78. Kawakami, N, et al. "Effects of smoking on incidence of non-insulin dependence diabetes mellitus." *Am J Epidemiology,* Jan. 15, 1997, 145(2):103–109.

79. Will, J C, et al. "Cigarette smoking and diabetes mellitus: Evidence of a positive association from a large prospective cohort study." *Int J Epidemiol,* 2001, 30:554–555.

80. Mitchell, B, Hawthorne, V, and Vinik, A. "Cigarette smoking and neuropathy in diabetic patients." *Diabetes Care,* 1990, 13:434–447.

81. Sands, M, et al. "Incidence of distal symmetric (sensory) neuropathy in NIDDM: The San Luis Diabetes Study." *Diabetes Care,* 1997, 20:322–329.

82. "Diabetes and Periodontal Disease Fact Book," http://www.healthnewsflash.com/conditions/diabetes_and_periodontal_disease.php

83. "Diabetes and Its Awful Toll Quietly Emerge as a Crisis," *New York Times,* January 9, 2006.

84. *Annals of Internal Medicine,* 136(3):130.

85. Humphries, S E, Gable, D, Cooper, J A, et al. "Common variants in the TCF7L2 gene and predisposition to type 2 diabetes in UK European whites, Indian Asians and Afro Carribean men and women." *J Molecular Medicine,* Dec. 2006, 84(12):1005–1014.

86. Murray, M, and Pizzorno, J. *Encyclopedia of Natural Medicine.* Rocklin, Calif.: Prima Publishing, 1998.

87. De Mattia, G, Bravi, M C, Laurenti, O, Cassone-Faldetta, M, Proietti A, De Luca, O, Armiento, A, and Ferri, C. "Reduction of oxidative stress by oral N-acetyl-L-cysteine treatment decreases plasma soluble vascular cell adhesion molecule-I concentrations in non-obese, non-dyslipidaemic, normotensive, patients with non-insulin-dependent diabetes." *Diabetologia,* 1998, 41(11):1392–1396.

88. Kaufman, F R. "Type diabetes in children and young adults: A 'new epidemic.'" *Clinical Diabetes,* 2002, 20:217–218.

89. Ibid.

90. Ibid.

91. Ibid.

92. Wang, Y. "Cross-national comparison of childhood obesity: the epidemic and the relationship between obesity and socioeconomic status." *Intl J Epidemiology,* October 2001, 30:1129–1136.

93. Adams, M. "Campaign for Commercial-Free Childhood blasts TV promotion of junk foods to children." http://www.newstarget.com/021835.html

94. Enos, W F, Holmes, R H, and Beyer, J. "Coronary disease among United States soldiers killed in action in Korea." *JAMA,* 1953, 152:1090–1093.

95. McNamara, J J, Molot, M A, Stremple, J F, and Cutting, R T. "Coronary artery disease in combat casualties in Vietnam." *JAMA,* 1971, 216:1185–1187.

96. Berenson, G, Srinivasan, S, Bau, W, Newman, W P, Tracy, R E, and Wattingney, W A. "Association between multiple cardiovascular risk factors and atherosclerosis in children and young adults." *N Engl J Med,* 1998, 338:1650–1656.

97. Strong, J P, Malcolm, G T, McMahan, C, Tracy, R, Newman, W, Hederick, E, and Cornhill, J. "Prevalence and extent of atherosclerosis in adolescents and young adults." *JAMA,* 1999, 281:727–735.

98. Berenson, G S, Wattigney, W A, Tracey, R E, et al. "Atherosclerosis of the aorta and coronary arteries and cardiovascular risk factors in persons aged 6 to 30 years and studied at necropsy (the Bogalusa heart study)." *Am J Cardiol,* 1992, 70:851–858.

99. Huerta, M G, et al. "Magnesium deficiency is associated with insulin resistance in obese children," *Diabetes Care,* 2005, 28:1175–1181.

100. Bircher-Brenner, M. *Food Science for All, New Sunlight Theory of Nutrition.* Health Research, 1928.

101. Wigmore, A. The Hippocrates Diet and Health Program. Avery Press, 1984.

102. Hughes, J H, and Latner, A L. "Chlorophyll and Hemoglobin Regeneration After Hemorrhage," *Journal of Physiology,* University of Liverpool, 1936, 86, #388.

103. Grimm, J J. "Interaction of physical activity and diet: implications for insulin-glucose dynamics." *Public Health Nutr,* 1999, 2:363–368.

104. Moore, M A, Park, C B, and Tsuda, H. "Implications of the hyperinsulinaemia-diabetes-cancer link for preventive efforts." *Eur J Cancer Prev,* 1998, 7:89–107.

105. Arthur, L S, Selvakumar, R, Seshadri, M S, and Seshadri, L. "Hyperinsulinemia in polycystic ovary disease." *J Reprod Med,* 1999, 44:783–787.

106. Pugeat, M, and Ducluzeau, P H. "Insulin resistance, polycystic ovary syndrome and metformin." *Drugs,* 1999, 58:41–46.

107. Baranowska, B, Radzikowska, M W, et al. "Neuropeptide Y, leptin, galanin and insulin in women with polycystic ovary syndrome." *Gynecol Endocrinol,* 1999, 13:344–351.

108. Kotake, H, and Oikawa, S. "Syndrome X." *Nippon Rinsho,* 1999, 57:622–626. (Article in Japanese.)

109. Watanabe, K, Sekiya, M, Tsuruoka, T, et al. "Relationship between insulin resistance and cardiac sympathetic nervous function in essential hypertension." *J Hypertens,* 1999, 17:1161–1168.

110. Lender, D, Arauz-Pacheco, C, Adams-Huet, B, and Raskin, P. "Essential hypertension is associated with decreased insulin clearance and insulin resistance." *Hypertension,* 1997, 29:111–114.

111. Stubbs, P J, Alaghband-Zadeh, J, Laycock, J F, et al. "Significance of an index of insulin resistance on admission in nondiabetic patients with acute coronary syndromes." *Heart,* 1999, 82:443–447.

112. Lempiainen, P, Mykkanen, L, Pyorala, K, et al. "Insulin resistance syndrome predicts coronary heart disease events in elderly nondiabetic men." *Circulation,* 1999, 100:123–128.

113. Misra, A, Reddy, R B, Reddy, K S, et al. "Clustering of impaired glucose tolerance, hyperinsulinemia and dyslipidemia in young north Indian patients with coronary heart disease: A preliminary case-control study." *Indian Heart J,* 1999, 51:275–280.

114. Davis, C L, Gutt, M, Llabre, M M, et al. "History of gestational diabetes, insulin resistance and coronary risk." *J Diabetes Complications,* 1999, 13:216–223.

115. Despres, J P, Lamarche, B, Mauriege, P, et al. "Hyperinsulinemia as an independent risk factor for ischemic heart disease." *N Engl J Med,* 1996, 334:952–957.

116. Tiihonen, M, Partinen, M, and Narvanen, S. "The severity of obstructive sleep apnea is associated with insulin resistance." *J Sleep Res,* 1993, 2:56–61.

117. Moore, Park, and Tsuda. Op. cit.

118. Pujol, P, Galtier-Dereure, F, and Bringer, J. "Obesity and breast cancer risk." *Hum Reprod,* 1997, 12:116–125.

119. Stoll, B A. "Essential fatty acids, insulin resistance, and breast cancer risk." *Nutr Cancer,* 1998, 31:72–77.

120. Grundy, S M. "Hypertriglyceridemia, insulin resistance, and the metabolic syndrome. *Am J Cardiol,* 1999, 83:25F–29F.

121. Belfiore, F, and Iannello, S. "Insulin resistance in obesity: Metabolic mechanisms and measurement methods." *Mol Genet Metab,* 1998, 65:121–128.

122. Samaras, K, Nguyen, T V, Jenkins, A B, et al. "Clustering of insulin resistance, total and central abdominal fat: Same genes or same environment? *Twin Res,* 1999, 2:218–225.

123. Benzi, L, Ciccarone, A M, Cecchetti, P, et al. "Intracellular hyperinsulinism: A metabolic characteristic of obesity with and without type 2 diabetes: Intracellular insulin in obesity and type 2 diabetes." *Diabetes Res Clin Pract,* 1999, 46:231–237.

124. Norbiato, G, Bevilacqua, M, Meroni, R, et al. "Effects of potassium supplementation on insulin binding and insulin action in human obesity: Protein modified fast and refeeding." *Eur J Clin Invest,* 1984, 14:414–419.

125. Reddi, A, DeAngelis, B, Frank, O, et al. "Biotin supplementation improves glucose and insulin tolerances in genetically diabetic KK mice." *Life Sci,* 1988, 42:1323–1330.

126. Brandi, L S, Santoro, D, Natali, A, et al. "Insulin resistance of stress: Sites and mechanisms." *Clin Sci (Colch),* 1993, 85:525–535.

127. Nilsson, P M, Moller, L, and Solstad, K. "Adverse effects of psychosocial stress on gonadal function and insulin levels in middle-aged males." *J Intern Med,* 1995, 237:479–486.

128. Hamann, A, and Matthaei, S. "Regulation of energy balance by leptin." *Exp Clin Endocrinol Diabetes,* 1996, 104:293–300.

129. *Alternative Medicine,* February 2007, p. 61.

130. Kuhl, C, and Holst, J J. "Plasma glucagon and insulin: Glucagon ratio in gestational diabetes." *Diabetes,* 1976, 25:16.

131. Freinkel, N. "Banting Lecture 1980: Of pregnancy and progeny." *Diabetes,* 1980, 29:1023–35.

132. Coustan, D R, Carpenter, M W, O'Sullivan, P S, and Carr, S R. "Gestational diabetes mellitus: Predictors of subsequent disordered glucose metabolism." *Am I Obstet Gynecol,* 1993, 168:1139–1145.

133. O'Sullivan and Mahan. Op. cit.

134. Mestman, Anderson, and Guadalupe. Op. cit.

135. O'Sullivan, J B. "Subsequent morbidity among GDM women." In *Carbohydrate Metabolism* in *Pregnancy and the Newborn.* Sutherland and Stowers, eds. New York: Churchill Livingstone, 1984.

136. O'Sullivan, J B, Charles, O, Mahan, C M, and Dandrow, R V. "Gestational diabetes and perinatal mortality rate." *Am I Obstet Gynecol,* 1973, 116:901–904.

137. Screening for gestational diabetes is technical and should be done with your doctor, who knows how to do it, but it is usually performed with a 50g oral glucose dose given between 20 and 28 weeks, followed by a one-hour venous glucose dose. A test result of above 140 at one hour suggests a gestational diabetes problem.

138. "Research Reveals Deepening Connections Between Diabetes and Alzheimer's: Existing diabetes therapies may help fight Alzheimer's." Alzheimer's Association, 2006. http://www.alz.org/icad/ newsreleases/071606_noon_diabtesandad.asp

139. Rivera, E J, Goldin, A, Fulmer, N, Tavares, R, Wands, J R, and de la Monte, S M. "Insulin and insulin-like growth factor expression and function deteriorate with progression of Alzheimer's disease: Link to brain reductions in acetylcholine." *J Alzheimers Dis,* Dec. 2005, 8(3):247–268.

140. "Alzheimer's Disease." *Alternative Medicine,* February 2007, p. 66.

141. Takeuchi, M, Kikuchi, S, Sasaki, N, et al. "Involvement of advanced glycation end products in Alzheimer's disease." *Curr Alzheimer Res,* Feb 2004, 1(1):39–46.

142. Rosick, E R. "The Deadly Connection Between Diabetes and Alzheimer's." *Life Extension,* Dec. 2006, pp. 33–41.

143. Ramasamy, R., Vannucci, S J, Yan, S S, et al. "Advanced glycation end products and RAGE: A common thread in aging, diabetes, neurodegeneration, and inflammation." *Glycobiology,* July 2005, 15(7):16R–28R.

144. Opara, E C. "Oxidative stress, micronutrients, diabetes mellitus and its complications." *J R Soc Health,* March 2002, 122(1):28–34.

145. Houstis, N, Rosen, E D, and Lander, E S. "Reactive oxygen species have a causal role in multiple forms of insulin resistance." *Nature,* April 2006, 440(7086):944–948.

146. Moreira, P I, Smith, M A, Zhu, X, et al. "Oxidative stress and neu-rodegeneration." *Ann NY Acad Sci,* June 2005, 1043:545–452.

147. Arivazhagan, P, and Panneerselvam, C. "Alpha-lipoic acid increases Na+K+ATPase activity and reduces lipofuscin accumulation in dis-crete brain regions of aged rats." *Ann NY Acad Sci.,* June 2004, 1019:350–354.

148. Lovell, M A, Xie, C, Xiong, S, and Markesbery, W R. "Protection against amyloid beta peptide and iron/hydrogen peroxide toxicity by alpha lipoic acid." *J Alzheimer's Dis,* June 2003, 5(3):229–239.

149. Hitti, M. "Fruit, Veggie Juices May Cut Alzheimer's Risk Antioxidants May Be the Key, Say Researchers." WebMD Medical News. June 20, 2005. http://my.webmd.com/content/Article/107/108607.htm

150. Nagamani, M, Hannigan, E V, Dinh, T V, and Stuart, C A. "Hyperinsulinemia and stromal luteinization of the ovaries in post-menopansal women with endometrial cancer."

151. Parazzini, F, La Vecchia, C, Negri, E, Riboldi, G L, Surace, M, Benzi, G, Maina, A, and Chiaffarino, F. "Diabetes and endometrial cancer: An Italian case-control study." *Int J Cancer,* 1999, 81(4):539–542.

152. Nagamani, et al. Op. cit.

153. Vishnevsky, A S, Bobrov, J F, Tsyrlina, E V, and Dilman, V M. "Hyperinsulinemia as a factor modifying sensitivity of endometrial carcinoma to hormonal influences." *Eur J Gynaecol Oncol,* 1993, 14(2):127–130.

154. Schoen, R E, Tangen, C M, Kuner, L H, Burke, G L, Cushman, M, Tracy, R P, Dobs, A, and Savage, P. "Increased blood glucose and insulin, body size, and incident colorectal cancer." *J Natl Cancer Inst,* 1999, 91(13):1147–1154.

155. Larsson, S C, Bergkvist, L, and Wolk, A. "Consumption of sugar and sugar-sweetened food and the risk of pancreatic cancer in a prospec-tive study." *Am J Clin Nutr,* Nov. 2006, 84(5):1171–1176.

Chapter 3: A Comprehensive Theory of Diabetes

1. Himsworth, H P. *ProcR Soc Med,* 1949, 42(3):323.

2. Campbell, G D. *Congr Abstr, S Afr Med Ass,* East London, 45. Cape Town: South African Medical Association, 1959.

3. *S Afr Med J,* 1960, 34:332.

4. Albertson, V. *Diabetes,* 1953, 2:1184.

5. Cohen, A M. *Israel Med J,* 1960, 19:6137.

6. Cook, C E. Personal communication with Dr. Cleave, 1963.

7. Campbell, C H. Personal communication with Dr. Cleave, 1963.

8. Prior, J A M, and Davidson, F. *N Z Med J,* 1966, 65:375.

9. Ascherio, A, and Willet, W C. "Health effects of trans-fatty acids." *Am J Clin Nutr,* Oct. 1997, 66(suppl. 4):S1006–S1010.

10. Norris, S. "Trans Fats: The Health Burden." http://www.parl.gc.ca/information/library/PRBpubs/prb0521-e.htm

11. Bluher, M, Kahn, B B, and Kahn, C R. "Extended longevity in mice lacking the insulin receptor in adipose tissue." *Science,* Jan. 24, 2003, 299(5606):572–574.

12. Lane, M A, Ingram, D K, and Roth, G S. "Calorie restriction in non-human primates: Effects on diabetes and cardiovascular risk." *Toxicol Sci,* Dec. 1999, 52(2 Suppl):41–48.

13. Kemnitz, J W, Roecker, E B, Weindruch, R, Elson, D F, Baum, S T, and Bergman, R N. "Dietary restriction increases insulin sensitivity and lowers blood glucose in rhesus monkeys." *Am J Physiol,* April 1994, 266(4, Pt.1):E540–E547.

14. Kent, S. "BioMarker pharmaceuticals develops anti-aging therapy." *Life Extension,* June 2003, 9(6):56–67. Ft. Lauderdale: Life Extension Foundation.

15. Suh, Y, Lee, K A, Kim, W H, Han, B G, Vijg, J, and Park, S. "Aging alters the apoptotic response to genotoxic stress." *Nat. Med,* Jan. 2002, 8(1):3–4.

16. Mukherjee, P, El-Abbadi, M M, Kasperzyk, J L, Ranes, M K, and Seyfried, T N. "Dietary restriction reduces angiogenesis and growth in an orthotopic mouse brain tumour model." *BI:* 1 *Cancer,* May 20, 2002, 86(10):1615–1621.

17. Kritchevsky, D. "Caloric restriction and cancer." *J Nutr Sci Vitaminol,* Feb. 2001, 47(1):13–19.

18. Moreschi, C. "The connection between nutrition and tumor promotion." *Z Immunitaetsforsch.,* 1909, 2:651.

19. Spindler, S R. "Reversing aging rapidly with short-term calorie restriction." *Life Extension Magazine,* 2001, 7(12):40–61. Ft. Lauderdale: Life Extension Foundation. www.lef.org/magazinc/mag2001/dec2001cover_spindler - 04.html

20. Yoshida, K, Inoue, T, Hirabayashi, Y, Nojima, K, and Sado, T "Calorie restriction and spontaneous hepatic tumors in C3H1He mice." *J Nutr Health Aging,* 1999, 3(2):121–126.

21. Widmer, S, Mauriz, M, and Gottesmann, S. "Posttranslational quality control: Folding, refolding, and degrading proteins." *Science,* Dec. 3, 1999, 286(5446):1888–1893.

22. Kritchevsky, D. "The effect of over- and undernutrition on cancer." *Eur J Cancer Prev,* Dec. 1995, 4(6):445–451.

23. Bjornholt, H V, Erikssen, G, Aaser, E, et al. "Fasting blood glucose: An underestimated risk factor for cardiovascular death. Results from a 22-year follow-up of healthy nondiabetic men." *Diabetes Care,* 1999, 22:45–49.

24. *Harrison's Principles of Internal Medicine,* thirteenth edition. New York: McGraw-Hill, 1994, p. 2001. "In one study in normal persons (arterialized venous samples), insulin secretion ceased at a 4.6 nmol/L glucose (83mg/dl)."

25. Ibid., p. 2004. "Plasma insulin concentration generally reaches background levels for the assay when plasma glucose falls below 4.6 nmol/L (83mg/dl)."

26. Ibid., table 328-4, Mean plasma glucose and insulin during fasting. (Zero values obtained after overnight fast. Results are mean values for twenty normal men and sixty normal women.)

27. Walford, R L, Harris, S B, and Gunion, M W. "The calorically restricted low-fat nutrient-dense diet in Biosphere 2 significantly lowers blood glucose, total leukocyte count, cholesterol, and blood pressure in humans." *Proc Natl Acad Sci USA,* Dec. 1, 1992, 89(23):11533–11537.

28. Heller, R F. "Hyperinsulinemic obesity and carbohydrate addiction: The missing link is the carbohydrate frequency factor." *Med Hypotheses,* May 1994, 42(5):307–312.

29. Goodpaster, B H, Katsiaras, A, and Kelley, D E. "Enhanced fat oxidation through physical activity is associated with improvements in insulin sensitivity in obesity." *Diabetes,* Sept. 2003, 52(9):2191–2197.

30. "An insulin index of foods: the insulin demand generated by 1000-kJ portions of common foods." *Am J Clin Nutr,* Nov. 1997, 66(5):1264–1276

31. Holt, S H A, et al. *European J Clin Nutr* 1995, 49:675–690.

32. Furber, J D. "Extracellular glycation crosslinks: Prospects for removal." *Rejuvenation Res,* Summer 2006, 9(2):274–278.

33. Peppa, M, Uribarri, J, and Vlassara, H. "Glucose, advanced glycation end products, and diabetes complications: What is new and what works." *Clinical Diabetes,* 2003, 21:186–187.

34. Werman, M J, et al. "The chronic effect of dietary fructose on glycation and collagen cross-linking in rats." *Am J Clin Nutr,* 1997, 66:219.

35. McCarty, M F. "The low AGE content of low-fat vegan diets could benefit diabetics, though concurrent taurine supplementation may be needed to minimize endogenous AGE production." *Med Hypotheses,* 2005, 64(2):394–398.

36. Qian, P, Cheng, S, Guo, J, and Niu, Y. "Effects of Vitamin E and Vitamin C on nonenzymatic glycation and peroxidation in experimental diabetic rats." *Wei Sheng Yan Jiu,* July 2000, 29(4):226–228.

37. Ceriello, A, Quatraro, A, and Giugliano, D. "New insights on nonenzymatic glycosylation may lead to therapeutic approaches for the prevention of diabetic complications." *Diabet Med,* 1992, 9:297–299.

38. Davie, S J, Gould, B J, and Yudkin, J S. "Effect of vitamin C on glycosylation of proteins." *Diabetes,* 1992, 41:167–173.

39. Ceriello, Quatraro, and Giugliano. Op. cit.

40. Davie, Gould, and Yudkin. Op. cit.

41. Jain, S K, McVie, R, Jaramillo, J J, et al. "Effect of modest vitamin E supplementation on blood glycated hemoglobin and triglyceride levels and red cell indices in Type-1 diabetic patients." *J Am Coll Nutr,* 1996, 15:458–461.

42. Fife, B. *The Healing Miracles of Coconut Oil.* Colorado Springs: Health Wise, 2003, p. 110.

43. Nicholson, A S, et al. "Toward Improved Management of NIDDM: A Randomized, Controlled, Pilot Intervention Using a Low-Fat, Vegetarian Diet." *Preventive Medicine,* 1999, 29: 87–91.

44. Barnard, N D, et al. "The Effects of a Low-Fat, Plant-Based Dietary Intervention on Body Weight, Metabolism, and Insulin Sensitivity." *Amer J Medicine,* 2005, 118:991–997.

45. Stratton, I M, Adler, A L, and Neil, H A. "Association of Glycaemia with Macrovascular and Microvascular Complications of Type 2 Diabetes (UKPDS 35): Prospective Observational Study." *BMJ,* 2000, 321: 405–412.

46. Ornish, D, et al. "Can Lifestyle Changes Reverse Coronary Heart Disease?" *The Lancet,* 1990, 336):129–133.

47. Petersen, K F, et al. "Impaired Mitochondrial Activity in the Insulin-Resistant Offspring of Patients with Type 2 Diabetes." *New England J Med,* 2004, 350:664–671.

48. Goff, L M, et al. "Veganism and Its Relationship with Insulin Resistance and Intramyocellular Lipid." *Eur J Clin Nutr,* 2005, 59:291–298.

49. Keen, H, and Mattock, M D. "Complications of diabetes mellitus: Role of essential fatty acids." In: Horrobin, D F, ed. *Omega-6 Essential Fatty Acids. Pathophysiology and Roles in Clinical Medicine.* New York: Wiley-Liss; 1990, pp. 447–455.

50. Storlien, L H, Jenkins, A B, Chisolm, D J, et al. "Influence of dietary fat composition on development of insulin resistance in rats." *Diabetes,* 1991, 40:280–289.

51. Dutta-Roy, A K. "Insulin mediated processes in platelets, erythrocytes, and monocytes/ macrophages: effects of essential fatty acid metabolism." *Prostaglandins Leukot Essent Fatty Acids,* 1994, 51:385–399.

52. Ibid.

53. Hagve, T-A. "Effects of unsaturated fatty acids on cell membrane functions." *Scand J Clin Lab Inves,* 1988, 48:381–388.

54. Anderson, R A. "Chromium, glucose tolerance, diabetes and lipid metabolism." *J Advan Med,* 1995, 8:37–50.

55. Horrobin, D F. "Essential Fatty Acid (EFA) metabolism in patients with diabetic neuropathy." *Prostaglandins Leukot Essent Fatty Acids,* 1997, 57:256(abstr.)

56. Enig, M G, Atal, S, Keeny, M, and Sampunga, J. "Isometric *trans-fatty acids* in the U.S. diet." *J Am Coll Nutr,* 1990, 5:471–486.

57. Pan, D A, Lilliioja, S, Milner, M R, et al. "Skeletal muscle membrane lipid composition is related to adiposity and insulin action." *J Clin Invest,* 1995, 96:2802–2808.

58. Storlien, L H, Pan, D A, Kriketos, A D, et al. "Skeletal muscle membrane lipids and insulin resistance." *Lipids,* 1996, 31:S262–S265.

59. Eritsland, J, Delijeflot, I, Abdelnoor, M, et al. "Long-term effects of n-3 fatty acids on serum lipids and glycemic control." *Scand J Clin Lab Invest,* 1994, 54:73–80.

60. Clandinin, M T, Cheema, S, Field, C H, and Baracos, V E. "Impact of dietary fatty acids on insulin responsiveness in adipose tissue, muscle, and liver." In: Sinclair, A, and Gibson, R, eds. *Essential Fatty Acids and Ecosanoids: Invited Papers from the Third International Conference.* Champaign, Ill.: AOCS Press, 1993, pp. 416–420.

61. Storlien, Pan, Kriketos, et al. Op cit..

62. Eritsland, Delijeflot, Abdelnoor, et al. Op. cit.

63. Kissebah, A H, and Hennes, M M I. "Central obesity and free fatty acid metabolism." *Prostaglandins Leukot Essent Fatty Acids,* 1995, 52:209–211.

64. Foster, D W. "Diabetes Mellitus." In: Braunwald, E, Isselbacher, K J, Petersdorf, R G, et al, eds. *Harrison's Principles of Internal Medicine,* eleventh edition. New York: McGraw-Hill; 1988, pp. 1778–1781.

65. Heller, B, Burkart, V, Lampeter, E, and Kolb, H. "Antioxidant therapy for the prevention of Type-1 diabetes." *Adv Pharm,* 1997, 38:629–638.

66. Mijac, V, Arrieta, J, Mendt, C. et al. "Role of environmental factors in the development of insulin-dependent diabetes mellitus (IDDM) in insulin-dependent Venezuelan children." *Invest Clin,* 1995, 36:73–82.

67. Ibid.

68. Schmernthaner, G. "Progress in the immunointervention of Type-1 diabetes mellitus." *Horm Metab Res,* 1995, 27:547–554.

69. Ibid.

70. Mijac, Arrieta, Mendt, et al. Op. cit.

71. Karjalainen, J, Martin, J, Knip, M, et al. "A bovine albumin peptide as a possible trigger of insulin-dependent diabetes." *N Eng J Med,* 1992, 327:302–307.

72. Saukkonen, T, Savilahti, E, Madascsy, L, et al. "Increased frequency of IgM antibodies to cow's milk proteins in Hungarian children with newly diagnosed insulin-dependent diabetes mellitus." *Eur J Pediatr,* 1996, 155:885–889.

73. Saukkonen, T, Savilahti, E, Landin-Olsson, M, and Dahlquist, G. "IgA bovine serum albumin antibodies are increased in newly diagnosed patients with insulin-dependent diabetes mellitus, but the increase is not an independent risk factor for diabetes." *Acta Paediatr,* 1995, 84:1258–1261.

74 .Vahasalo, P, Petays, T, Knip, M, et al. "Relation between antibodies to islet cell antigens, other autoantigens and cow's milk protein in diabetic children and unaffected siblings at the clinical manifestation of IDDM." The Childhood Diabetes in Finland Study Group. *Autoimmunity,* 1996, 23:165–174.

75. Leslie, R D G, and Elliott, R B. "Early environmental events as a cause of IDDM." *Diabetes,* 1994, 43:843–850.

76. *Diabetes,* 1993, 42:288–295.

77. Karjalainen, et al. Op. cit.

78. Akerblom, H K, et al. "Dietary Manipulation of Beta Cell Autoimmunity in Infants at Increased Risk of Type-1 Diabetes: A Pilot Study." *Diabetologia,* 2005, 48:829–837.

79. Clyne, P S, and Kulczycki Jr., A. "Human Breast Milk Contains Bovine IgG: Relationship to Infant Colic?" *Pediatrics,* 1997, 87:439–444.

80. American Academy of Pediatrics Work Group on Cow's Milk Protein and Diabetes Mellitus. "Infant Feeding Practices and Their Possible Relationship to the Etiology of Diabetes Mellitus." *Pediatrics,* 1994, 94:752–754.

81. Brownlee, M, Vlassara, H, and Cerami, A. "Nonenzymatic glycosylation and the pathogenesis of diabetic complications." *Ann Int Med,* 1984, 101:527–537.

82. Whitaker, J. *Reversing Diabetes.* New York: Warner Books, 2001, p. 21.

83. American Diabetes Association. "Diabetes and Heart (Cardiovascular) Disease." http://www.diabetes.org/diabetes-statistics/heart-disease.jsp

84. Esselstyn, C B, Ellis, S G, Medendorp, S V, et al. "A strategy to arrest and revse coronary artery disease: A 5-year longitudinal study of a single physician's practice." *J Fam Prac,* 1995, 41:560–568.

85. Esselstyn, C B. *Prevent and Reverse Heart Disease.* www.heartattackproof.com

86. *World Health Statistics Annual 1994–1998.* Online version: www.who.int/whosis. Statistical database food balance sheets, 1961–1999. Available online at www.fao.org. Food and Agriculture Organization of the United Nations. National Institutes of Health. Global cancer rates, cancer death rates among 50 countries, 1986-1999. Available online at www.nih.gov.

87. Fuhrman, J. *Eat to Live.* New York: Little, Brown, and Company, 2003, pp. 51–52.

88. "Children of diabetics show signs of atherosclerosis." Accessed online July 2007. http://medicineworld.org/cancer/lead/6-2006/children-of-diabetics.html

89. Ross-Flanigan, N. "Diabetes and periodontal disease: A complex, two-way connection." http://www.umich.edu/~urecord/9899/Jan25_99/gums.htm

90. Wyngaarden, J B, Smith, L H, and Bennett, J C. *Cecil Textbook of Medicine.* Philadelphia: W B Saunders, 1992.

91. Cogan, D G, Kinoshita, J H, Kador, P F, et al. "Aldose reductase and complications of diabetes." *Ann Int Med,* 1984, 101:82–91.

92. Crane, M G, and Sample, C. "Regression of Diabetic Neuropathy with Total Vegetarian (Vegan) Diet." *J Nutritional Med,* 1994, 4:431–439.

93. Pecoraro, R E, Reiber, G E, and Burgess, E M. "Pathways to diabetic limb amputation: Basis for prevention." *Diabetes Care,* 1990, 13:513–521.

94. Lavery, L A, Ashry, H R, van Houtum, W, Pugh, J A, Harkless, L B, and Basu, S. "Variation in the incidence and proportion of diabetes-related amputations in minorities." *Diabetes Care,* 1996, 19:48–52.

95. Armstrong, D G, Lavery, L A, Quebedeaux, T L, and Walker, S C. "Surgical morbidity and the risk of amputation due to infected puncture wounds in diabetic versus nondiabetic adults." *South Med J,* 1997, 90:384–389.

96. Whitaker. Op. cit., pp. 6 and 146.

97. Thomas, S H, Wisher, M, Brandenberg, D, and Sonksen, P H. "Insulin action on adipocytes, evidence that the antilipolytic and lipogenic effects of insulin are mediated by the same receptor." *Biochem J,* 1979, 184:355–360.

98. Baskin, et al. "Insulin receptor substrate 1 (IRS-1) expression in rat brain." *Endocrin,* 1998, 134:1952–1955.

99. Zhao, W, Chen, H, Xu, H, Moore, E, Meiri, N, Quon, MJ, and Alkon, D. "Brain insulin receptors and spatial memory. Correlated changes in gene expression tyrosine phosphorylation and signaling molecules in the hippocampus of water maze trained rats." *J Biol Chem,* 1990, 274:34893–34902

100. Sonksen, P H. "Insulin, growth hormone and sport." *J Endocrinol,* 2001, 170:23–25.

101. Berkson, L. *Hormone Deception.* New York: Contemporary Books, 2000, p. 208.

102. Bertazzi, P A. "Long-Term Health Effects of Dioxin Exposure in a Residential Population," Talk at Keystone Symposium on Endocrine Disruptors (B5) in Tahoe City, Calif. (Jan 31–Feb 5, 1999).

103. Berkson. Op. cit. (312)

104. Moller, J, and Einfeldt, H. *Testosterone Treatment of Cardiovascular Diseases: Principles and Experiences.* Berlin: Springer-Verlag, 1984.

105. Anderson, D C. "Sex hormone binding globulin." *Clin Endocrin,* 1972, 3:69–96.

106. Haffner, S M, Shaten, J, Stern, M P, Smith, G D, and Kuller, L. "Low levels of sex hormone binding globulin and testosterone predict the development of non-insulin-dependent diabetes in men." MRFIT Research Group. Multiple Risk Factor Intervention Trial. *Am J Epidemiol*, 1996, 143(9):889–897.

107. Haffner, S M, Valdez, R A, Morales, P A, Hazuda, H P, and Stern, M O. "Decreased sex hormone binding globulin predicts non-insulin dependent diabetes mellitus in women but not in men." *J Clin Endocrin Metab*, 1993, 77:56–60.

108. Haffner, Shaten, Stern, Smith, and Kuller. Op. cit..

109. Haffner, Valdez, Morales, Hazuda, and Stern. Op. cit.

110. Tibblin, G, Alderberth, A, Lindstedt, G, and Bjorntorp, P. "The pituitary gonadal axis and health in elderly men: A study of men born in 1913." *Diabetes*, 1996, 45(11):1605–1609.

111. Kaplan, N M. "The Deadly Quartet. Upper body obesity, glucose intolerance, hypertriglyceridemia, and hypertension." *Arch Int Med*, 1989, 149:1514–1520.

112. Depres, J B, Lamarche, B, Mauriege, P, Cantin, P, et al. "Hyperinsulinemia as an independent risk factor for ischemic heart disease." *N Eng J Med*, 1996, 334(15):952–957.

113. Zmuda, J M, Cauley, J A, Kriska, A, Glynn, N W, et al. "Longitudinal relation between endogenous testosterone and cardiac disease risk factors in middle-aged men. A 13-year follow-up of former Multiple Risk Factor Intervention Trial Participants." *Am J Epidemiol*, 1997, 146(8):609–617.

114. Birkeland, K I, Hanssen, K F, Tojesen, P A, and Valler, S. "Level of sex hormone binding globulin is positively correlated with insulin sensitivity in men with Type-2 diabetes." *J Clin Endocrin Metab*, 1993, 76(2):275–278.

115. Haffner, S M, Valdrez, R A, Mykkanen, L, Stern, P, and Katz, M S. "Decreased testosterone and dehydroepiandrosterone sulfate concentrations are associated with increased insulin and glucose concentrations in nondiabetic men." *Metab Clin Experim*, 1994, 43(5):599–603.

116. Haffner, S M. "Sex hormone binding globulin, hyperinsulinemia, insulin resistance and non-insulin dependent diabetes mellitus." *Hormone Res*, 1996, 45(3–5):233–237.

117. Rosenthal and Ziegler. *Arch Int Med*, 1929, 44:344–350.

118. Howell, E. *Enzyme Nutrition*. New York: Penguin Putnam, 1985.

119. *Zeit Ges Exp Med,* 1930, 71:245–250.

120. *Am J Dig Dis & Nutr,* 1936, 3:159–161.

121. *Nederlands Tij v Geneesk,* 1934, 78:1529–1536.

122. *Am J Dig Dis & Nutr,* 1934–1935, vol 1.

123. *Br Med J,* 1923, 1:317–319.

124. Miehlke, Lopez, and Williams. *Enzymes the Fountain of Life.* Charleston, S.C.: The Neville Press, Inc., 1994.

125. Nobmann, E D, Byers, T, Lanier, A P, Hankin, J H, and Jackson, M. "The diet of Alaska Native adults 1987–1988." *Am J Clin Nutr,* 1992, 55:1024–1032.

126. Murphy, N J, Schraer, C D, Bulkow, L R, Boyko, E J, and Lanier, A P. "Diabetes mellitus in Alaskan Yupik Eskimos and Athabascan Indians after 25 years."

127. Shelton, H. *Getting Well.* San Antonio, Texas, 1946, pp. 233–234.

128. Shelton, H. *The History of Natural Hygiene and the Principles of Natural Hygiene.* Pp. 59–60.

129. Pecoraro, R E, Reiber, G E, and Burgess, E M. "Pathways to diabetic limb amputation. Basis for prevention." *Diabetes Care,* 1990, 13:513–521.

130. Lavery, L A, Ashry, H R, van Houtum, W, Pugh, J A, Harkless, L B, and Basu, S. "Variation in the incidence and proportion of diabetes-related amputations in minorities." *Diabetes Care,* 1996, 19:48–52.

131. Armstrong, D G, Lavery, L A, Quebedeaux, T L, and Walker, S C. "Surgical morbidity and the risk of amputation due to infected puncture wounds in diabetic versus nondiabetic adults." *South Med J,* 1997, 90:384–389.

Chapter 4: The Tree of Life 21-Day+ Program

1. Considine, R V, Sinha, M K, Heiman, M L, et al. "Serum Immunoreactive-Leptin Concentrations in Normal-Weight and Obese Humans." *New Eng J Med,* 1996, 334:292–295.

2. Spiller, G A, Jensen, C D, Pattison, T S, et al. "Effect of Protein Dose on Serum Glucose and Insulin Response to Sugars." *Amer J Clin Nutr,* 1987, 46:474–480.

3. Bland, J. *Genetic Nutritioneering.* Lincolnwood, Ill.: Keats, 1999.

4. Franz, M J. "Protein: Metabolism and Effect on Blood Glucose Levels." *Diabetes Education,* 1992, 18:1–29.

5. Block, G. "Dietary Guidelines and the Results of Food Consumption Surveys." *Amer J Clin Nutr,* 1991, 53:56S–57S.

6. Xu, Y X, Pindolia, K R, Janakiraman, N, et. al. "Curcumin, a compound with anti inflammatory and and antioxidant properties, down regulates chemokine expression in bone marrow stromal cells." *Exper Hematology,* 1997, 25:413–422.

7. Finch, C E, and Tanzi, R E. *Science,* October 17, 1997, 278(5337):407–411.

8. Barclay, L. "Growing Evidence Links Resveratrol to Extended Life Span." *Life Extension,* Spring 2007, pp. 33–40.

9. Heilbronn, L K, de Jonge, L, Frisard, M I, et al. "Effect of 6 month calorie restriction on biomarkers of longevity, metabolic adaptation, and oxidative stress in overweight individuals: A randomized controlled trial." *JAMA,* Apr. 5, 2006, 295(13):1539–1548.

10. Ku1vinskas, V. *Survival into the 21st Century.* Woodstock Valley, Conn. and Fairfield, Iowa: 21st Century Publications, 1975.

11. Howell, E. *Food Enzymes for Health and Longevity.* Woodstock Valley, Conn: Omangod Press, 1946.

12. Lee, C, Klopp, R, Weindruch, R, and Prolla, T. "Gene Expression Profile of Aging and its Retardation by Caloric Restriction." *Science,* 1999, 285(5432):1390–1393.

13. Kramer, P. "Health and Longevity: What Centenarians Can Teach Us." *Yoga Journal.* Berkeley: Goodfellow Publishers, Sept/Oct 1983, pp 26–30.

14. Cao, S X, Dhahbi, J M, Mote, P L, and Spindler, S R. "Genomic profiling of short- and long-term caloric restriction effects in the liver of aging mice." *Proc Natl Academy of Sciences,* 98(19):10630–10635. Cited in: Fahy, G, and Kent, S. "Reversing Aging Rapidly with Short-Term Calorie Restriction." *Life Extension,* May 2001.

15. Esselstyn, C B. www.heartattackproof.com

16. Grundy, S M, et al. "Implications of Recent Clinical Trials for the National Cholesterol Education Program Adult Treatment Panel III Guidelines." *Circulation,* 2004, 110:227–239.

17. Pradhan A D. "C-reactive protein, interleukin 6, and risk of developing type 2 diabetes mellitus." *JAMA,* 2001, 286:327–334.

18. Lopez-Garcia, E. "Consumption of Trans Fatty Acids Is Related to Plasma Biomarkers of Inflammation and Endothelial Dysfunction." *J Nutrition,* 2005, 135(3):562–566.

19. Shaw Dunn, J, Sheehan, H L, and McLetchie, N G B. "Necrosis of the islets of Langerhans produced experimentally." *The Lancet,* 1943, 244:484–487.

20. Braly, J, and Hoggan, R. *Dangerous Grains.* New York: Penguin Putnam, 2002, p. 126.

21. Berger, S. *Dr. Berger's Immune Power Diet.* New York: New American Library, 1986.

22. Daniel, K T. *The Whole Soy Story.* www.thewholesoystory.com

23. Ibid.

24. Casanova, M, et al. "Developmental effects of dietary phytoestrogens in Sprague: Dawley rats and interactions of genistein and daidzein with rat estrogen receptors alpha and beta in vitro." *Toxicol Sci,* Oct. 1999, 51(2):236–244.

25. Santell, L, et al. "Dietary genistein exerts estrogenic effects upon the uterus, mammary gland and the hypothalamic / pituitary axis in rats." *J Nutr,* Feb. 1997, 127(2):263–269.

26. Harrison, R M, et al. "Effect of genistein on steroid hormone production in the pregnant rhesus monkey." *Proc Soc Exp Biol Med,* Oct. 1999, 222(1):78–84.

27. Divi, R L, Chang, H C, and Doerge, D R. "Identification, characterization and mechanisms of anti-thyroid activity of isoflavones from soybeans." *Biochem Pharmacol,* 1997, 54:1087–1096.

28. Fort, P, Moses, N, Fasano, M, Goldberg, T, and Lifshitz, F. "Breast and soy formula feedings in early infancy and the prevalence of autoimmune disease in children." *J Am Coll Nutr,* 1990, 9:164–165.

29. Setchell, K D R, Zimmer-Nechemias, L, Cai, J, and Heubi, J E. "Exposure of infants to phytoestrogens from soy based infant formula." *The Lancet,* 1997, 350:23–27.

30. Ashton, E, and Ball, M. "Effects of soy as tofu vs. meat on lipoprotein concentrations." *Eur J Clin Nutr,* Jan. 2000, 54(1):14–19.

31. Madani, S, et al. "Dietary protein level and origin (casein and highly purified soybean protein) affect hepatic storage, plasma lipid transport, and antioxidative defense status in the rat." *Nutrition,* May 2000, 16(5):368–375.

32. White, L R, Petrovich, H, Ross, G W, and Masaki, K H. "Association of mid-life consumption of tofu with late life cognitive impairment and dementia: The Honolulu-Asia Aging Study." Fifth International Conference on Alzheimer's Disease, #487, 27 July 1996, Osaka, Japan.

33. White, L R, Petrovitch, H, Ross, G W, Masaki, K H, Hardman. J, Nelson. J, Davis. D, and Markesbery, W. "Brain aging and midlife tofu consumption." *J Am Coll Nutr,* April 2000, 19(2):242–255.

34. Nagata, C, et al. "Inverse association of soy product intake with serum androgen and estrogen in Japanese men." *Nutr Cancer,* 2000, 36(1):14–18.

35. Zhong, Ying, et al. "Effects of dietary supplement of soy protein isolate and low fat diet on prostate cancer." *FASEB J,* 2000, 14(4):a531.11.

36. Rapp, D J. *Is This Your Child's World?* New York: Bantam Books, 1996, p. 501.

37. Irvine, C H G, Fitzpatrick, M G, and Alexander, S L. "Phytoestrogens in soy based infant foods: Concentrations, daily intake and possible biological effects." *Proc Soc Exp Biol Med,* 1998, 217:247–253.

38. Levy, J R, Faber, F A, Ayyash, L, and Hughes, C L. "The effect of prenatal exposure to phytoestrogens genistein on sexual differentiation in rats." *Proc Soc Exp Biol Med,* 1995, 208:60–66.

39. Daniel, K T. Op. cit.

40. "Soy Infant Formula Could Be Harmful to Infants: Groups Want it Pulled." *Nutrition Week,* Dec 10, 1999, 29(46):1–2; see also www.soyonlineservice.co.nz.

41. Setchell, K D, Zimmer-Nechemias, L, Cai, J, and Heubi, J E. "Exposure of infants to phyto-oestrogens from soy-based infant formula." *The Lancet,* July 5, 1997, 350(9070):23–27.

42. Cassidy, A, Bingham, S, and Setchell, K D. "Biological effects of a diet of soy protein rich in isoflavones on the menstrual cycle of premenopausal women." *Am J Clin Nutr,* Sept. 1994, 60(3):333–340.

43. *J Clin Endocrinol Metab,* March 2003, 88(3):1048–1054.

44. Yu, H. "Role of the insulin-like growth factor family in cancer development and progression." *J Natl Cancer Inst,* Sept. 20, 2000, 92(18):1472–1489.

45. Ikonomidou, C, and Turski, L. "Glutamate in Neurode generative Disorders." In Stone, T W, ed., *Neurotransmitters and Neuromodulators: Glutamate.* Boca Raton: CRC Press, 1995, pp. 253–272.

46. Blaylock, R. *Excitotoxins: The Taste That Kills.* Santa Fe, N.M.: Health Press, 1997.

47. Whetsell, W O, and Shapira, N A. "Biology of Disease. Neuroexcitation, excitotoxicity and human neurological disease." *Lab Invest,* 1993, 68:372–387.

48. Kalaria, R N, and Harik, S I. "Reduced glucose transporter at the blood-brain barrier and in the cerebral cortex in Alzheimer's disease." *J Neurochem,* 1989, 53:1083–1088.

49. International Medical Veritas Association. "Chemical Causes of Diabetes." http://imva.info/diabetescauses.shtml

50. "The Bitter Truth about Artificial Sweeteners." http://www.curezone.com/foods/aspartame.html

51. Kataya, H A H, and Hamza, A A. "Red Cabbage (*Brassica oleracea*) Ameliorates Diabetic Nephropathy in Rats." Department of Biology, Faculty of Science, UAE University. Oxford Journals: Evidence Based Complementary and Alternative Medicine. http://ecam.oxfordjournals.org/cgi/content/abstract/nem029v1

52. Welihinda, J, Arvidson, G, Gylfe, E, et al. "The insulin-releasing activity of the tropical plant Momordica charantia." *Acta Bio Med Germ,* 1982, 41:1229–1240.

53. Welihinda, J, Karunanaya, E H, Sheriff, M H R, and Jayasinghe, K S A. "Effect of Momordica charantia on the glucose tolerance in maturity onset diabetes." *J Ethnopharmacol,* 1986, 17:277–282.

54. Srivastava, Y, Venkatakrishna-Bhatt, H, Verma, Y, et al. "Antidiabetic and adaptogenic properties of Momordica charantia extract: An experimental and clinical evaluation." *Phytotherapy Res,* 1993, 7:285–289.

55. Welihinda, Karunanaya, Sheriff, and Jayasinghe. Op. cit.

56. Srivastava, Venkatakrishna-Bhatt, Verma, et al. Op. cit.

57. Frati, A C, Jimenez, E, and Ariza, R C. "Hypogylcemic effect of *Opuntia ficus indica* in non insulin-dependent diabetes mellitus patients." *Phytother Res,* 1990, 4:195–197.

58. Trejo-Gonzales, A, Gabriel Ortiz, G, Puebla-Perez, A M, et al. "A purified extract from prickly pear cactus (*Opuntia fulignosa*) controls experimentally induced diabetes in rats." *J Ethnopharm,* 1996, 55:27–33.

59. Sheela, C G, and Augusti, K T. "Antidiabetic effects of S-allyl cysteine sulphoxide isolated from garlic Allium sativum Linn." *Ind J Exper Biol,* 1992, 30:523–526.

60. Sharma, K K, et al. "Antihyperglycemic effect on onion: Effect on fasting blood sugar and induced hyperglycemia in man." *Ind J Med Res,* 1977, 65:422–429.

61. Hu, F B, and Stampfer, M J. "Nut consumption and risk of coronary heart disease: A review of epidemiologic evidence." *Curr Atheroscler Rep,* 1999, 1(3):204–209.

62. Kris-Etherton, P M, Yu-Poth, S, Sabate, J, Ratcliffe, H E, Zhao, G, and Etherton, T D. "Nuts and their bioactive constituents: Effects on serum lipids and other factors that affect disease risk." *Am J Clin Nutr,* 1999, 70(3 Suppl):504S–511S.

63. Rivellese, A A, and Lilli, S. "Quality of dietary fatty acids, insulin sensitivity and Type-2 diabetes." *Biomed Pharmacother,* March 2003, 57(2):84–87.

64. Berger, A, Jones, P J, and Abumweis, S S. "Plant sterols: Factors affecting their efficacy and safety as functional food ingredients." *Lipids Health Dis,* 2004, 3(1):5.

65. Katan, M B, Grundy, S M, Jones, P, Law, M, Miettinen, T, and Paoletti, R. "Efficacy and safety of plant stanols and sterols in the management of blood cholesterol levels." *Mayo Clin Proc,* 2003, 78(8):965–978.

66. Nissinen, M, Gylling, H, Vuoristo, M, and Miettinen, T A. "Micellar distribution of cholesterol and phytosterols after duodenal plant stanol ester infusion." *Am J Physiol Gastrointest Liver Physiol,* 2002, 282(6):G1009–1015.

67. Guixiang, Z, Etherton, T D, Martin, K R, West, S G, Gillies, P J, and Kris-Etherton, P M. "Dietary -Linolenic Acid Reduces Inflammatory and Lipid Cardiovascular Risk Factors in Hypercholesterolemic Men and Women." *Amer Soc for Nutr Sci J Nutr,* Nov. 2004, 134:2991–2997. See also:

68. Sabate, J, Fraser, G E, Burke, K, Knutsen, S, Bennett, H, and Lindsted, K D. "Effects of walnuts on serum lipid levels and blood pressure in normal men." *N Engl J Med,* 1993, 328:603–607.

69. *Stroke,* 1993, 26:778–782. These results were first published in *The Lancet* in 1994 (343:1454–1459), and then subsequently in other reputable journals, such as *Preventative Medicine* (28:333–339), *American Journal of Clinical Nutrition* (74:72–79), and *Annals of Internal Medicine* (132(7):538–546.

70. World's Healthiest Foods. "Walnuts." http://www.whfoods.com/genpage.php?tname=foodspice&dbid=99

71. Ros, E, Nunez, I, Perez-Heras, A, Serra, M, Gilabert, R, Casals, E, and Deulofeu, R. "A walnut diet improves endothelial function in hypercholesterolemic subjects: A randomized crossover trial." *Circulation,* 2004 109:1609–1614.

72. Abbey, M, Noakes, M, Belling, G B, and Nestel, P J. "Partial replacement of saturated fatty acids with almonds or walnuts lowers total plasma cholesterol and low-density-lipoprotein cholesterol." *Am J Clin Nutr,* 1994, 59:995–999.

73. Iwamoto, M, Sato, M, Kono, M, Hirooka, Y, Sakai, K, Takeshita, A, and Imaizumi, K. "Walnuts lower serum cholesterol in Japanese men and women." *J Nutr,* 2000, 130:171–176.

74. Lavedrine, F, Zmirou, D, Ravel, A, Balducci, F, and Alary, J. "Blood cholesterol and walnut consumption: A cross-sectional survey in France." *Prev Med,* 1999, 28:333–339.

75. Lovejoy, J C, Most, M M, Lefevre, M, Greenway, FL, and Rood, J C. "Effects of diets enriched in almonds on insulin action and serum lipids in adults with normal glucose tolerance in type 2 diabetes." *Am J Clin Nutr,* 2002, 76:1000–1006.

76. *J Medical Hypothesis,* 2005, 65:953.

77. Keen, H, Payan, J, Allawi, J, et al. "Treatment of diabetic neuropathy with gamma-linoleic acid." The Gamma Linoleic Acid Multicenter Trial Group. *Diabetes Care,* 1993, 16:8–15.

78. Schwartz, et al. "Inhibition of experimental oral carcinogenesis by topical beta carotene." Harvard School of Dental Medicine. *Carcinogenesis,* 1986, 7(5):711–715.

79. Annapurna, V, et al. "Bioavailability of Spirulina carotenes in pre-school children." National Institute of Nutrition, Hyderabad, India. *J Clin Biochem Nutrition,* 1991, 10:145–151.

80. Oviedo, et al. "Hypoglycaemic Action of Stevia rebaudiana Bertoni (Kaa-he-e)." *Exerpta Medica* (International Congress Series), 1971, 208–292.

81. Suzuki, et al. "Influence of Oral Administration of Stevioside on Levels of Blood Glucose and Liver Glycogen in Intact Rats." *Nippon Nogei Kagaku,* 1977, 51(3):171–173.

82. Ishii, et al. "Inhibition of Monosaccharide Transport in the Intact Rat Liver by Stevioside," *Biochem Pharmacology,* 1987, 36(9):1417–1433.

83. Alvarez, et al. "Effect of Aqueous Extract of Stevia rebaudiana Bertone on Biochemical Parameters of Normal Adult Persons." *Brazilian J Med Biol Res,* 1986, 19:771–774.

84. Boeckh, E A. "Stevia Rebaudiana (Bert.) Bertoni: Clinical Evaluation of its Acute Action on Cardio-Circulatory, Metabolic and Electrolitic Parameters in 60 Healthy Individuals." *Third Brazilian Seminar on Stevia Rebaudiana (Bert.),* July 1986, pp. 22–23.

85. Lazarow, A, Liambies, J, and Tausch, A J. "Protection against Diabetes with Nicotinamide." *J Lab Clin Med,* 1950, 36:249–258..

86. *Diabetologia,* 1989, 32(3):160–162. *The Lancet,* 1987, 1(8533):619–620.

87. *Diabetologia*, 1991, 34(5):362–365.

88. *Diabetes*, 1994, 43:770–777.

89. *Diabetologia*, 1993, 36:675–677.

90. Karjalainen, J, Martin, J, Knip, M, et al. "A bovine albumin peptide as a possible trigger of insulin-dependent diabetes." *N Eng J Med*, 1992, 327:302–307.

91. Gale, E A. "Theory and practice of nicotinamide trials in pre-Type-1 diabetes." *J Pediatr Endocrinol Metab*, 1996, 9:375–379.

92. Cleary, J P. "Vitamin B3 in the treatment of diabetes mellitus: Case reports and review of the literature." *J Nutr Med*, 1990, 1:217–225.

93. Murray, M. *How to Prevent and Treat Diabetes with Natural Medicine*. New York: Riverhead Books, 2003, p. 176.

94. Jones, C L, and Gonzalez, V. "Pyridoxine deficiency: A new factor in diabetic neuropathy." *J Am Pod Assoc*, 1978, 68:646–653.

95. Solomon, L R, and Cohen, K. "Erythrocyte O_2 transport and metabolism and effects on vitamin B-6 therapy in type-2 diabetes mellitus." *Diabetes*, 1989, 38:881–886.

96. Coelingh-Bennick, H J T, and Schreurs, W H P. "Improvement of oral glucose tolerance in gestational diabetes." *BMJ*, 1975, 3:13–15.

97. Takahishi, Y, Takayama, S, Itou, T, Owada, K, and Omori, Y. "Effect of Glycemic Control on Vitamin B12 Metabolism in Diabetes Mellitus." *Diabetes Res and Clin Practice*, 1994, 25:13–17.

98. Zhang, H, Osada, K, Sone, H, and Furukawa, Y. "Biotin administration improves the impaired glucose tolerance of streptozotocin-induced diabetic Wistar rats." *J Nutr Sci Vitaminol* (Tokyo), 1997, 43(3):271–280.

99. Maebashi, M, Makino, Y, Furukawa, Y, Ohinata, K, Kimura, S, and Sato, T. "Therapeutic evaluation of the effect of biotin on hyperglycemia in patients with non-insulin dependent diabetes mellitus." *J Clin Biochem Nutr*, 1993, 14:211–218.

100. Coggeshall, J C, Heggers, J P, Robson, M C, and Baker, H. "Biotin status and plasma glucose levels in diabetics." *Ann NY Acad Sci*, 1985, 447:389–392.

101. Romero-Navarro, G, Cabrera-Valladares, G, German, M S, et al. "Biotin regulation of pancreatic glucokinase and insulin in primary cultured rat islets and in biotin-deficient rats." *Endocrinology*, 1999, 140(10):4595–4600.

102. Murray, M, and Pizzorno, J. *Encyclopedia of Natural Medicine*. Rocklin, Calif.: Prima Publishing, 1998.

103. Coggeshall, et al. Op. cit.

104. Cunningham, J. "Reduced mononuclear leukocyte ascorbic acid content in adults with insulin-dependent diabetes mellitus consuming adequate dietary vitamin C." *Metabolism,* 1991, 40:146–149.

105. Davie, S J, Gould, B J, and Yudkin, J S. "Effect of vitamin C on glycosylation of proteins." *Diabetes,* 1992, 41:167–173.

106. Vinson, J A, et al. "In vitro and in vivo reduction of erythrocyte sorbitol by ascorbic acid." *Diabetes,* 1989, 38:1036–1041.

107. Cunningham, J J, Mearkle, P L, and Brown, R G. "Vitamin C: An aldose reductase inhibitor that normalizes erythrocyte sorbitol in insulin-dependent diabetes mellitus." *J Am Coll Nutr,* 1994, 4:344–350.

108. Hobday, R. *The Healing Sun.* Scotland: Findhorn Press, 1999, p. 78.

109. Need, AG, et al. "Relationship between fasting serum glucose, age, body mass index and serum 25 hydroxyvitamin D in postmenopausal women." *Clin Endocrinol,* 2005, 62(6):738–741.

110. *Cancer Epidemiol Biomarkers Prev,* 2004, 13:1502–1508.

111. *Alternatives for the Health Conscious Individual,* April 2007, 169:176.

112. Fontana, L, et al. "Low Bone Mass in Subjects on a Long-Term Raw Vegetarian Diet." *Arch Intern Med,* 2005, 165:684–689

113. *Alternatives for the Health Conscious Individual,* April 2007, 169:172.

114. Paolisso, G, et al. "Daily Vitamin E supplements improve metabolic control but not insulin secretion in elderly Type-2 diabetic patients." *Diabetes Care,* 1993, 16:1433–1437.

115. Davi, G, Ciabattoni, G, Consoli, A, et al. "In vivo formation of 8-iso-prostaglandin f2alpha and platelet activation in diabetes mellitus: Effects of improved metabolic control and vitamin E supplementation." *Circulation,* 1999, 99(2):224–229.

116. Jain, S K, McVie, R, Jaramillo, J J, Palmer, M, and Smith, T. "Effect of modest vitamin E supplementation on blood glycated hemoglobin and triglyceride levels and red cell indices in type I diabetic patients." *J Am Coll Nutr,* 1996, 15(5):458–461.

117. *Vitamin Research News,* April 2000, Footnote 30.

118. Salonen, J T, et al. "Increased risk of Non-Insulin Diabetes Mellitus at Low Plasma Vitamin E Concentrations: A Four-Year Follow-up Study in Men." *BMJ,* 1995, 311:1124–1127.

119. Cody, V, Middleton, E, and Harborne, J B. *Plant Flavonoids in Biology and Medicine—Biochemical, Pharmacological, and Structure-Activity Relationships.* New York: Alan R Liss, 1986.

120. Cody, V, Middleton, E, Harborne, J B, and Beretz, A. *Plant Flavonoids in Biology and Medicine—Biochemical, Pharmacological, and Structure-Activity Relationships.* Volume II. New York: Alan R Liss, 1988.

121. Chaudhry, P S, Cabera, J, Hector, R, et al. "Inhibition of human lens aldose reductase by flavonoids, sulindac, and indomethacin." *Biochem Pharmacol,* July 1, 1983, 32(13):1995–1998.

122. Varma, S D, Schocket, S S, and Richards, R D. "Implications of aldose reductase in cataracts in human diabetes." *Invest Ophthalmol Vis Sci,* 1979, 18:237–241.

123. Varma, S D, Mizuno, A, and Kinoshita, J H. "Diabetic cataracts and flavonoids." *Science,* 1977, 195:205–206.

124. Nakai, N, Fujii, Y, Kobashi, K, and Nomura, K. "Aldose reductase inhibitors: Flavonoids, alkaloids, acetophenones, benzophenones, and spirohydantoins of chroman." *Arch Biochem Biophys,* 1985, 239:491–496.

125. Varma, D. "Inhibition of aldose reductase by flavonoids: Possible attenuation of diabetic complications." *Prog Clin Biol Res,* 1986, 213:343–358.

126. Kuhnau, J. "The flavonoids: A class of semi-essential food components: Their role in human nutrition." *Wld Rev Nutr Diet,* 1976, 24:117–191.

127. Keen, H, Payan, J, Allawi, J, et al. "Treatment of diabetic neuropathy with gamma-linoleic acid. The Gamma Linoleic Acid Multicenter Trial Group." *Diabetes Care,* 1993, 16:8–15.

128. Fuller, C J, Chandalia, M, Garg, A, et al. "RRR-alpha-tocopheryl acetate supplementation at pharmacologic doses decreses low-density lipoprotein oxidative susceptibility but not protein glycation in patients with diabetes mellitus." *Am J Clin Nutr,* 1996, 63:753–759.

129. Packer, L, Witt, E H, and Tritschler, H J. "Alpha-lipoic acid as a biological antioxidant." *Free Radic Biol Med,* 1995, 19:227–250.

130. Estrada, D E, Ewart, H S, Tsakiridis, T, et al. "Stimulation of glucose uptake by the natural coenzyme alpha lipoic acid/thioctic acid: Participation of elements of the insulin signaling pathway." *Diabetes,* 1996, 45:1798–1804.

131. Packer, L. "Antioxidant properties of lipoic acid and its therapeutic effects in prevention of diabetes complications and cataracts." *Ann N Y Acad Sci,* 1994, 738:257–264.

132. Nagamatsu, M, et al. "Lipoic acid improves nerve blood flow, reduces oxidative stress, and improves distal nerve conduction in

experimental diabetic neuropathy." *Diabetes Care*, 1995, 18:1160–1167.

133. Jacob, S, et al. "Enhancement of glucose disposal in patients with Type-2 diabetes by alpha-lipoic acid." *Arzneim Forsch*, 1995, 45:872–874.

134. Kawabata, T, and Packer, L. "Alpha-lipoate can protect against glycation of serum albumin, but not low-density lipoprotein." *Biochem Biophys Res Commun*, 1994, 203:99–104.

135. Suzuki, Y J, Tsuchiya, M and Packer, L. "Lipoate prevents glucose induced protein modifications." *Free Rad Res Commun*, 1992, 17:211–217.

136. Jacob, S, Ruus, P, Hermann, R, et al. "Oral administration of RAC-alpha lipoic acid modulates insulin sensitivity in patients with Type-2 diabetes mellitus: A placebo controlled pilot trial." *Free Radic Biol Med*, Aug. 1999, 27(3–4):309–314.

137. Houtsmuller, A J, van Hal-Ferwerba, J, Zahn, K J, and Henkes, H E. "Favorable influences of linoleic acid on the progression of diabetic micro and macroangiopathy." *Nutr Metab*, 1980, 24:S105–S118.

138. Lubec, B, Hayn, M, Kitzmuller, I, Vierhapper, H, and Lubec, G. "L-Arginine Reduces Lipid Peroxidation in Patients with Diabetes Mellitus." *Free Radical Biol & Med*, 1997, 22:355–357.

139. Bosia, S, Burdino, E, Grignola, F, and Ugazio, G. "Protective effect on nephropathy and on cataract in the streptozotocin-diabetic rat of the vanadium-lazaroid combination." *G Ital Med Lav*, 1995, 17:71–75.

140. Shamberger, R J. "The insulin-like effects of vanadium." *J Adv Med*, 1996, 9:121–131.

141. Tosiello, L. "Hypomagnesemia and diabetes mellitus. A review of clinical implications." *Arch Intern Med*, 1996, 156(11):1143–1148.

142. White, J R, and Campbell, R K. "Magnesium and diabetes: A review." *Ann Pharmacother*, 1993, 27:775–780.

143. Nadler, J L, Buchanan, T, Natarajan, R, et al. "Magnesium deficiency produces insulin resistance and increased thromboxane synthesis." *Hypertension*, 1993, 21:1024–1029.

144. Humphries, S, Kushner, H, and Falkner, B. "Low dietary magnesium is associated with insulin resistance in a sample of young, nondiabetic Black Americans." *Am J Hypertens*, 1999, 12:747–756.

145. Paolisso, G, Sgambato, S, Gambardella, A, et al. "Daily magnesium supplements improve glucose handling in elderly subjects." *Am J Clin Nutr*, 1992, 55(6):1161–1167.

146. Van Dam, R M, et al. "Dietary Calcium and Magnesium, Major Food Sources, and Risk of Type 2 Diabetes in U.S. Black Women." *Diabetes Care,* 2006, 29:2238–2243.

147. Song, Y, Ridker, P M, Manson, J E, Cook, N R, Buring, J E, and Liu, S. "Magnesium Intake, C-Reactive Protein, and the Prevalence of Metabolic Syndrome in Middle-Aged and Older U.S. Women." *Diabetes Care,* 2005, 28:1438–1444.

148. Klatz, R, and Goldman, R. *Stopping the Clock.* New Canaan, Conn.: Keats Publishing, 1996, p. 129.

149. Chausmer, A B. "Zinc, insulin and diabetes." *J Am Coll Nutr,* April 1998, 17(2):109–115.

150. Blostein-Fujii, A, DiSilvestro, R A, Frid, D, Katz, C, and Malarkey, W. "Short-term zinc supplementation in women with non-insulin-dependent diabetes mellitus: Effects on plasma 5'-nucleotidase activities, insulin-like growth factor I concentrations, and lipoprotein oxidation rates in vitro." *Am J Clin Nutr,* 1997, 66(3):639–642.

151. Hegazi, S M, et al. "Effect of zinc supplementation on serum glucose, insulin, glucagon, glucose-6-phosphatase, and mineral levels in diabetics." *J Clin Biochem Nutr,* 1992, 12:209–215.

152. DiSilvestro, R A. "Zinc in relation to diabetes and oxidative disease." *J Nutr,* May 2000, 130(5S Suppl):1509S–1511S.

153. Barri, Y M, and Wingo, C S. "The effects of potassium depletion and supplementation on blood pressure: A clinical review." *Am J Med Sci,* 1997, 314(1):37–40.

154. Hajjar, I M, Grim, C E, George, V, and Kotchen, T A. "Impact of diet on blood pressure and age-related changes in blood pressure in the U.S. population: Analysis of NHANES III." *Arch Intern Med,* 2001, 161(4):589–593.

155. Appel, L J, Moore, T J, Obarzanek, E, et al. "A clinical trial of the effects of dietary patterns on blood pressure." DASH Collaborative Research Group. *N Engl J Med,* 1997, 336(16):1117–1124.

156. Wimhurst, J M, and Manchester, K L. "Comparison of ability of Mg and Mn to activate the key enzymes of glycolysis." *FEBS Letters,* 1972, 27:321–326.

157. Editorial: "Manganese and glucose tolerance." *Nutr Rev,* 1968, 26:207–210.

158. el-Yazigi, A, Hannan, N, and Raines, D A. "Urinary excretion of chromium, copper, and manganese in diabetes mellitus and associated disorders." *Diabetes Res,* 1991, 18(3):129–134.

159. Nath, N, Chari, S N, and Rathi, A B. "Superoxide dismutase in diabetic polymorphonuclear leukocytes." *Diabetes,* 1984, 33(6):586–589.

160. Food and Nutrition Board, Institute of Medicine. *Chromium. Dietary reference intakes for vitamin A, vitamin K, boron, chromium, copper, iodine, iron, manganese, molybdenum, nickel, silicon, vanadium, and zinc.* Washington, D.C.: National Academy Press, 2001:197–223.

161. Jeejeebhoy, K N. "The role of chromium in nutrition and therapeutics and as a potential toxin." *Nutr Rev,* 1999, 57(11):329–335.

162. Morris, B W, MacNeil, S, Hardisty, C A, Heller, S, Burgin, C, and Gray, T A. "Chromium homeostasis in patients with type II (NIDDM) diabetes." *J Trace Elem Med Biol,* 1999, 13(1–2):57–61.

163. Kobla, H V, and Volpe, S L. "Chromium, exercise, and body composition." *Crit Rev Food Sci Nutr,* 2000, 40(4):291–308.

164. Goldman, L, and Bennett, J C. *Cecil Textbook of Medicine,* twenty-first edition. Philadelphia: W. B. Saunders Co., 2000.

165. Anderson, R A, Cheng, N, Bryden, N A, Polansky, M M, Chi, J, and Feng, J. "Elevated intakes of supplemental chromium improve glucose and insulin variables in individuals with type 2 diabetes." *Diabetes,* 1997, 46(11):1786–1791.

166. Lukaski, H C. "Chromium as a supplement." *Ann Rev Nutr,* 1999, 19:279–302.

167. Jovanovic-Peterson, L, and Peterson, C M. "Vitamin and mineral deficiencies which may predispose to glucose intolerance of pregnancy." *J Am Coll Nutr,* 1996, 15(1):14–20.

168. Airola, P. *How to Get Well.* Phoenix: Health Plus Publishers, 1984, p. 72.

169. "Bean Pod Tea: The Miracle Tea for Diabetics." www.Beanpodtea.com

170. Heinerman, J. *Heinerman's Encyclopedia of Healing Herbs and Spices.* New York: Penguin Putnam, 1996, pp. 52–53.

171. Ibid., p. 200.

172. Shanmugasundarum, E R, Rajeswari, G, Baskaran, K, et al. "Use of Gymnema sylvestre leaf in the control of blood glucose in insulin-dependent diabetes mellitus." *J Ethnopharmacol,* 1990, 30:281–294.

173. Prakash, A O, Mathur, S, and Mathur, R. "Effect of feeding Gymnema sylvestre leaves on blood glucose in beryllium nitrate treated rats." *J Ethnopharmacol,* 1986, 18:143–146.

174. Baskaran, K, Ahamath, BK, Shanmugasundaram, K R, and Shanmugasundaram, E R B. "Antidiabetic effect of a leaf extract from Gymnema sylvestre in non-insulin dependent diabetes mellitus patients." *J Ethnopharmacol,* 1990, 30:295–305.

175. Bordia, A, et al. "Effect of ginger (*Zingibwe officinale Rosc.*) and fenugreek (*Trigonella foenum graecum L.*) on blood lipids, blood sugar, and platelet aggregation in patients with coronary artery disease." *Prost Leuko EFA,* 1997, 56:379–384.

176. Sharma, R D, Raghumram, T C, and Rao, N S. "Effect of fenugreek seeds on blood glucose and serum lipids in type-1 diabetes." *Eur J Clin Nutr,* 1990, 44:301–306.

177. Sharma, R D. "Effect of fenugreek seeds and leaves on blood glucose and serum insulin responses in human subjects." *Nutr Res,* 1986, 6:1353–1364.

178. Madar, Z, et al. "Glucose-lowering effect of fenugreek in non-insulin dependent diabetes." *Eur J Clin Nutr,* 1988, 42:51–54.

179. Bordia A, et al. Op. cit.

180. Sharma, Raghumram, and Rao. Op. cit..

181. Anderson, R A, Broadhurst, C L, Polansky, M M, et al. "Isolation and characterization of polyphenol type-A polymers from cinnamon with insulin-like biological activity." *J Agric Food Chem,* Jan. 2004, 52(1):65–70.

182. Broadhurst, C L, Polansky, M M, and Anderson, R A. "Insulin-like biological activity of culinary and medicinal plant aqueous extracts in vitro." *J Agric Food Chem,* March 2000, 48(3):183–188.

183. Imparl-Radosevich, J, Deas, S, Polansky, M M, et al. "Regulation of PTP-1 and insulin receptor kinase by fractions from cinnamon: Implications for cinnamon regulation of insulin signaling." *Horm Res,* Sept. 1998, 50(3):177–182.

184. Khan, A, Safdar, M, Muzaffar Ali Khan, M, Nawak Khattak, K, and Anderson, R A. "Cinnamon improves glucose and lipids of people with Type-2 diabetes." *Diabetes Care,* Dec. 2003, 26(12):3215–3218.

185. Shibib, B A, Khan, L A, and Rahman, R. "Hypoglycemic activity of Coccinia indica and Momordica charantia in diabetic rats: Depression of the hepatic gluconeogenic enzymes glucose-6-phosphatase and fructose-1,6 bisphosphatase and elevation of both liver and red-cell shunt enzyme glucose-6-phosphate dehydrogenase." *Biochem J,* 1993, 292:267–270.

186. Day, C, Cartwright, T, Provost, J, and Bailey, C J. "Hypoglycemic effect of Momordica charantia extracts." *Planta Med,* 1990, 56:426–429.

187. Droy-Lefaix, M T, Vennat, J C, Besse, G, and Doly, M. "Effect of Ginkgo biloba extract (EGb 761) on chloroquine induced retinal alterations." *Lens Eye Toxic Res,* 1992, 9:521–528.

188. Vuksan, V, Stavro, M P, Sievenpiper, J L, Beljan-Zdravkovic, U, Leiter, L A, Josse, R G, and Xu, Z. "Similar postprandial glycemic reductions with escalation of dose and administration time of American ginseng in type-2 diabetes." *Diabetes Care,* Sept. 2000, 23(9):1221–1226.

189. Vuksan, V, Sievenpiper, J L, Koo, V Y Y, Francis, T, Beljan-Zdravkovic, U, Xu, Z, and Vidgen, E. "American ginseng (*Panax quinquefolius L*) reduces postprandial glycemia in nondiabetic and diabetic individuals with type-2 diabetes mellitus." *Arch Int Med,* 2000, 160:1009–1013.

190. Petricic, J, and Kalodera, Z. "Galegin in the goat's rue herb: Its toxicity, antidiabetic activity, and content determination." *Ata Pharm Jugosl,* 1982, 32(3):219–223.

191. Muller, H, and Reinwein, H. "Pharmacology of galegin." *Arch Expll Path Pharm,* 1927, 125:212–228.

192. Cignarella, A, Nastasi, M, Cavalli, E, and Puglisi, L. "Novel lipid-lowering properties of Vaccinium myrtillus L. leaves, a traditional antidiabetic treatment, in several models of rat dyslipidaemia: A comparison with ciprofibrate." *Thromb Res,* 1996, 84:311–322.

193. Boniface, R, and Robert, A M. "Effect of anthocyanins on human connective tissue metabolism in the human." *Klin Monatsbl Augenheilkd,* 1996, 209:368–372.

194. Detre, Z, Jellinek, H, Miskulin, M, and Robert, A M. "Studies on vascular permeability in hypertension: Action of anthocyanosides."

195. Boniface and Robert. Op. cit..

196. Lagrue, G, Robert, A M, Miskulin, M, et al. "Pathology of the microcirculation in diabetes and alterations of the biosynthesis of intracellular matrix molecules." *Front Matrix Bio,* 1970, 7:324–335.

197. Challem, J, et al. *Syndrome X.* New York: John Wiley and Sons, 2002, p. 220.

198. Knowler, W C, Barrett-Connor, E, Fowler, S E, Hamman, R F, Lachin, J M, Walker, E A, and Nathan, D M. Diabetes Prevention Program Research Group. "Reduction in the Incidence of Type 2 Diabetes with Lifestyle Intervention or Metformin." *New Eng J Med,* February 7, 2002, 346:393–403.

199. Pederson, O, Beck-Nielsen, H, and Heding, L. "Increased insulin receptors after exercise in patients with insulin-dependent diabetes mellitus." *N Eng J Med,* 1980, 302:886–892.

200. Williams, D G. "The World's First Diabetes Cure." *Alternatives for the Health-Conscious Individual,* 2005, p. 4. www.drdavidwilliams.com

201. King, D E, Mainous, II, A G, and Pearson, W S. "C-reactive protein, diabetes, and attendance at religious services." *Diabetes Care,* 2002, 25:1172–1176.

202. Pollack, A. "Skincare." *Alternative Medicine,* Feb. 2007, p. 63.

Chapter 5: Happy Continuation: Living in the Culture of Life and Juice Feasting

1. Pollan, M. "You Are What You Grow." *New York Times,* April 22, 2007.

2. *Am J Cardiol,* 2002, 90(Suppl):S551–S621.

3. Jensen, B. *Dr. Jensen's Guide to Better Bowel Care.* New York: Penguin-Putnam, 1999, p. 118.

4. U.S. Department of Health and Human Services. *Dietary Guidelines for Americans 2005.* http://www.health.gov/dietaryguidelines/dga2005

Chapter 6: Culture of Life Cuisine

1. Williams, D E, et al. "Frequent salad vegetable consumption is associated with a reduction in the risk of diabetes mellitus." *J Clin Epidemiol,* 1999, 52(4):329–335.

INDEX